Lipids and Women's Health

Geoffrey P. Redmond
Editor

Lipids and Women's Health

With 28 Illustrations

Springer-Verlag
New York Berlin Heidelberg London
Paris Tokyo Hong Kong Barcelona

Geoffrey P. Redmond, MD
President
Foundation for Developmental Endocrinology, Inc.
23200 Chagrin Boulevard
Cleveland, Ohio 44122
USA

Library of Congress Cataloging-in-Publication Data
Lipids and women's health / Geoffrey P. Redmond, editor.
    p.   cm.
  Includes bibliographical references.
  Includes index.
  ISBN 0-387-97318-4 (alk. paper).—ISBN 3-540-97318-4 (alk.
paper)
    1. Lipid—Metabolism—Disorders—Sex factors.   2. Women—Diseases.
3. Women—Health and hygiene.   4. Cardiovascular system—Diseases—
Risk factors.   I. Redmond, Geoffrey P.
  [DNLM: 1. Cardiovascular Diseases. 2. Lipids. QU 85 L765225]
RC632.L5L57   1990
616.3'997'0082—dc20
DNLM/DLC
for Library of Congress   90-9816

Printed on acid-free paper.

Typeset by Asco Trade Typesetting Ltd., Quarry Bay, Hong Kong.
Printed and bound by Edwards Brothers, Inc., Ann Arbor, Michigan.
Printed in the United States of America.

9 8 7 6 5 4 3 2 1

ISBN 0-387-97318-4 Springer-Verlag New York Berlin Heidelberg
ISBN 3-540-97318-4 Springer-Verlag Berlin Heidelberg New York

Acknowledgments

Science is a collaborative enterprise and any contribution to it, however modest, is the result of the efforts of many individuals. The present book is no exception. I have had stimulating conversations with many individuals regarding the unique aspects of lipid metabolism in women. These include Drs. Byron Hoogwerf, Jeffrey Chang, Steven Miller, and Robert Wild. While I was at the University of Vermont I benefited greatly from my interactions with members of the Division of Endocrinology and Metabolism, notably Drs. Elliot Danforth, Edward Horton, David Robbins, and Ethan A.H. Simms. Mrs. Dorothea Simms was an inspiration to me as she has been to many others. Teachers in medical school who provided essential guidance included Drs. George Curran, Gerald Cohen, and Albert Grokoest.

Anyone interested in androgenic disorders owes a great debt of gratitude to Dr. Wilma Bergfeld. Her pioneering interest in this field and her willingness to take her patients' concerns seriously is an inspiration. I have learned much from her and have greatly enjoyed our clinical and research collaboration.

Without the support, suggestions, and hard work of my present team this book could not have become a reality. Ms. Joyce O'Meara utilized her considerable tact and persistence in working with contributors. Ms. Carol Siverd helped prepare the manuscripts for publication and Ms. Nita Bedocs, RN, BSN, provided much useful advice and encouragement. The staff at Springer-Verlag was also most patient and encouraging.

Finally, I would like to acknowledge the important role of our patients in the androgenic disorders program. The many women whose active interest in their own health led them to pose sometimes difficult questions have been a great stimulant to recognizing *lacunas* and attempting to fill them in.

It goes without saying that none of these individuals are to be held to account for any faults in my contributions to this book.

Contents

Contributors

DAVID W. BILHEIMER, MD, Professor of Medicine, Department of Internal Medicine, University of Texas Southwestern Medical Center, Dallas, Texas 75235, USA

TRUDY L. BUSH, MHS, PHD, Associate Professor, Department of Epidemiology, The Johns Hopkins University, School of Hygiene and Public Health, Baltimore, Maryland 21205, USA

DAVID A. CHAPPELL, MD, Assistant Professor, Department of Medicine, University of Iowa, Iowa City, Iowa 52242, USA

ERICA FRANK, MD, MPH, Post-Doctoral Fellow, Stanford Center for Research and Disease Prevention, Stanford University, Palo Alto, California 94304-1885, USA

RICHARD E. GARCIA, MD, Department of Primary Care/Pediatrics, The Cleveland Clinic Foundation, Cleveland, Ohio 44195-5223, USA

BYRON J. HOOGWERF, MD, FACP, Chairman, Department of Endocrinology, The Cleveland Clinic Foundation, Cleveland, Ohio 44195, USA

JOHN C. LAROSA, MD, Dean for Clinical Affairs; Director, Lipid Research Clinic, The George Washington University Medical Center, Washington, DC 20037, USA

VALERY T. MILLER, MD, Associate Research Professor in Medicine; Medical Director, Lipid Research Clinic, The George Washington University Medical Center, Washington, DC 20037, USA

DOUGLAS S. MOODIE, MD, Chairman, Pediatric and Adolescent Medicine; Pediatric Cardiologist, The Cleveland Clinic Foundation, Cleveland, Ohio 44106, USA

GEOFFREY P. REDMOND, MD, President, Foundation for Developmental Endocrinology, Inc., Cleveland, Ohio 44122, USA

DAVID P. ROSE, MD, PHD, DSC, Associate Director and Chief of the Division of Nutrition and Endocrinology, American Health Foundation, Valhalla, New York 10595, USA

ARTHUR A. SPECTOR, MD, Professor of Biochemistry and Internal Medicine, University of Iowa, Iowa City, Iowa 52242, USA

EVAN A. STEIN, MD, PHD, Medical Research Laboratories and The Christ Hospital Cardiovascular Research Center; Clinical Professor of Pathology and Laboratory Medicine, University of Cincinnati Medical Center, Cincinnati, Ohio 45219, USA

LIAN G. ULRICH, MD, Director, Medical Department, Pharmaceuticals Division, Novo Industri A/S, Bagsvaerd, Denmark

1
Introduction

GEOFFREY P. REDMOND

An astute student of the human mind, psychologist James Hillman observed that "the mind doesn't necessary work in steps; it fills out *lacunas*; we become aware because a *lacuna*, and it's the *lacuna* that's hungry and then begins to eat something."[1] Thus addition to human knowledge does not advance in a linear, systematic way. Rather, we become aware of unexpected gaps, important matters about which we should know but do not. When such an area is recognized there is initial shock followed by intense research activity to fill in the gap. In medicine this pattern has been particularly evident in women's health. Until recently it went almost unnoticed that heart disease is a major killer of women as well as men. As a result, our knowledge of cardiovascular risk factors and means of intervention in women is surprisingly limited. The major studies have been done in men, the justification for which has sometimes been the confounding effects of hormonal changes during the menstrual cycle and menopause and the lower incidence of coronary heart heart disease in the young age group under study. Belatedly it has been appreciated that these are the very factors mandating that studies be done in women. Indeed it has been known for some time that sex steroids are important determinants of the levels of the low density (LDL) and high (HDL) density lipoprotein cholesterol subfractions, which are the lipid parameters clearly related to cardiovascular risk. Because levels of androgens and estrogens vary more in women than in men they may be more significant in determining differences in lipid levels and therefore differences in cardiovascular risk in women. This greater role of endocrine factors presents not only a challenge to understand the complexity of lipid and lipoprotein regulation in women but also an opportunity, as hormonal alteration might be an additional therapeutic mode in female patients.

This book is an attempt to feed the hungry lacuna by synthesizing existing knowledge of lipids in women and their relation to health. A few preliminary comments may be helpful in directing the reader's attention to the important scientific and clinical issues. All the authors herein have exerted themselves to present up-to-date surveys of their fields of expertise. This task is not easily done in a field in which many uncertainties remain. Human lipid studies are inherently difficult because the endpoint —a decreased incidence of cardiovascular disease—requires long-term follow-up of large numbers of subjects. The purist approach of abstaining from treatment decisions until double-blind clinical trials have established the efficacy and safety of a particular treatment is less favored than formerly as the public becomes more aware of issues affecting their health. The public expects, and is entitled to, rapid practical application of current therapeutic information about diseases of major concern such as cancer, heart disease, and acquired immunodeficiency syndrome (AIDS). A patient concerned about a high cholesterol level can hardly be told to wait 5 to 10 years for the outcome of definitive studies. Nor is it always better to use older, better studied treatments if the new ones seem, on the basis of preliminary results, to be superior. In the absence of a clear consensus, the individual clinician must make critical decisions based on his or her own assessment of the evidence. It is the editor's hope that this book will provide the necessary background to make these difficult decisions.

The state of the art regarding lipid disorders in women does not permit generation of a "how to" manual. Instead, the editor has attempted to assemble an up-to-date, critical review of the pertinent scientific issues. Each of the contributors is a respected authority in his or her field, although each may have an individual viewpoint regarding controversial issues. When a consensus does not exist, it is important that all major positions be stated and the issues engaged. The discussion of these controversies in this book should equip the clinician or scientist to read the current literature in critical fashion so as to interpret new developments.

The first chapter establishes the public health significance of cardiovascular disease in women. Some readers may be surprised to learn from Bush's discussion that more women than men die of cardiovascular disease. The death rate from cardiovascular disease is higher in men than in women in all ages (Fig. 2–5); however, because of the longer survival of women the cumulative total is larger. Breast and uterine cancer account for far fewer deaths in women than heart disease despite greater fear associated with these conditions in the public mind. Bush presents the view that HDL rather than LDL is the cholesterol subfraction most strongly related to cardiovascular risk in women. For a contrasting view, the reader is referred to Bilheimer's chapter.

The division of medical specialties by patient age accounts in part for lack of awareness of this epidemiologic pattern. Female patients are cared for initially by pediatricians, whose concerns in the past have not been oriented toward the reproductive system or lipid metabolism. Concern during the early and midadult years has been mainly with reproductive function and care by obstetrician-gynecologists. The success of medicine in reproductive health care has greatly prolonged life expectancy for women and thereby created the need for a more long-term perspective. In later life women are cared for by internists, who see the effects of the risk factors but not their earliest appearance.

It is also possible that many physicians have avoided the topic of lipo-protein and lipid metabolism because of its reputation, not entirely unde-served, for being an impenetrable subject. Here the reader of this book is fortunate in having the review by Spector and Chapell, which summarizes in lucid but rigorous fashion the current understanding of lipoprotein and lipid metabolism. Although many steps in the process are still not well understood, it is clear that cholesterol deposition in the arterial wall is the net result of a balance of processes that deliver cholesterol to that site and others that remove it and transport it back to the liver. LDL appears to be the principal lipoprotein involved in transport to the arterial wall and HDL in the reverse transport away from it. Lipid biochemists are starting to look at these processes in more detail so as to better understand how individual differences in lipoprotein structure result in different degrees of risk for coronary heart disease. An additional factor is the response of the arterial wall. Atheromas occur as a result of scarring, and the tissue response to injury may be important for determining whether occlusive lesions appear and progress. Lipid levels by themselves do not explain differences in the occurrence of heart disease. Although it has been assumed that the effects of estrogens and androgens are entirely on lipid transport, these hormones may exert other effects on atheroma formation. For example, androgens in women can produce hyperinsulinism, which may be a factor in athero-genesis.

Laboratory determination of lipid and lipoprotein levels is of fun-damental importance, as most patients with abnormalities have no signs or symptoms. Although the quantities of lipid are in the milligram per deciliter rather than the nanogram per deciliter level, the endocrinologist should realize that there are nonetheless serious problems with precision and re-peatability of lipid measurements. Stein's chapter discusses these consid-erations. A national program for standardization does exist, and the clini-cian should be satisied himself that the laboratory employed is performing up to these standards.

The effects of estrogens and progestins on lipid metabolism are discussed by LaRosa and Miller. It is well known that estrogens have a positive effect on HDL cholesterol, and some progestins have an unfavorable effect. Pre-scribing decisions regarding these agents should be informed by a thorough knowledge of these actions. Sufficient information exists to guide these prescribing practices, although important uncertainties remain—notably the possible different effects of oral and transdermal estrogens and the effects of long-term progestin use after menopause. Most investigators be-lieve that the unfavorable action of progestins on lipoproteins may be clini-cally more important than the favorable effect of preventing endometrial cancer.

Androgens are also important in hormonal regulation of lipid and lipoprotein levels; moreover, they may produce insulin resistance through an as yet not understood mechanism. Many women have increased androgen action either as a primary disorder or as a result of hormonal treatment. Because androgens account for the less favorable lipid profile of men it is plausible that increased androgen action predisposes to cardiovascular disease in women. Evidence that this situation is the case is discussed in Chapter 7.

Menopause is a dramatic event in the life of a woman not only psychologically but metabolically as well. This process is now being intensively investigated, although many questions remain to be answered. The relative effects of menopause itself, in contrast to advancing age, are controversial. Divergent views on this point are presented by Ulrich (Chapter 6) and Bush (Chapter 2).

Despite the near universality of dieting, obesity continues to increase in the American population. Most people with unfavorable lipid patterns are obese. The paradox of obesity, a curable disease that is rarely cured, is discussed in Chapter 9. Adult-onset diabetes mellitus is the obesity complication that is most important in terms of producing lipid abnormalities and heart attacks. Diabetic women may lose their female advantage with respect to cardiovascular disease. Although some forms of diabetes are the same in men and women, it now appears that abnormalities of carbohydrate metabolism may also be a result of specific endocrine abnonnalities in women. Because the physician concerned with lipid disorders must have a good knowledge of diabetes, a review of this subject by Hoogwerf is included. Hoogwerf's chapter presents the advances in conceptional understanding of this condition that have clarified diagnosis and possibly improved treatment.

Diet and lipid intake may have particular importance in women's health because of their possible relations to the development of breast and uterine cancer. Evidence in this regard is subject of a detailed review by Rose. This chapter should have considerable interest for physicians, as the literature in this area has been voluminous and not always consistent. Rose presents the case regarding the role of fat intake in the etiology of breast cancer. A more skeptical view is expressed by Hoogwerf in his chapter on diet.

One of the reasons for the increased interest in lipid disorders is the introduction of new and effective agents for their treatment, which underlines the need for clinicians who treat women to have a good background in lipid disorders. Many of the women seen by clinicians have total cholesterol or cholesterol subfraction levels above the treatment threshold. The use of dietary alteration for treatment is discussed by Hoogwerf and drug treatment by Bilheimer.

The chapter on drug treatment is detailed, with a comprehensive discussion of the clinical pharmacology of lipid-lowering drugs. Knowledge of this aspect of therapeutics up to now has been confined to lipidologists and a few internists who have maintained an interest in the field. With the new recommendations that more moderate degrees of hypercholesterolemia be treated, physicians involved in primary care must be able to treat lipid disorders. In many cases such treatment means drug therapy because dietary alteration is not always effective or achievable.

Many patients, perhaps women more often than men, are interested in the effects of life style on their health. This area is one in which there have been many enthusiasms but not always good science. Studies in this area and their limitations are reviewed by Frank.

Another area in which reproductive medicine and lipidology interact is treatment of the family. A woman with a just-diagnosed lipid disorder is likely to ask her physician about the implications for her family. She needs to be informed about the possible role of genetics for any abnormalities detected, the significance of lipid levels in children, and the impact of diet on lipid levels. The relevant information in this areas is reviewed by Garcia and Moodie.

As physicians, we tend to be most interested in information we can put to practical use. Because treatment has been difficult and results often disappointing, lipid disorders have until recently mainly interested researchers. This situation is changing rapidly. A variety of effective drugs have been introduced, and widespread availability of lipid subfraction measurements makes treatment easier to institute and monitor. Although a prevented heart attack cannot be detected, the decrease in risk can be determined by measuring cholesterol subfractions. Although this is a substitute endpoint, it can motivate patient and physician.

It is the hope of the editor that the present work will be useful to gynecologists, internists, family practitioners, pediatricians, and others with a major concern for the health of female patients. Although the lacuna is still hungry, it is likely that those interested in reproductive physiology and in lipids will combine their forces to fill it up during the next decade.

Reference

1. Hillman J. Interviews: Conversations with Laura Pozzo on Psychotherapy, Biography, Love, Soul, Dreams, Work, Imagination and the State of the Culture. Harper & Row: New York, 1983:94.

2
Epidemiology of Cardiovascular Disease in Women

Trudy L. Bush

Cardiovascular disease, broadly defined to include coronary heart disease and stroke, is the major killer of women in the United States. In terms of absolute number of deaths, the total is staggering. For example, in 1984 nearly 500,000 women died from cardiovascular disease, including 250,000 from ischemic heart disease and 100,000 from cerebrovascular disease.[1] It is an insufficiently appreciated fact that each year in the United States more women die from cardiovascular diseases than from all of the following conditions combined: cancers, respiratory conditions, digestive conditions, endocrine disorders, accidents, suicide, and infectious diseases (Fig. 2–1).

It is well accepted by both medical and lay persons that cardiovascular disease is the major health problem for men. There are numerous studies that have assessed the antecedents of cardiovascular disease in men, and there are many clinical trials of cardiovascular disease prevention in men. Despite the magnitude of the problem of cardiovascular disease in women, relatively few studies (either descriptive or experimental) have been conducted in women. However, more women than men actually die from cardiovascular diseases (Fig. 2–2).

A historical reason for this apparent lack of attention to cardiovascular disease in women is that early efforts at preventing cardiovascular disease have focused nearly exclusively on "premature" disease, i.e., that occurring before the age of 50 or 60 years. Cardiovascular mortality before age 50 is relatively rare in women. However, that definition of "premature" death is being challenged, and now many public health practitioners consider a death before age 70 or 75 to be "premature." Additionally, it was thought in the not too distant past that atherosclerosis (and thus cardiovascular disease) was an inevitable consequence of normal aging and not necessarily a separate, preventable disease process. Because cardiovascular disease occurs primarily in older women (> 50 years) we now are beginning to look more carefully at this condition in women and in older men.

Given the magnitude of the problem of cardiovascular disease in

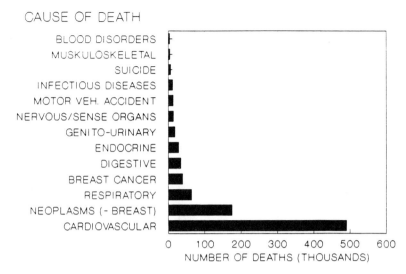

FIGURE 2–1. Number of deaths in women (in thousands) by cause, United States, 1984.

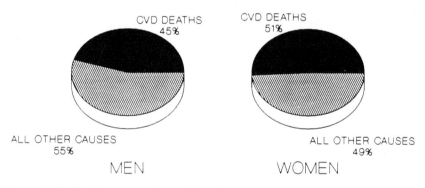

FIGURE 2–2. Cardiovascular disease (CVD) deaths as a proportion of all deaths in men and women, United States, 1984. (From *Vital Statistics of the United States*, 1983.[1])

women, the purpose of this chapter is threefold: (1) to briefly describe the occurrence of cardiovascular diseases in women by immutable personal characteristics; (2) to review the evidence on modifiable risk factors and cardiovascular disease in women; and (3) to describe and review the evidence on risk factors for cardiovascular disease that are unique to women. This chapter is mainly limited to studies and data accrued from the United States and focuses primarily on cardiovascular death rather than incidence.

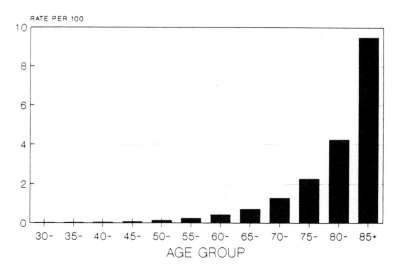

FIGURE 2–3. CVD death rates (per 100) in women by 5-year age groups, United States, 1984. (From *Vital Statistics of the United States*, 1983.[1])

Immutable Risk Factors

Age

Age is the strongest predictor of cardiovascular disease mortality in women. As seen in Figure 2–3, mortality from cardiovascular disease is approximately 50% higher for each succeeding 5-year age group.[1] The death rates from cardiovascular disease in women under 50 years of age are low, which has prompted some investigators to infer that premenopausal women are protected against the development of cardiovascular disease and that menopause per se increases the risk of cardiovascular disease. However, there is no evidence from vital statistics data that it is, in fact, the case. The rate of increase in mortality from cardiovascular disease between the ages of 30 to 49 is nearly identical to the rate of increase between the ages of 50 to 69 (Fig. 2–4), suggesting that age, not menopause, is determining the risk of cardiovascular disease.

Cardiovascular disease rates by 5-year age groups and sex are presented in Figure 2–5. As can be seen, the shape of the mortality curves are similar for both men and women (mortality from cardiovascular disease is approximately 50% higher for each succeeding 5-year age group in men also). However, death rates from cardiovascular disease in women lag approximately 7 to 8 years behind that in men. For example, women 52 years of age have approximately the same mortality rate due to cardiovascular disease as men 60 years of age, and women 65 years of age have cardiovascular disease death rates similar to those of men 73 years of age. However, at

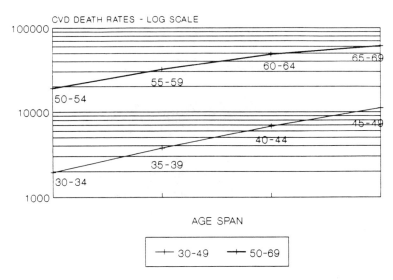

FIGURE 2–4. CVD death rates, women aged 30 to 49 years and 50 to 69 years, United States, 1984. (From *Vital Statistics of the United States*, 1983.[1])

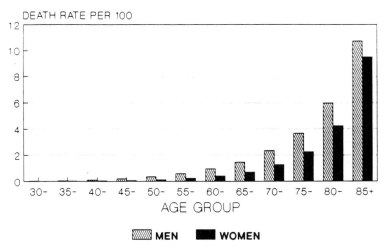

FIGURE 2–5. CVD death rates (per 100) in women and men by 5-year Age Groups, United States, 1984. (From *Vital Statistics of the United States*, 1983.[1])

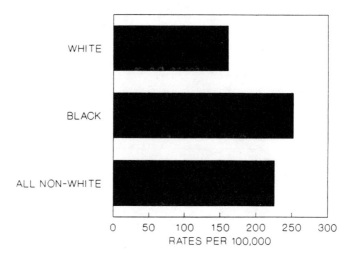

FIGURE 2–6. Age-adjusted CVD death rates in women by racial group, United States, 1984. (From *Vital Statistics of the United States*, 1983.[1])

every age, even the oldest ages (85+ years) women have lower cardiovascular disease mortality rates than do men.

Race

Mortality rates from all cardiovascular diseases are presented by racial group in Figure 2–6.[1] Before age 75, cardiovascular disease death rates are nearly twice as high in black women as in white women, whereas over age 75 death rates are somewhat higher among white women.[1] Death rates for specific cardiovascular diseases by race is presented in Figure 2–7. Compared to white women, black women have a 35% increased risk of dying from myocardial infarction and are three times as likely to die from cerebrovascular disease (stroke).

The lowest cardiovascular disease mortality rates among women are seen in those whose racial identity is neither black nor white (primarily Oriental women and non-black Hispanics). Women identified in this manner have death rates from cardiovascular disease that are approximately one-half that of white women.[2]

Family History

A family history of early cardiovascular disease has been clearly demonstrated to be a risk factor in men. Although data are not as plentiful for women, there is consistent evidence that a family history of cardiovascular

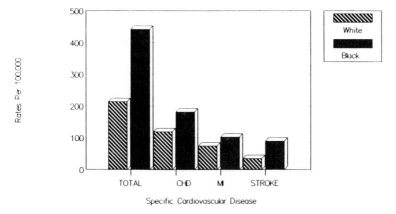

FIGURE 2–7. Age-adjusted specific cardiovascular death rates by race, women 35 to 74 years, United States, 1983. CHD = coronary heart disease; MI = mycordial infarction. (From Thom,[2] with permission.)

disease is a strong risk factor for young women particularly. Slack and Evans reported that female relatives of women with coronary disease under 55 years of age have an increased risk (risk ratio = 4.6) of early coronary death compared to the general population.[3] Rosenberg et al. found an increased risk (odds ratio = 1.5) of a maternal history of cardiovascular disease in women under age 50 with a myocardial infarction.[4] It is currently unknown whether a familial aggregation of specific cardiovascular disease risk factors (i.e., hyperlipidemia) or some as yet unidentified genetic factors account for these observed associations.

The association of a family history of cardiovascular disease with cardiovascular death in women over 50 years of age is unclear at this time. One large prospective study (Tecumseh Community Health Study) found a strong association between family history of cardiovascular disease and cardiovascular disease occurrence in women under 50 years of age (risk ratio = 5.7) but no association in those over 50 years of age.[5] In another prospective study (Rancho Bernardo Study), the family history of heart disease was only modestly (relative risk = 1.2) related to the risk of death from cardiovascular disease among women over 50 years of age.[6]

Modifiable Risk Factors

Blood Pressure

Elevated levels of either diastolic or systolic blood pressure have been documented to increase the risk of cardiovascular disease in women at all ages. In the Lipid Research Clinics' Follow-Up Study, women in the highest quartile of systolic blood pressure compared to women in the lowest quartile had a sevenfold increased risk of cardiovascular death.[7] In this 8-year prospective study, each 10 mm Hg increase in level of systolic blood pressure was associated with a 30% increase in risk of cardiovascular death, after adjustment for other cardiovascular disease risk factors.

A similar magnitude of effect has been shown in other studies. For example, in the Charleston Heart Study, a 10 mm Hg increase in the level of systolic blood pressure was associated with a 20% increase in risk of cardiovascular death in both black and white women.[8] In the Tecumseh Study, a 20 mm Hg increase in level of systolic blood pressure was associated with 70 to 80% increase in risk of coronary disease in women over age 50 years.[5] In the Framingham Study, a 10 mm Hg increase in level of systolic blood pressure was associated with a 20% increase in risk of cardiovascular disease occurrence in women age 50 to 59 years.[9]

Data from both the Hypertension Detection and Follow-Up Program[10] and the Australian Trial of Mild Hypertension[11] have clearly demonstrated that treating hypertension in women of all ages is both safe and effective.

Smoking

Cigarette smoking is also clearly a risk factor for cardiovascular disease among women.[12,13] The actual degree of risk varies from study to study and is dose dependent. It has been reported that women smoking as few as 10 cigarettes per day have a 50% increased risk of cardiovascular death, and among women smoking a pack or more per day the risk is increased more than 100% compared to nonsmokers.[13,14] There is currently some controversy as to whether cigarette smoking at the oldest ages (>65 years) remains a significant determinant of cardiovascular mortality in women. This issue can not be resolved until we have studied sufficient numbers of older women to adequately assess the question.

There is evidence, however, suggesting that quitting smoking for women reduces their risk of subsequent cardiovascular disease. In the Framingham Study the risk of developing cardiovascular disease after quitting smoking declined, over time, to that of nonsmokers.[15] Furthermore, as has been demonstrated in the Göteborg Study, women who quit smoking after a myocardial infarction have a significantly better survival than women who continued to smoke.[16]

Lipids and Lipoproteins

The association of lipids and lipoproteins with cardiovascular disease in women has been reviewed in detail elsewhere,[17] and only a summary is presented here. Overall, the data currently show that total cholesterol and high density lipoprotein (HDL) cholesterol are significant predictors of cardiovascular disease in women. The association of elevated LDL cholesterol levels has not been clearly documented to increase the risk of

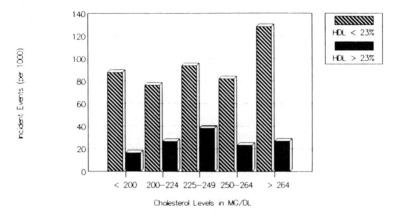

FIGURE 2–8. Incidence of coronary disease in women in the Donolo-Tel Aviv Study by levels of total cholesterol and percent of cholesterol in HDL. (From Brunner et al.,[19] with permission.)

cardiovascular disease in women, although this may be due to statistical considerations.

Women with elevations of total cholesterol over 260 mg/dl clearly appear to be at the highest risk for cardiovascular disease. In the Framingham Study, women with levels greater than 265 mg/dl had a relative risk of developing new cardiovascular disease that was two to three times higher than that of women with cholesterol levels less than 205 mg/dl.[18] A similar magnitude in increased risk was seen in other studies; i.e., women with total cholesterol levels greater than 264 mg/dl had a relative risk of 3.3 compared to women with concentrations less than 200 mg/dl in the Donolo-Tel Aviv Study.[19] In the Lipid Research Clinics Study, women with total cholesterol levels over 235 mg/dl had a 70% higher risk of cardiovascular disease death than women with levels less than 200 mg/dl.[7]

Although the total cholesterol level is a significant predictor of cardiovascular disease in women, HDL appears to be the more important lipid determinant in women. In the Framingham and Lipid Research Clinics Studies, a 10 mg/dl change in HDL levels in women was associated with a 45 to 50% risk difference in cardiovascular disease. Furthermore, in the Donolo-Tel Aviv Study, total cholesterol levels did not predict cardiovascular disease in women with high levels of HDL. That is, women with elevated total cholesterol levels and high HDL concentrations were not at increased risk of coronary disease (Fig. 2–8).

Diet

No studies of how diet may directly influence the risk of cardiovascular disease in women exist. However, diet can indirectly influence a woman's risk of cardiovascular disease in two major ways: (1) by contributing to

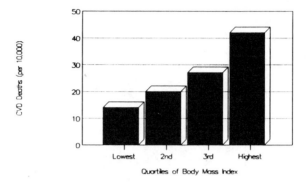

FIGURE 2–9. Age-adjusted cardiovascular mortality rates in women by quartiles of body mass index: results from the Lipid Research Clinics' Follow-Up Study. (From Bush et al.,[7] with permission.)

obesity and perhaps diabetes via excess total calories; and (2) by effecting changes in lipid and lipoprotein levels via fat composition/content. These indirect mechanisms are briefly reviewed below.

Obesity

There is evidence that obesity may significantly increase a woman's risk of developing cardiovascular disease. Current evidence suggests that obesity alone may not confer any additional risk, but obesity associated with hypertension and hyperlipidemia is causally related to cardiovascular disease risk.

In a univariate analysis of data from the Lipid Research Clinics Study, women in the highest quartile of body mass had a threefold excess risk of developing fatal cardiovascular disease compared to women in the lowest quartile of body mass.[7] Furthermore, there was a consistent dose-response relationship between body mass and cardiovascular death in this cohort (Fig. 2–9). Adjustment for other cardiovascular disease risk factors (i.e., blood pressure and cholesterol) attenuated the effect of body mass on cardiovascular risk, suggesting that some of the adverse effects of obesity are mediated through increased blood pressure and cholesterol levels.

Similar patterns of associations were seen in the Framingham Study,[9] the Alameda County Study,[20] and the Rancho Bernardo Study.[6] In the Framingham Study, a high relative weight was significantly associated with risk of developing cardiovascular disease in women aged 40 to 59 years. However, after adjustment for other cardiovascular disease risk factors, including hypertension, hyperlipidemia, and glucose intolerance, relative weight was no longer independently associated with an increased risk of disease.

In the Alameda County Study, women over 40 years of age in the highest quintile of body weight had a 2.5 excess risk of cardiovascular mortality compared to those in the middle quintile. Statistical adjustment for physical health status (blood pressure, chest pain, heart trouble, diabetes), resulted in weight no longer being a significant predictor of death. Likewise, in the Rancho Bernardo Study, women 50 to 64 years with a high body mass had a significant excess risk of cardiovascular mortality (risk ratio = 4.7), although after adjustment for other factors body mass was no longer a significant predictor.

The fact that most studies show that excess body weight is a significant predictor of cardiovascular disease only before statistical adjustment for other risk factors does not mean that obesity is unimportant in the pathogenesis of cardiovascular disease in women. Rather, it suggests that obesity may be one of the most important modifiable risk factors in women, as obesity usually precedes (and probably causes) such potent risk factors such as hypertension, hyperlipidemia, and hyperglycemia. In this regard, obesity could be considered the most important risk factor for cardiovascular disease in women and, from a public health perspective, should be targeted for significant intervention.

Diabetes

The association of diabetes and cardiovascular disease in women has been reviewed elsewhere,[21] and so only a brief overview is presented here. Two major points need to be emphasized. First, diabetes is a significant predictor of cardiovascular disease in women. Adult women with diabetes have rates of cardiovascular disease two to five times higher than those of women without diabetes. Second, women with diabetes lose the advantage of being female. That is, at every level of any other cardiovascular disease risk factor, women always have lower cardiovascular disease rates than men. (For example, women with systolic blood pressure levels of more than 160 mm Hg have lower cardiovascular disease rates than men with levels of more than 160 mm Hg, and women with total cholesterol values of more than 300 mg/dl have lower rates than men with values of more than 300 mg/dl.) However, women with diabetes tend to have the same rates of cardiovascular disease occurrence as men with diabetes. This loss of female protection is currently unexplained.

Lipids and Lipoproteins

Numerous components of diet, including dietary cholesterol, saturated and unsaturated fatty acids, complex carbohydrates, and fiber have been suggested to alter serum lipids and lipoproteins. Unfortunately, relatively few studies of dietary effects on lipids and lipoproteins have been conducted in women; the studies that have been performed are reviewed elsewhere.[17]

In women, the overall impact of a diet low in total fat (< 30% of total calories), a diet high in polyunsaturated fatty acids, or both is to modestly lower all lipids and lipoproteins, including HDL. Reductions for total cholesterol, LDL, and HDL have been reported to range between 7% and 12%. For some unknown reason, women tend to respond to dietary intervention less well than men; i.e., they appear to be somewhat resistant. This resistance may be due to high levels of circulating hormones, which among women may be more important determinants of serum lipid levels than diet.

Exercise

Most epidemiological data demonstrate a protective effect of physical activity on the risk for cardiovascular disease in men. Unfortunately, few studies have prospectively evaluated the association of regular physical activity and risk of cardiovascular disease among women. In men, the apparent protective effect of physical activity has been suggested to occur through two major mechanisms: (1) beneficial changes in other cardiovascular disease risk factors; and (2) improved physiologic functioning of the heart and vascular system.

Three prospective studies have evaluated the impact of physical activity on the risk of fatal cardiovascular disease among women. In the Lipid Research Clinics Study,[7] there was no association between regular physical activity and risk of dying from cardiovascular disease. However, in both the Framingham Study[9] and the Alameda County Study,[20] in univariate analysis physical activity was associated with a significantly lower risk of cardiovascular death. However, after statistical adjustment for other risk factors, physical activity was no longer significantly related to cardiovascular disease mortality in either study.

These findings suggest that physical activity, like obesity, may exert a beneficial effect on cardiovascular disease risk by operating through other risk factors. Indeed, physical activity has been demonstrated in men to decrease body fat, lower blood pressure, beneficially influence glucose and insulin levels, and modify lipid and lipoprotein levels. There is some evidence that exercise may modify lipid and lipoprotein levels in women.[17] However, the magnitude of the effect of physical activity on cardiovascular disease risk and other mechanisms by which physical activity may lower risk in women remain unclear.

Risk Factors Unique to Women

Parity

It has been suggested that endogenous hormonal factors may be related to both fertility and the subsequent development of cardiovascular disease in women. However, although some studies have reported an excess risk of cardiovascular disease among women with an increased number of pregnancies and abortions, others have found no such relation.[22] This issue is confounded by the fact that women with lower educational levels are more likely to have more children at an earlier age than educated women. Thus it may be education rather than number of pregnancies that influences the risk of cardiovascular disease.

Menopause

There is currently controversy as to whether natural menopause per se increases a woman's risk of cardiovascular disease. Certainly vital statistics data do not support such a conclusion, as the mortality rates from cardiovascular disease in women during the menopausal age parallel those of women prior to that age (Fig. 2–4). That is, if menopause did increase the risk of cardiovascular disease, we should see a change in the shape of the mortality curve for women aged 50 to 69 years.

Methodological problems also confuse the picture. For example, data from case-control studies suggest that early natural menopause is associated with an increased risk of cardiovascular disease. However, cigarette smoking is associated with both early natural menopause and an increased risk of cardiovascular disease; thus it is likely that the association between early menopause and disease risk is due to smoking.

Although the relationship between natural menopause and cardiovascular disease risk remains uncertain, there is an abundance of evidence suggesting that early surgical menopause is associated with an increased risk of cardiovascular disease.[22] It is unclear at this time if this increase in risk is due to the early loss of ovarian hormones or if factors associated with the reasons for the surgery affect the development of cardiovascular disease.

Exogenous Hormone Use

Oral Contraceptives

It is well documented and generally accepted that women using high-dose oral contraceptives have an increased risk of cardiovascular disease,[23,24] although other interpretations of those data are available.[25] Generally, increased risks of cardiovascular disease have been shown to be directly related to the dose of estrogen used, with users generally having rates two to four times higher than nonusers. The major adverse effects of oral contraceptive use appear to be concentrated in two groups of women: those over 35 years of age and those who smoke cigarettes. Currently, there are few studies on the effect of low-dose oral contraceptives on cardiovascular disease risk. However, a major initiative by the National Institutes of Health is being launched in 1990 to examine the effect of low-dose oral contraceptives on cardiovascular disease.

Estrogen Replacement Therapy

Most studies assessing the effects of estrogen replacement therapy on cardiovascular risk show that estrogen users have about one-half the risk of developing cardiovascular disease as non-users.[26] It has been demonstrated that much of the cardioprotective effect of estrogen use may be mediated through estrogen-induced increases in HDL levels,[27] although other mechanisms have been postulated.

It is currently unknown if the addition of a progestin to an estrogen regimen, as is currently done to protect the endometrium, influences the risk of cardiovascular disease in women receiving hormonal replacement therapy. This issue is of particular concern, as progestins generally adversely affect lipid and lipoprotein concentrations and thus may negate or overwhelm any beneficial estrogen effects. A multicenter clinical trial (Postmenopausal Estrogen and Progestin Intervention, or PEPI) which is assessing the relative effects of various estrogen and estrogen/progestin regimens on cardiovascular disease risk factors, is currently under way in the United States.

Summary

This chapter has provided an overview of the occurrence of cardiovascular disease in women in the United States and briefly has reviewed the evidence for selected risk factors for cardiovascular disease in women. Three general conclusions can be drawn from the data presented here.

First, the traditional male risk factors for cardiovascular disease (smoking, elevated blood pressure, elevated cholesterol) also predict cardiovascular disease in women. Thus women as well as men should be evaluated and treated for the presence of these risk factors.

Second, although obesity and physical activity are not independently associated with risk of cardiovascular disease, it seems prudent, given their impact on other powerful determinants of cardiovascular disease, to encourage women to maintain an appropriate body weight and to engage in regular physical activity.

Third, given the magnitude of the protective effect shown in most studies, the use of estrogen replacement therapy in postmenopausal women ought to be considered as prophylactic therapy for cardiovascular disease, particularly in women at high risk of cardiovascular disease.

References

1. Vital statistics of the United States 1983. II. Mortality part B. Washington, DC: US Department of Health and Human Services Publication 87-1114, 1987.
2. Thom TJ. Cardiovascular disease mortality in U.S. women. In: Eaker E, Pac-

kard B, Wenger N, et al, eds. Coronary Heart Disease in Women. New York: Haymarket Doyma, 1987:33–41.

3. Slack J, Evans KA. The increased risk of death from ischemic heart disease in first degree relatives of 121 men and 96 women with ischemic heart disease. J Med Genet 1966;3:239–257.

4. Rosenberg L, Miller DR, Kaufman DW, et al. Myocardial infarction in women under 50 years of age. JAMA 1983;250:2801–2806.

5. Higgins M, Keller JB, Ostrander LD. Risk factors for coronary heart disease in women: Tecumseh Community Health Study, 1959 to 1980. In: Eaker E, Packard B, Wenger N, et al, eds. Coronary Heart Disease in Women. New York: Haymarket Doyma, 1987:83–89.

6. Barrett-Connor E, Khaw KT, Wingard DL. A ten-year prospective study of coronary heart disease mortality among Rancho Bernardo women. In: Eaker E, Packard B, Wenger N, et al, eds. Coronary Heart Disease in Women. New York: Haymarket Doyma, 1987:117–21.

7. Bush TL, Criqui MH, Cowan LD, et al. Cardiovascular disease mortality in women: results from the Lipid Research Clinics Follow-up Study. In: Eaker E, Packard B, Wenger N, et al, eds. Coronary Heart Disease in Women. New York: Haymarket Doyma, 1987:106–11.

8. Keil JE, Gazes PC, Loadbolt CB, et al. Coronary heart disease mortality and its predictors among women in Charleston, South Carolina. In: Eaker E, Packard B, Wenger N, et al, eds. Coronary Heart Disease in Women. New York: Haymarket Doyma, 1987:90–98.

9. Eaker ED, Castelli WP. Coronary heart disease and its risk factors among women in the Framingham Study. In: Eaker E, Packard B, Wenger N, et al, eds. Coronary heart disease in women. New York: Haymarket Doyma, 1987:122–130.

10. Hypertension Detection and Follow-up Program Cooperative Group. Five-year findings of the Hypertensive Detection and Follow-up Program. II. Mortality by race, sex and age. JAMA 1979;242:2572–2577.

11. Management Committee of the Australian Therapeutic Trial in Mild Hypertension. Untreated mild hypertension: a report by the Management Committee of the Australian Therapeutic Trial in Mild Hypertension. Lancet 1982;1:185–91.

12. Johansson S, Vedin A, Wilhelmsson C. Myocardial infarction in women. Epidemiol Rev 1983;5:67–95.

13. Bush TL, Comstock GW. Smoking and cardiovascular mortlity in women. Am J Epidemiol 1983;118:480–488.

14. Doll R, Gray R, Hafner B, et al. Mortality in relation to smoking: 22 years' observations on female British doctors. Br Med J 1980;1:967–971.

15. Kannel WB, Castelli WP, McNamara PM. Cigarette smoking and risk of coronary heart disease; epidemiologic clues to pathogenesis: The Framingham Study. In: Wynder EL, Hoffman D, eds. Toward a Less Harmful Cigarette. Bethesda: National Cancer Institute Monograph 28, 1968:9–21.

16. Wilhelmsson C, Johansson S, Vedin A. Stopping smoking after myocardial infarction in women. In: Oliver MF, Vedin A, Wilhelmsson C, eds. Myocardial Infarction in Women. New York: Churchill Livingstone, 1986:160–165.

17. Bush TL, Fried LP, Barrett-Connor E. Cholesterol, lipoproteins, and coronary heart disease in women. Clin Chem 1988;34:B60–B70.

18. Kannel WB, Gordon T, eds. The Framingham Study: An Epidemiological Investigation of Cardiovascular Disease. Section 30. Some Characteristics Related to the Incidence of cardiovascular Disease and Death: Framingham Study, 18-Year Follow-up. DHEW publication NIH 74-599. Washington, DC: US Government Printing Office, February 1974.

19. Brunner D, Weisbort J, Meshulam N, et al. Relation of serum total cholesterol and high-density lipoprotein cholesterol percentage to the incidence of definite coronary events: twenty year follow-up of the Donolo-Tel Aviv Prospective Coronary Artery Disease Study. Am J Cardiol 1987;59:1271–276.

20. Wingard DL, Cohn BA. Coronary heart disease mortality among women in Alameda County, 1965 to 1973. In: Eaker E, Packard B, Wenger N, et al, eds. Coronary Heart Disease in Women. New York: Haymarket Doyma, 1987:99–105.

21. Barrett-Connor E, Wingard DL. Diabetes and heart disease in women. In: Eaker E, Packard B, Wenger N, et al, eds. Coronary Heart Disease in Women. New York: Haymarket Doyma, 1987:190–194.

22. Bush TL, Barrett-Connor E. Noncontraceptive estrogen use and cardiovascular disease. Epidemiol Rev 1985;7:80–104.

23. Stadel B. Oral contraceptives and cardiovascular disease. N Engl J Med 1981;305:612–618, 672–677.

24. Vessey MP. Oral contraceptives and cardiovascular disease: some questions and answers. Br Med J 1982;284:615–619.

25. Realini JP, Goldzieher JW. Oral contraceptives and cardiovascular disease: a critique of the epidemiologic studies. Am J Obstet Gynecol 1985;152:729–798.

26. Bush TL. Non-contraceptive estrogen use and risk of cardiovascular disease: an overview and critique of the literature. In: Korenman SG, ed. Menopause: Biological and Clinical Consequences of Ovarian Failure—Evaluation and Management, New York, Plenum Publishing. Second Symposium, USA, 1990.

27. Bush TL, Barrett-Connor E, Cowan LD, et al. Cardiovascular mortality and noncontraceptive use of estrogen in women: results from the Lipid Research Clinics Program Follow-up Study. Circulation 1987;75:1102–1109.

3
Lipoprotein and Lipid Metabolism: Basic and Clinical Aspects

DAVID A. CHAPPELL and ARTHUR A. SPECTOR

Lipoproteins are complexes of lipid and specialized proteins called apoproteins. Apoproteins have physical properties that allow them to bind lipids that are insoluble in water and transport them in the plasma and interstitial fluid. The lipids consist of phospholipids and cholesterol, which are required for cell membrane synthesis, and triglycerides, which are the primary form of energy storage in mammals. In addition, cholesterol is a precursor for steroid hormone and bile acid synthesis. Lipoproteins are synthesized predominantly in two tissues, the liver and the intestine. Upon entering the circulation, lipoproteins undergo a complicated series of modifications. Abnormalities in the synthesis or metabolism of lipoproteins may lead to hyperlipidemia and accelerated atherosclerosis.

Plasma lipoproteins mediate the flux of lipids among the intestine, liver, and extrahepatic tissues, as illustrated in a simplified form in Figure 3–1. The metabolism of triglycerides and cholesterol is different. Dietary triglycerides and cholesterol initially are transported to extrahepatic tissues, e.g., adipose tissue and skeletal muscle, where most of the triglycerides are taken up and metabolized. The remainder of the triglycerides and most of the cholesterol are then removed from the plasma by the liver. In addition, cholesterol that accumulates in extrahepatic tissues may be transferred by plasma lipoproteins to the liver, where it is either resecreted into the plasma in newly synthesized lipoproteins or excreted in the bile. The liver also synthesizes triglycerides and secretes them in lipoproteins that are metabolized by extrahepatic tissues.

Lipoprotein Structure and Classification

Lipoproteins are exceedingly heterogeneous.[1] In fact, despite 60 years of research in this area, new species of lipoproteins are still in the process of being identified and characterized. Historically, lipoproteins have been divided into four broad classes according to their density: very low density lipoproteins (VLDL), intermediate density lipoproteins (IDL), low density

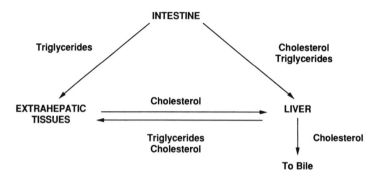

FIGURE 3–1. Lipid transport among tissues.

lipoproteins (LDL), and high density lipoproteins (HDL). Chylomicrons may be considered as a separate class of lipoproteins, but they resemble VLDL in many respects. VLDL are synthesized in the liver, whereas chylomicrons are synthesized in the intestine.[2] Because chylomicrons transport dietary fats, they are found only in low concentrations in the plasma in the fasted state. Chylomicrons and VLDL have the highest lipid content per particle and consequently are the least dense lipoproteins, whereas HDL have the lowest lipid content per particle and are the most dense lipoproteins. The properties of the major classes of lipoproteins are listed in Table 3–1. The distribution of plasma triglycerides and cholesterol in the fasted state among the major lipoprotein classes is illustrated in Figure 3–2. Most of the triglycerides in the plasma are carried in VLDL, whereas LDL carry most of the cholesterol.

All plasma lipoproteins have the same basic structure.[1] The most hydrophilic components—nonesterified cholesterol (i.e., cholesterol that does not contain a covalently bound fatty acid), phospholipids, and apoproteins—form a spherical surface that surrounds a hydrophobic core consisting of cholesteryl esters and triglycerides. With some exceptions, the content of nonesterified cholesterol and phospholipids in VLDL, IDL, LDL, and HDL is similar. However, the apoprotein content and the relative proportion of cholesteryl esters and triglycerides differ among the lipoprotein classes.

Chylomicrons and VLDL have a density less than that of the background plasma salt density (i.e., $d < 1.006$ g/ml). These lipoproteins are triglyceride-rich and contain relatively little cholesteryl ester. They range in molecular weight from about 12 million to over 200 million. On average, chylomicrons are larger than VLDL. In the plasma, the large triglyceride-rich lipoproteins are converted to smaller, more cholesteryl ester-rich lipoproteins through the action of lipases.[3] During this process, IDL are formed from VLDL. IDL, which have a density (d) intermediate between that of VLDL and LDL ($d = 1.006–1.019$ g/ml), are similar to VLDL ex-

TABLE 3–1. Plasma lipoproteins

Class	Abbreviation	Density (g/ml)	Electrophoretic mobility	Major lipid(s)	Major apoprotein(s)	Origin	Physiological function
Chylomicrons	None	<1.006	Origin[a]	Triglycerides	B48 A-I, A-IV	Intestine	Absorption of dietary fat and transport to tissues
Chylomicron remnants	None	<1.006	Pre-β to β	Cholesteryl esters, triglycerides	E B48	Plasma	Delivery of dietary fat to the liver
Very low density lipoproteins	VLDL	<1.006	Pre-β	Triglycerides	B100 E C-I, C-II, C-III	Liver	Transport of triglycerides from the liver to other tissues
Intermediate density lipoproteins	IDL	1.006–1.019	β to pre-β	Triglycerides, cholesteryl, esters	B100 E	Plasma	Initial product formed in VLDL catabolism
Low density lipoproteins	LDL	1.019–1.063	β	Cholesteryl esters	B100	Plasma	Cholesteryl ester transport
High density lipoproteins	HDL	1.063–1.210	α	Cholesteryl esters, phospholipids	A-I, A-II	Liver, intestine	Removal of excess cholesterol from tissues and lipoproteins; remodeling of lipoproteins

[a]Chylomicrons have pre-β mobility by free electrophoresis; but because of their size they are trapped at the origin when electrophoresis is performed on agarose, cellulose acetate, or paper supports.

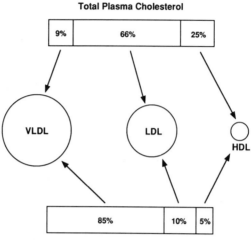

FIGURE 3–2. Distribution of plasma lipids among the major lipoprotein classes. This figure illustrates the distribution in the fasting state when the amounts of chylomicrons and remnant particles are negligible.

cept that IDL are smaller and are more enriched in cholesteryl esters. Further modification of IDL gives rise to LDL, which have a density of 1.019 to 1.063 g/ml and contain a core consisting predominantly of cholesteryl esters. Subclasses of LDL have been identified; their physiological significance is unclear. HDL have a density of 1.063 to 1.210 g/ml. HDL have been divided into three subclasses by density and into more than five subclasses using other techniques.[4] HDL_2 have an average density of about 1.075 g/ml, whereas HDL_1 are less dense, and HDL_3 are more dense. HDL_2 concentrations in plasma vary with different physiological states to a greater degree than do the other HDL subclasses. HDL_2 concentrations are higher in premenopausal women than in men and are increased by the administration of estrogens and by exercise.

Apoprotein Structure and Function

The apoproteins direct the metabolic fate of the lipoproteins on which they are carried.[5] They may act as recognition sites for cell-surface receptors or as cofactors for enzyme activation, or they may have a structural role in maintaining the integrity of the lipoproteins. The genes for the major plasma apoproteins have been cloned and the amino acid sequences determined.[6] All apoproteins contain hydrophobic amino acids that bind to lipids and hydrophilic amino acids that are exposed to the aqueous en-

TABLE 3–2. Apolipoproteins

Type	Lipoprotein class(es)	Molecular weight	Origin	Metabolic function
A-I	HDL, nascent chylomicrons	28,000	Liver, intestine	LCAT cofactor
A-II	HDL	17,400	Liver, intestine	Unknown
A-IV	Nascent chylo-microns, HDL	44,500	Intestine	Unknown
B48	Chylomicrons, chylo-micron remnants	265,000	Intestine	Chylomicron syn-thesis and secretion
B100	VLDL, IDL, LDL	550,000	Liver	Recognition by the LDL receptor; up-take of LDL by tis-sues
C-I	VLDL, HDL	6,630	Liver	Unknown
C-II	VLDL, HDL	8,900	Liver	Lipoprotein lipase cofactor
C-III	VLDL, HDL	8,800	Liver	Unknown
D	HDL	22,000	Unknown	Unknown
E	VLDL, IDL, chylo-micron remnants	34,100	Liver, macro-phages	Recognition by the LDL receptor; up-take of remnants by the liver

vironment in the plasma. Table 3–2 lists the apoproteins and their properties.

Apoprotein B100 (apo B100) and apo B48 are the largest apoproteins. A single gene encodes both apo B100 and apo B48.[7] However, because of tissue-specific intracellular processing in humans, apo B100 is produced only in the liver, whereas apo B48 is produced only in the intestine. Apo B48 has an amino acid sequence identical to that of the amino-terminal 48% of apo B100. Apo B100 contains a recognition site for cell-surface lipoprotein receptors, but apo B48 does not. As is discussed later, the ability of apo B100 to bind to cell-surface lipoprotein receptors permits receptor-mediated removal of apo B100-containing lipoproteins from the plasma. VLDL, IDL, and LDL contain apo B100, whereas chylomicrons and chylomicron remnants contain apo B48. The function of apo B48 is unknown. Because of its large size, apo B48 may play a structural role in maintaining the integrity of chylomicrons.

The other apoproteins are much smaller than apo B100 and apo B48 (molecular weights that range from 6,630 to 44,500), which may account for their ability to exchange freely between the various lipoprotein classes in the plasma. Like apo B100, apo E has a recognition site for cell-surface lipoprotein receptors,[8] which allows cells to bind and internalize lipoproteins that contain apo E. Apo E is found in chylomicron remnants, VLDL, IDL, and some HDL. There are three common isoforms of apo E called E2, E3, and E4, that differ by a single amino acid substitution.[9] Apo E3 and apo E4 have 50-fold higher affinity for LDL receptors than does apo E2. Apo E is important in the normal receptor-mediated clearance of triglyceride-rich lipoproteins and their remnants. Defective apo E-mediated binding of lipoproteins from individuals homozygous for apo E2 is associated with type III hyperlipoproteinemia, also called dysbetalipoproteinemia.

Two apoproteins, apo CII and apo AI, serve as cofactors for important enzymes in lipoprotein metabolism.[5] Apo CII is essential for activation of lipoprotein lipase. Apo AI is the predominant, but not the sole, activator of lecithin: cholesterol acyltransferase (LCAT). The function of the other apoproteins is not well established. Apo CI, apo CII, and apo CIII exist predominantly in chylomicrons, VLDL, and HDL, whereas apo AI, apo AII, and apo AIV exist predominantly in HDL.

Lipoprotein Formation

Chylomicron Synthesis

Dietary triglycerides and cholestryl esters are emulsified by the bile and then digested to cholesterol, fatty acids, and 2-monoglyceride by pancreatic enzymes.[10,11] The mucosal cells in the small intestine absorb the products of lipid digestion by passive diffusion. Triglycerides are resynthesized from the absorbed fatty acids and monoglycerides in the smooth endoplasmic reticulum, and cholesterol and phospholipids are added to form a micelle.[2] Apo B48, apo AI, apo AII, and apo AIV are synthesized in the rough endoplasmic reticulum and are combined with the lipid as the components move from the rough and smooth endoplasmic reticulum into the Golgi apparatus, where additional glycosylation occurs. The newly assembled chylomicrons then enter secretory vesicles and move to the basolateral plasma membrane, where they are secreted into the lateral intercellular space and then into the lymph. Apo B48 is required for chylomicron synthesis. Individuals with congenital abetalipoproteinemia cannot synthesize apo B48 or chylomicrons.

The size of the chylomicrons formed depends on the amount of triglyceride available in the enterocyte. When more dietary triglycerides are available, larger chylomicrons are formed. When chylomicrons enter the plasma, apo AI and apo AIV are transferred to HDL, and apo C is acquired from HDL. Immediately after secretion, modification begins to occur through the action of enzymes and the exchange of apoproteins, so that the mature chylomicrons present in the plasma have a somewhat different lipid and apoprotein composition than the newly secreted particles. For example, chylomicrons in the lymph contain little apo C.

VLDL Synthesis

VLDL are triglyceride-rich particles that are produced in the liver.[2] The fatty acids used for triglyceride synthesis in the liver are derived from two sources: dietary carbohydrates that are converted into fatty acids in the hepatocytes, and fatty acids that are removed from the plasma by the liver. The latter are derived from either free fatty acids that are released into the plasma by extrahepatic tissues, primarily adipocytes, or the triglycerides contained in plasma lipoproteins taken up by the liver. Lipoprotein assembly in the liver occurs in a manner similar to that in the intestine. Triglycerides, phospholipids, and cholesterol present in the smooth endoplasmic reticulum are combined into a micelle and are then further combined with apolipoproteins B100, E, CI, CII, and CIII, which are synthesized in the rough endoplasmic reticulum. The mechanism whereby the apoproteins are combined with the lipids during lipoprotein assembly is not understood. It is known, however, that apo B100 is required for VLDL synthesis because individuals with congenital abetalipoproteinemia, who cannot synthesize apo B100, do not produce VLDL. Apo B100 is partially glycosylated in the rough endoplasmic reticulum, and additional glycosylation occurs in the Golgi apparatus. After the particle enters the secretory vesicle, it is released into the space of Disse and then enters the plasma. As described earlier for the chylomicron, the nascent VLDL undergo enzymatic modification and apoprotein exchanges immediately after they enter the plasma.

HDL Synthesis

Nascent HDL are formed by the liver and small intestine, but little is known about this process or its regulation.[2,12,13] The liver secretes a discoid particle containing phospholipid, nonesterified cholesterol, and apo E. These discoid HDL are remodeled into the spherical HDL after secretion.[2] During this process cholesterol is esterified enzymatically and apo E is exchanged with apo AI from other lipoproteins. Some evidence indicates that the intestine also secretes similar discoid particles, except that they contain apo AI instead of apo E. Other data suggest that the intestine does not secrete nascent HDL directly; rather, the HDL may be derived from the catabolism of chylomicrons. More work is needed to determine the extent to which each of these two mechanisms operate.

Factors Regulating Lipoprotein Synthesis

Chylomicron and VLDL synthesis may be affected by both the quantity and type of fatty acids that are available for lipoprotein assembly. Chylomicron synthesis increases as the dietary triglyceride intake increases; VLDL synthesis increases as the liver triglyceride content increases. Unsaturated fatty acids are more effective than saturated fatty acids in stimulating VLDL synthesis. In addition, long-chain fatty acids stimulate VLDL more than do medium- or short-chain fatty acids. Increased dietary carbohydrate intake also increases VLDL production by stimulating hepatic fatty acid synthesis. Likewise, alcohol increases VLDL production by making more fatty acid available for triglyceride synthesis in the liver. Insulin, glucagon, and other hormones also regulate fatty acid synthesis.

The effects of dietary cholesterol on lipoprotein formation are complicated and not fully understood. In experimental animals, a high dietary cholesterol intake may alter the type of particle that is formed, rather than increasing the production of normal lipoproteins. For example, in some species the liver produces a modified form of VLDL that is rich in cholesteryl esters, called β-VLDL. In others, a large HDL particle rich in cholesterol and apo E, called either HDL_1 or HDL_c, is produced in response to excess dietary cholesterol. In humans, LDL concentrations are often elevated when the diet is high in cholesterol. Both experimental animals and humans manifest individual variability in the severity of hypercholesterolemia induced by a high-cholesterol diet. The cause of this variability is unknown.

Lipoprotein Metabolism in Plasma

Enzymatic Modifications and Apoprotein Exchanges

Enzymatic modifications and apoprotein exchanges occur continuously in the plasma. Several enzymes that are involved in the modification and metabolism of lipoproteins are listed in Table 3–3 and illustrated in Figure 3–3. Lipoprotein lipase and hepatic lipase catalyze the hydrolysis of triglycerides and phospholipids. Both enzymes are bound to heparin-like sites on capillary endothelium in various tissues and the liver, respectively.[3] However, lipoprotein lipase appears to be most important in triglyceride hydrolysis, as a deficiency of this enzyme or its cofactor, apo CII, is associated with severe hypertriglyceridemia. The absence of hepatic lipase has been reported in two brothers who have increased plasma concentrations of remnant lipoproteins called β-VLDL. Other evidence suggests that hepatic lipase is important in the conversion of HDL_2 to HDL_3. Hepatic lipase is increased by androgens and decreased by estrogens. Lipoprotein lipase is increased in the fed versus the fasted state and is regulated by insulin and other hormones.

TABLE 3–3. Enzymes mediating lipoprotein metabolism

Enzyme	Substrate(s)	Reaction	Site of action	Metabolic role
Lipoprotein lipase	Triglycerides and phospholipids	Hydrolysis	Capillary surface	Release of fatty acids from VLDL and chylomicrons
Hepatic lipase	Triglyceride and phospholipids	Hydrolysis	Liver sinusoids	Unknown, possibly HDL$_2$ catabolism
Lecithin: cholesterol acyltranferase (LCAT)	Cholesterol and phosphatidyl-choline	Cholesterol esterifica-tion	Plasma lipopro-teins, especial-ly HDL	Reverse cholesterol transport
Acid lipase	Triglycerides and cholesteryl esters	Hydrolysis	Lysosomes	Catabolism of lipoproteins incorporated into tissues by receptor-mediated endo-cytosis

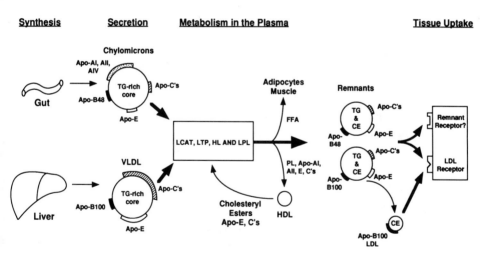

FIGURE 3–3. Metabolism of the triglyceride-rich lipoproteins and LDL. TG = triglycerides; LCAT = lecithin: cholesterol acyltransferase; LTP = lipid transfer protein; HL = hepatic lipase; LPL = lipoprotein lipase; FFA = free fatty acid; PL = phospholipids; CE = cholesteryl esters.

Other enzymes that are involved in lipoprotein metabolism include LCAT and lysosomal acid lipase. LCAT, which catalyzes cholesteryl ester formation in the plasma,[14] plays an important role in reverse cholesterol transport. In this process, excess nonesterified cholesterol in extrahepatic tissues is transferred to plasma lipoproteins, predominantly HDL, where it is esterified through the LCAT reaction. The resulting cholesteryl esters are subsequently taken up by the liver. LCAT deficiency causes a variety of lipid abnormalities, including a decrease in the plasma cholesteryl ester content and an increase in the nonesterified cholesterol content of erythrocyte and tissue membranes.

Lysosomal acid lipase is an intracellular enzyme; it is not found in the plasma. This lipase mediates the lysosomal degradation of triglycerides and cholesteryl esters that have been taken up by cells through receptor-mediated endocytosis.[15] Wolman's disease, which is characterized by massive intracellular lipid accumulation, is caused by a deficiency of the lysosomal acid lipase.

Apoprotein exchanges among plasma lipoproteins are important in normal lipid metabolism (Fig. 3–3). For example, following ingestion of a fatty meal, apo E and the C apoproteins exchange from HDL to the triglyceride-rich lipoproteins. This exchange is associated with the hydrolysis of triglycerides by lipases. The effect of hydrolysis on the structure of chylomicrons and VLDL is analogous to letting air out of a balloon. As triglycerides are lost, the surface material becomes greater than that needed to surround the contents, which causes the lipoproteins to transiently acquire a floppy appearance. Excess nonesterified cholesterol, phospholipids, apo E, and the C apoproteins are partially transferred to HDL. In contrast, apo B100 and apo B48 are retained on the particles. Little is known about the relative affinities of different apoproteins for different lipids. As a result, the mechanism whereby apoproteins partition among the various lipoprotein classes is unknown.

Lipoprotein Remnants

Chylomicrons and VLDL that have undergone hydrolysis by the lipases are called *remnants*.[16] The remnants of triglyceride-rich lipoproteins comprise an ill-defined class of lipoproteins consisting of small VLDL and IDL that are relatively enriched in cholesteryl esters due to the selective loss of triglycerides during lipolysis (Fig. 3–3). Except in certain diseases, such as type III hyperlipoproteinemia, the plasma concentration of remnant lipoproteins is low in the fasted state. Most VLDL remnants and virtually all of the chylomicron remnants undergo receptor-mediated clearance by the liver. Current evidence suggests that this clearance is mediated by apo E.[17] A small portion of VLDL remnants undergo further hydrolysis of triglycerides and further loss of apo E and the C apoproteins to form LDL, which contain apo B100 as the sole apoprotein. The conversion of VLDL

TABLE 3–4. Lipoprotein receptors

Receptor	Recognition factor	Lipoprotein-bound	Tissue	Metabolic role
LDL	Apo B100, Apo E	LDL, IDL	Liver, many other tissues	Removal for LDL, IDL from circulation
Scavenger	Chemically modified lipoproteins	Modified lipoproteins	Macrophages, endothelium	Unknown; probably removal of damaged lipoproteins
HDL	Unknown	HDL	Liver, possibly other tissues	Existence and function are questionable

to LDL is the major, if not the only, pathway for the synthesis of LDL. The metabolism of VLDL and chylomicrons—including hydrolysis of triglycerides by lipases, loss of excess surface material to HDL, receptor-mediated clearance of remnants by the liver, and conversion of a small fraction of VLDL to LDL—takes place during a few hours. In contrast to the relatively rapid clearance of triglyceride-rich lipoproteins, LDL and HDL have more prolonged residence times in the plasma (>2 days).

Receptor-Mediated Clearance of Lipoproteins

The interaction of lipoproteins with cell-surface receptors is a major determinant of the metabolic fate of the lipoproteins.[18,19] Hereditary mutations that disrupt the interaction between lipoproteins and cell-surface receptors may decrease the rate of clearance from the plasma of certain lipoproteins.[18,20] The receptors and their characteristics are listed in Table 3–4.

Two apoproteins are known to have receptor recognition sites: apo B100 and apo E. They bind with high affinity and specificity to LDL receptors. Because LDL receptors recognize both apo B100-containing and apo E-containing lipoproteins, they are also called apo B,E receptors. Individuals with familial hypercholesterolemia have abnormalities in the LDL receptor that prevent normal binding of LDL and cause elevated plasma LDL concentrations. Abnormalities in apo E that disrupt its binding to the LDL receptor are strongly associated with type III hyperlipoproteinemia. Defective binding of apo E-containing lipoproteins to LDL receptors may cause delayed clearance of chylomicron and VLDL remnants, thereby causing elevated plasma cholesterol and triglyceride concentrations. Furthermore, a mutation in apo B100 has been implicated as a cause of hypercholesterolemia due to defective binding of LDL to the LDL receptor.

As triglyceride-rich lipoproteins undergo lipolysis, they become progressively smaller and enriched in cholesterol. Almost all of the intestinal (apo

B48-containing) and hepatic (apo B100-containing) remnant particles are removed rapidly from the plasma (Fig. 3–3). However, a small fraction of the apo B100-containing remnant particles are converted to LDL. The removal of triglyceride-rich lipoproteins and their remnants from the plasma during lipolysis is thought to occur by receptor-mediated clearance. There is some evidence for the existence of a remnant receptor that is distinct from the LDL receptor, but it is unproved. It is clear that triglyceride-rich lipoproteins and their remnants may bind to LDL receptors in vitro. Large VLDL bind to LDL receptors via apo E, whereas small VLDL and LDL bind to the LDL receptor via apo B100.

Virtually every tissue in the body may express LDL receptors, but the largest reservoir of this receptor is the liver. Normally, about 70% of the plasma LDL is removed by the liver. Although virtually every cell can synthesize cholesterol, cells preferentially use their LDL receptors to obtain cholesterol by taking up plasma lipoproteins. The expression of LDL receptors is regulated by the intracellular demand for cholesterol. For example, depletion of bile acids by the oral administration of bile acid binding resins increases hepatic demand for cholesterol and causes an increase in the number of hepatic LDL receptors. Conversely, if cells have too much cholesterol, they decrease their LDL receptor number. For example, feeding a high-cholesterol diet to experimental animals causes suppression of hepatic LDL receptors. Lipoproteins that are incorporated into tissues via the LDL receptor are degraded in lysosomes by several enzymes, including acid lipase, which hydrolyzes both triglycerides and cholesteryl esters (Table 3–3). The nonesterified cholesterol released into the cell by this hydrolysis decreases expression of the LDL receptor.

Although the regulation of LDL receptors is understood to some degree in vitro, we cannot measure LDL receptors noninvasively in human tissues. Therefore, with the exception of subjects with familial hypercholesterolemia who have a deficiency or abnormality in LDL receptors, we can only speculate about how LDL receptors govern the variability in plasma cholesterol concentrations in humans. Pharmacological doses of estrogens increase hepatic LDL receptor expression in experimental animals. However, similar data are not available in humans; we do not know how physiological variations in estrogen levels affect the expression of LDL receptors. We also cannot measure how variations in dietary fats affect the expression of LDL receptors in humans.

Two other lipoprotein receptors have been described, but their function is unknown. The scavenger receptor of macrophages recognizes a variety of chemically modified proteins, including modified lipoproteins. It is possible that scavenger receptors are important in the removal of damaged proteins and lipoproteins from the plasma. Receptors that specifically recognize HDL have been identified by some investigators; however, their role in lipid metabolism is not established.

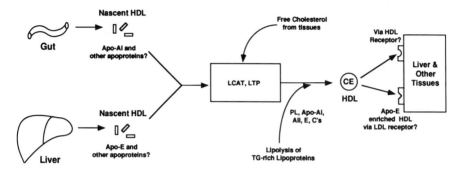

FIGURE 3–4. HDL metabolism. The abbreviations are the same as those in Figure 3–3.

Reverse Cholesterol Transport

Reverse cholesterol transport refers to the process of removal of cholesterol from extrahepatic tissues.[21,22] The physiological significance, magnitude, and regulation of reverse cholesterol transport are not completely understood. Nonesterified cholesterol is a structural component of biological membranes. In addition, it exists on the surface of lipoproteins. LCAT catalyzes the esterification of cholesterol by a fatty acid donated from phospholipids. This reaction may occur in a variety of lipoproteins but appears to be most prevalent in HDL. The metabolism of HDL is illustrated in Figure 3–4. Apo AI contained in HDL is the most potent activator of LCAT in the plasma. After esterification, the cholesteryl ester moves to the hydrophobic core of the lipoprotein, which causes the conversion of nascent discoid HDL to the spherical HDL that are found in the plasma. Normally, there may be a chemical gradient whereby nonesterified cholesterol moves from cell membranes to the plasma. The esterification of cholesterol and its transport to the core of lipoproteins may maintain this chemical gradient. Cholesteryl esters may be exchanged for triglycerides in chylomicrons, VLDL, or IDL through the action of a lipid transfer protein (LTP).[23] Most cholesteryl esters in VLDL probably are transferred there from HDL by LTP. The removal of cholestryl esters contained in the VLDL, IDL, and LDL through uptake by tissues expressing LDL receptors completes the reverse cholesterol transport pathway. The cholesterol taken up by liver may be excreted in bile as nonesterified cholesterol or after conversion to a bile acid. Alternatively, the liver may secrete cholesterol back into the circulation in nascent lipoproteins. Some HDL may become enriched in apo E and be cleared from the plasma by LDL receptors. In addition, there is some evidence for a distinct HDL receptor that does not bind apo E. However, the physiological significance of lipoprotein receptors in HDL metabolism is currently unknown.

The plasma HDL cholesterol concentration may be an indicator for the activity of the reverse cholesterol transport pathway. High plasma HDL cholesterol concentrations are associated with low risk for atherosclerosis. Presumably, the high HDL concentration is a reflection of the ability of the reverse cholesterol transport pathway to remove cholesterol from tissues, but we do not know enough yet about the regulation of this pathway. In general, premenopausal women have higher HDL cholesterol concentrations than do men, suggesting that sex hormones may regulate this pathway to some extent.

Lipid Disorders

Overview of Atherosclerosis

Atherosclerosis is a complicated disease process involving platelets, macrophages, smooth muscle cells, clotting factors, growth factors, and lipoproteins.[24] The plasma LDL cholesterol concentration is positively correlated with atherosclerotic risk.[25] High concentrations of other cholesterol-rich lipoproteins such as β-VLDL are also associated with increased risk for atherosclerosis. The endothelial surface provides a barrier between the plasma and the arterial wall. Hypertension, cigarette smoking, and other factors may injure the endothelium, resulting in extravasation of plasma into the arterial wall. The details of atherogenesis are beyond the scope of this chapter. However, it should be noted that, of all the plasma constituents that may accumulate in the arterial wall after endothelial injury, cholesterol is the most difficult substance to metabolize. Cholesterol is virtually indestructible in the arterial wall because this tissue does not contain any enzymatic machinery to break it down into smaller fragments. Therefore if delivery of cholesterol to the arterial wall exceeds the capacity of the reverse cholesterol transport pathway to remove it, progressive cholesterol deposition results. This situation ultimately may cause arterial occlusion.

Phenotypic Classification of Hyperlipoproteinemia

The hyperlipoproteinemias are classified phenotypically by the lipoprotein constituent that is elevated in the plasma, as is shown in Table 3–5. The type I, IV, and V patterns are due to elevations in triglyceride-rich lipoproteins that are derived from the intestine, liver, or both, respectively. The type IIa and IIb patterns result from an elevation of plasma LDL or both LDL and VLDL, respectively. The type III pattern is due to elevation of

TABLE 3–5. Phenotypic classification of hyperlipoproteinemia

Phenotype	Elevated lipoproteins	Plasma lipid elevations
I	Chylomicrons	Triglycerides
IIa	LDL	Cholesterol
IIb	LDL, VLDL	Cholesterol, triglycerides
III	β-VLDL, IDL	Cholesterol, triglycerides
IV	VLDL	Triglycerides
V	Chylomicrons, VLDL	Triglycerides, cholesterol

β-VLDL, a lipoprotein not normally found in the plasma. Several environmental and genetic factors may give rise to each of the various lipoprotein phenotypes. In other words, no lipoprotein phenotype is specifically caused by only a single underlying metabolic defect.

Lipid Disorders Associated with Single-Gene Mutations

The molecular basis of lipid disorders associated with several single gene defects is now understood.[26] These diseases are listed in Table 3–6. Familial hypercholesterolemia is a single gene mutation that is most commonly associated with a IIa phenotype. However, most individuals with a IIa phenotype probably have multifactorial hypercholesterolemia, not the single gene defect.

Familial hypercholesterolemia is a fairly common lipid disorder. Heterozygous individuals occur with a frequency of about 1 in 500 and often have myocardial infarctions in their forties and fifties. Homozygous individuals are rare; they may have plasma cholesterol concentrations of 1000 mg/dl and myocardial infarctions during infancy or childhood. Familial hypercholesterolemia results from a mutation in the gene encoding the LDL receptor. Mutations in the LDL receptor gene may cause abnormal intracellular processing of the receptor, production of a receptor that binds lipoproteins defectively, or loss of the production of any receptor protein at all.[18]

Familial combined hyperlipidemia is another single gene defect that is associated with a IIa, IIb, or IV phenotype. Individuals with familial combined hyperlipidemia have overproduction of apo B100-containing lipoproteins. The molecular basis for this overproduction and for the variability in phenotypic expression is unknown.

Another single gene mutation that is strongly associated with hyperlipidemia involves apo E.[27] Mutations in the apo E gene that cause defective binding of apo E-containing lipoproteins to the LDL receptor may lead to the accumulation of β-VLDL and IDL. The presence of β-VLDL in the plasma is the hallmark of type III hyperlipoproteinemia (also called dysbetalipoproteinemia). Because type III hyperlipoproteinemic subjects often

TABLE 3–6. Diseases of lipoprotein metabolism due to single gene defects

Disease	Lipoprotein abnormality	Lipid abnormality	Metabolic basis	Clinical implications
Familial hypercholesterolemia	LDL elevated	Cholesterol elevated	Decreased clearance of LDL from plasma due to a genetic deficiency or abnormality in LDL receptor	Risk factor for atherosclerosis
Familial hypertriglyceridemia	VLDL elevated	Triglyceride elevated	Uncertain; VLDL overproduction or decreased catabolism	Exacerbated by diabetes, obesity, alcoholism
Familial combined hyperlipidemia	LDL and VLDL elevated	Cholesterol and/or triglyceride elevated	Uncertain; overproduction of apo B100	Risk factor for atherosclerosis
Type III hyperlipoproteinemia (familial dysbetalipoproteinemia)	β-VLDL and IDL elevated	Cholesterol and triglyceride elevated	Decreased clearance of remnants; defective binding of apo E to the LDL receptor	Risk factor for atherosclerosis
Familial lipoprotein lipase deficiency	VLDL and chylomicrons elevated	Triglyceride elevated	Deficiency of lipoprotein lipase or apo C-II	Acute pancreatitis
Hypoalphalipoproteinemia	HDL reduced	None	Uncertain; occasionally due to genetic apo A-I/C-III deficiency	Risk factor for atherosclerosis

have accelerated atherosclerosis, β-VLDL and IDL, like LDL, probably are atherogenic.

Single gene mutations may cause low plasma HDL concentrations. Low HDL, also called hypoalphalipoproteinemia, may be associated with accelerated atherosclerosis. LCAT deficiency is a rare autosomal recessive disorder in which HDL are abnormal and premature atherosclerosis occurs. Tangier disease is also a rare autosomal recessive disorder characterized by an extremely low concentration of apo AI and the virtual absence of HDL. Subjects with Tangier disease have an abnormal ratio of the isoforms of apo AI in their plasma due to faulty conversion of pro-apo AI to the mature isoform. Pro-apo AI does not bind normally to lipids.

Rare individuals have been described with severe deficiency of both apo AI and apo CIII. The apo AI and apo CIII genes are closely linked in the human genome, which may account for both genes being affected in this disorder.[28] Single gene mutations involving lipoprotein lipase and apo CII have also been described, but these mutations are not associated with increased atherosclerosis.

Acknowledgements. Supported by Arteriosclerosis Specialized Center of Research grant HL 14230 and by Clinical Investigator Award HL 02024 from the National Heart, Lung and Blood Institute, National Institutes of Health.

References

1. Gotto AM Jr, Pownall HJ, Havel RJ. Introduction to the plasma lipoproteins. Methods Enzymol 1986;128:3–41.
2. Hay R, Driscoll, D, Getz G. The biogenesis of lipoproteins. In: Scanu AM, Spector AA, eds. Biochemistry and Biology of Plasma Lipoproteins. New York: Marcel Dekker, 1986:11–51.
3. Nilsson-Ehle P, Garfinkel AS, Schotz MC. Lipolytic enzymes and plasma lipoprotein metabolism. Annu Rev Biochem 1980;667–693.
4. Nichols AV, Krauss RM, Musliner TA. Nondenaturing polyacrylamide gradient gel electrophoresis. Methods Enzymol 1986;128:417–431.
5. Mahley RW, Innerarity TL, Rall SC Jr, et al. Plasma lipoproteins: apolipoprotein structure and function. J Lipid Res 1984;25:1277–1294.
6. Li W-H, Tanimura M, Luo C-C, et al. The apolipoprotein multigene family: biosynthesis, structure, structure-function relationships, and evolution. J Lipid Res 1988;29:245–271.
7. Innerarity TL, Young SG, Poksay KS, et al. Structural relationship of human apolipoprotein B48 to apolipoprotein B100. J Clin Invest 1987;80:1794–1798.
8. Mahley RW. Apolipoprotein E: cholesterol transport protein with expanding role in cell biology. Science 1988;24:622–630.
9. Weisgraber KH. The role of apo E in cholesterol metabolism. In: Scanu AM, Spector AA, eds. Biochemistry and Biology of Plasma Lipoproteins. New York: Marcel Dekker, 1986:301–329.

10. Tso P. Gastrointestinal digestion and absorption of lipid. Adv Lipid Res 1985;21:143–186.
11. Carey MC, Small DM, Bliss CM. Lipid digestion and absorption. Annu Rev Physiol 1983;45:651–577.
12. Tall AR, Small DM. Plasma high-density lipoproteins. N Engl J Med 1978;299:1232–1236.
13. Gotto AM Jr. High-density lipoproteins: biochemical and metabolic factors. Am J Cardiol 1983;52:2B–4B.
14. Fielding CJ. Mechanism of action of lecithin-cholesterol acyltransferase. Methods Enzymol 1986;129:783–790.
15. Sando GN, Rosenbaum LM. Human acid lipase/cholesteryl ester hydrolase: purification and properties of the form secreted by fibroblasts in microcarrier culture. J Biol Chem 1985;260:15186–15193.
16. Eisenberg S. Plasma lipoprotein conversions. Methods Enzymol 1986;129:347–366.
17. Gregg RE, Brewer HB Jr. In vivo metabolism of apolipoprotein E in humans. Methods Enzymol 1986;129:482–497.
18. Brown MS, Goldstein JL. A receptor-mediated pathway for cholesterol homeostasis. Science 1986;232:34–47.
19. Goldstein JL, Brown MS, Anderson RGW, et al. Receptor-mediated endocytosis: concepts emerging from the LDL receptor system. Annu Rev Cell Biol 1985;1:1–39.
20. Russell DW, Esser V, Hobbs HH. Molecular basis of familial hypercholesterolemia. Arteriosclerosis 1989;9:I9–I13.
21. Rothblat GH, Bamberger M, Phillips MC. Reverse cholesterol transport. Methods Enzymol 1986;129:628–644.
22. Tall AR, Small DM. Body cholesterol removal: role of plasma high density lipoproteins. Adv Lipid Res 1980;17:1–51.
23. Tall AR. Plasma lipid transfer proteins. J Lipid Res. 1986;27:361–367.
24. Stary HC. Evolution and progression of atherosclerotic lesions in coronary arteries of children and young adults. Arteriosclerosis 1989;9:I19–I32.
25. Rudel LL, Parks JS, Johnson FL, et al. Low density lipoproteins in atherosclerosis. J Lipid Res 1986;27:465–474.
26. Zannis, VI, Breslow JL. Genetic mutations affecting human lipoprotein metabolism. Adv Hum Genet 1985;14:125–215.
27. Zannis VI. Genetic polymorphism in human apolipoprotein E. Methods Enzymol 1986;128:823–851.
28. Karathanasis SK, Zannis VI, Breslow JL. Characterization of the apolipoprotein A-I–C-III gene complex. Methods Enzymol 1986;128:712–726.

4
Use of the Clinical Laboratory for Lipid Evaluation

Evan A. Stein

Hyperlipidemia, like many other metabolic and endocrine disorders, is almost totally dependent on laboratory analysis of plasma or serum for its detection, evaluation, and therapy. Most subjects have few if any clinical signs, and the clinician is therefore "hostage" to the quality of the lipid and lipoprotein analysis. This fact was well recognized by the National Cholesterol Education Program (NCEP)[1], in that the initial Expert Panel report dealing with treatment of adults[2] was published simultaneously with a detailed report from the NCEP Lipid Standardization Panel.[3] These reports focused on total cholesterol, triglyceride, and high and low density lipoprotein (HDL and LDL) cholesterol. It is anticipated that, despite the growing ability by clinical laboratories to measure apolipoproteins, the lipid parameters just listed will, for the next few years, remain the cornerstone of clinical lipidology.

The clinician involved in the practice of effective lipid management has a right and an obligation to demand detailed and ongoing information from the laboratory to ensure proper evaluation of lipid disorders and monitoring of ongoing therapy. The laboratory is as crucial for dealing with hyperlipidemia as it is for detecting and evaluating potential fetal neural tube defects by maternal serum α-fetoprotein screening.

It is not the intention of this chapter to discuss in detail the specifics of laboratory analysis unless they are germane to the information base needed by the clinician to assess laboratory performance or to converse confidently with the laboratory professional. Although laboratories can and do respond to regulatory agencies in terms of improving performance, often the most rapid and influential motivating factor for enhancing performance is physician feedback and the free market forces that enable physicians to seek alternative suppliers of quality laboratory analysis. Such decisions, however, can occur only with a well informed, demanding clinician.

TABLE 4–1. Routine lipid analysis

Screening mode
    Total cholesterol (fingerstick sample)
Diagnostic mode
    Total cholesterol
    Triglyceride
    HDL cholesterol
    LDL cholesterol (calculated)
Special circumstances
    Familial hyperchylomicronemia
        Naked eye appearance
        Lipoprotein electrophoresis
    Dysbetalipoproteinemia
        Preparative ultracentrifugation combined with lipoprotein electrophoresis of
        d = 1.006 top and bottom
        VLDL cholesterol/triglyceride ratio
        Apo E isoforms
    Familial combined hyperlipidemia/hyperapobetalipoproteinemia
        Total apo B
    Severe hyperchylomicronemia
        Lipoprotein lipase estimation
        Apo C-II analysis
    Familial hypercholesterolemia
        LDL receptor analyses
    Early atherosclerosis with no obvious lipid abnormality
        LP(a) quantitation

Parameters to Be Measured

The array of lipid, lipoprotein, and apolipoprotein analyses that are available today in sophisticated lipid laboratories is large and continually growing. For most routine clinical purposes, however, detection, evaluation, and therapy of hyperlipidemia remains firmly dependent on measurement of the following: total cholesterol, triglycerides, HDL cholesterol, and calculated LDL cholesterol using the formula of Friedewald et al.[4] The information obtained from these parameters should suffice for most potential lipid disorders with additional specific tests being indicated in special circumstances. As an adjunct or precursor to these analyses, one could utilize a total cholesterol variant based on fingerstick screening in what are known as desp-top analyzers. The major part of this chapter deals with these basic analyses, but brief mention is made of potential additional measurements that may be needed to properly evaluate and treat specific patients with fairly rare lipid disorders. The routine and specialized testing is outlined in Table 4–1. The analyses shown in Table 4–1 are rarely necessary even in the largest clinical lipid centers. As few of these tests are offered by routine hospital or commercial laboratories, it is often necessary to contact well established lipid research core laboratories when such

TABLE 4–2. "Preanalytic variables"

Fasting: 12–14 hours overnight, water only
Stable weight, diet, and activity over last 3–6 weeks
No recent illness, surgery, or injury; at least 12 weeks after myocardial infarction or coronary artery bypass surgery
Not currently pregnant and at least 12 weeks postpartum
Stable (4–8 weeks) postmenopausal or after oral contraceptive hormone therapy
Stable doses of, or no other medications known to affect, lipid and lipoproteins, e.g., corticosteroids, androgenic steroids, thyroid hormone, thiazide and other loop diuretics, nonselective β-blockers, carbamazepine
Menstrual cycle
Phlebotomy position, e.g., sitting vs. recumbent
Prolonged venous occlusion
Sample handling prior to plasma/serum isolation
Biological variation

---

clinical disorders are suspected and detailed lipid, lipoprotein, or apolipoprotein analysis is required.

Preanalytical Variables

Less-than-optimal laboratory performance and lack of repeat sampling are two major factors resulting in incorrect diagnosis and therapy. A third important factor, i.e., improper sampling, is often just as important. In addition, this parameter is directly under the control of the clinician. These "preanalytical" variables are listed in Table 4–2. Although nonfasting samples are acceptable for total cholesterol screening,[3] it is important that, for further evaluation, confirmation of a previously diagnosed abormality, or monitoring therapy, patients be evaluated in a fasting (12-hour overnight) state. During this time only water may be consumed (to maintain hydration). Even though total cholesterol is minimally affected by the nonfasting state, there are significant alterations in the very low density lipoprotein (VLDL) fraction, which carries triglyceride. This point has two important ramifications for complete lipid profiling. First, the Friedewald formula,[14] which is dependent on triglycerides to estimate VLDL cholesterol, is substantially altered in the nonfasting state due to the presence of chylomicrons and chylomicron remnants. Second, the presence of chylomicrons and other triglyceride-rich lipoprotein particles may have an adverse impact on the ability of the laboratory to accurately isolate HDL for its cholesterol measurement. To isolate HDL prior to its cholesterol quantitation, it is necessary to precipitate the other lipoprotein fractions. In the fasting state, it usually depends only on precipitating VLDL and LDL with a specific reagent. This precipitate forms a compact mass on centrifugation. In the nonfasting state triglyceride-rich lipoproteins with densities lower than that of VLDL (e.g., chylomicrons and remnant particles) are often difficult to precipitate cleanly and can contaminate the HDL-containing supernatant. The relative cholesterol contribution of these non-HDL lipoproteins can be significant even in small amounts and can therefore produce potentially large errors in HDL cholesterol estimation.

It is important that subjects maintain stable diet, exercise, and weight at the time of initial evaluation, as fluctuations in any of these parameters may significantly and temporarily alter certain lipoproteins. For example, sudden weight gain or weight loss can cause large alterations in fasting triglyceride levels; extreme calorie-deficient diets can result in sudden and temporary reductions in both HDL and LDL cholesterol, and variations in alcohol may produce major alterations in triglyceride and HDL levels. Obviously, once a definitive diagnosis has been established and therapy implemented, progress may be monitored by lipid evaluation while weight, diet, activity, and alcohol are manipulated. However, before determining if final lipid goals have been met or additional therapy, especially drug therapy, is warranted, the patient should again achieve stability in these areas for at least 3 to 6 weeks.

The efforts of recent illness, even acute viral illness, major surgery, or trauma on lipoproteins are variable and often significant. As the diagnosis of hyperlipidemia is potentially serious in terms of committing patients to life-long therapy and protracted and expensive investigations and a short delay is not life-threatening, it is *essential* that evaluation and diagnosis *not* be undertaken in subjects where the underlying long-term lipoprotein pattern is likely to be clouded. Thus it is recommended that at least 12 weeks elapse after any major adverse health experience before embarking on evaluation for hyperlipidemia.

There are specific preanalytical variables that apply to the female segment of the population. Some studies have demonstrated that lipoprotein levels vary with the menstrual cycle. However, these variations appear to be due mainly to hemodilutory effects; and if lipoprotein concentrations are corrected for the fluctuations in total protein, less variation is seen. It is also important to assess subjects taking postmenopausal estrogens of oral contraceptives when they are stable on these preparations, which in practice occurs after 1 to 2 months of therapy. It may be advisable prior to starting such therapy to assess the baseline lipid levels in these subjects. This practice has two clinically important ramifications. First, it allows the physician to detect previously undiagnosed hyperlipidemias and select an appropriate hormone preparation, one that is likely to have minimal adverse impact on atherogenesis; and second, it allows one to avoid the pitfalls of attempting to interpret lipoprotein abnormalities in subjects already taking hormonal preparations. In humans, pregnancy produces significant lipid alterations, with LDL increasing significantly in many subjects. As there is no clinical indication for treatment of gestational hyperlipidemia, it is not recommended that lipid levels be measured during pregnancy. Furthermore, is often takes 8 to 12 weeks for lipid levels to return to their prepregnancy state following childbirth. This return to pregestational levels may be prolonged in subjects continuing to breastfeed for extended periods.

It is important to ensure that there is consistency in the method by which the blood sample is obtained. Hemodilution or hemoconcentration can occur with rapid changes in patient position (e.g., recumbent to sitting or vice versa) and by prolonged occlusion of the anticubital vein during the phlebotomy process. These two factors alone may cause fluctuations of up to 10% in lipoprotein concentrations in the blood sample. If plasma is to be utilized, it is important that the collection tube be filled to the prescribed levels as the anticoagulant ethylenediamine tetraacetic acid (EDTA) can exert a considerably hemodilutory effect on the final lipid concentrations due to an osmotic action that increases the movement of water from cells into plasma. The speed at which samples are processed to isolate either plasma or serum is also important, as is the temperature at which samples are stored prior to cell separation. Prolonged storage at room temperature, which is often the case in many clinical settings, can result in slightly falsely elevated cholesterol levels due to movement of cellular cholesterol into the plasma or serum. Samples should therefore be kept at 4 °C (common household refrigerator temperature) until separated. Hemolysis due to poor phlebotomy techniques may also cause analytical errors in the laboratory and should be avoided whenever possible.

Laboratory and Analytical Considerations

Once the sample has reached the laboratory, the reliability of results centers around two important performance characteristics: accuracy and precision. It is important that clinicians understand the meaning of these two terms, as it allows them to assess the performance of any laboratory.

Accuracy, or bias, is defined as deviation from the true value. It is usually expressed by the laboratory as a percentage of the true value. For example, if the true value was 200 and a laboratory obtained a value of 190, it would have a *negative* bias of 5%. Conversely, a laboratory that obtained a value of 220 would have a *positive* bias of 10%. Given the fact that some methods, especially those involving reflectance spectrophotometry and so-called dry chemistry, are not rectilinear (i.e., measurements over a wide range of concentrations do not follow a straight line), it is also important to know the accuracy, or bias, at specific concentrations. For example, a particular method may be accurate (0 bias) at a value of 200, whereas it has a significant positive bias (i.e., reads too high) at a value of 300. Similarly, the same method may have a negative bias (i.e., gives results below the true value) at a value of 100.

Although inaccuracies, or biases, for other biochemical analytes exist among laboratories, they are corrected for by each laboratory or method when it develops its own reference range. This situation was, in fact, the case with lipid measurements until the guidelines established by the National Cholesterol Education Program (NCEP) appeared. For the first time in the clinical chemistry arena, a specific series of cutoff points have been defined above which certain interventions, including drug therapy, are recommended. Thus it is no longer acceptable for individual laboratories or manufacturers of particular methods to compensate for biased procedures by defining a new set cutoff points or reference ranges. The advantages of this type of *true value system* is well described and discussed in the series of articles by Naitos[5] and the Lipid Standardization Panel[3] of the NCEP.

The true value for cholesterol is based on results obtained using either the *reference* method carried out the Centers for Disease Control (CDC)[6] or the *definitive* method of the National Institutes of Standards and Technology (formerly National Bureau of Standards). Fortunately, these methods agree closely. It is now possible through a national reference system for cholesterol[7] for laboratories to ensure that not only are their methods accurate but that they are also traceable back to values obtained by the CDC reference method.

Regarding expectations clinicians should have from their local laboratory in terms of accuracy or bias, the NCEP Lipid Standardization Panel recommended that all laboratories should, in 1988, be within 5% of the true cholesterol value as designated by the CDC reference method. The bias should be reduced by 0.5% per year, and that by 1992 all laboratories should be within 3% of the true value. These recommendations and their potential impact at a cholesterol concentration of 200 and 240 mg/dl are shown in Table 4–3.

Precision, or reproducibility, is defined as the ability to obtain the same result on repeated analyses. It is distinctly different from accuracy in that a method can be totally inaccurate but precise (i.e., the method could obtain an average result of 160 when the true value is 200 and, if the sample was analyzed ten times, achieve results between 158 and 162). Alternatively, another method may be accurate but have poor precision: obtaining an average result of 200 when the true result was 200, but on repeated measurements, e.g., 10 days, the range of results would be 180–220. Precision, although it does to some extent determine accuracy for any given single determination, is most important for monitoring therapy. For example, in a situation where a laboratory is slightly biased but precise, it is considerably easier to monitor the effects of various interventions, such as diet or drug, than when utilizing a laboratory where the results may be more accurate but the precision is less than optimal, resulting in marked fluctuation of patient results, even without therapeutic interventions.

Precision is generally reported by most laboratories as the coefficient of variation (CV), which is derived by two common procedures. Within-run

TABLE 4–3. Accuracy (bias) recommendations of U.S. clinical laboratories performing cholesterol measurements

Parameter	1988	1989	1990	1991	1992
Maximum bias (%)	5.0	4.5	4.0	3.5	3.0
Range at 200 mg/dl	190–210	191–209	192–208	193–207	194–206
Range at 240 mg/dl	228–252	229–251	230–250	231–249	233–247

precision is obtained by analyzing the same sample, usually at least 10 times, in the same analytic batch. Between-run or between-day precision is obtained by analyzing the same sample over 10 different working days. The means and standard deviations for both of these 10-run studies are obtained, and the precision is expressed as standard deviation/the mean × 100/1. Thus the better the precision, the lower is the CV and vice versa. As for assessing accuracy or bias, it is important to know the precision at specific concentration points, as the performance characteristics of many systems differ depending on the concentration of the analyte. For example, the precision at 100 mg/dl for total cholesterol could be 8% on a particular system, whereas at 300 mg/dl it could be 2%. Thus the astute clinician should be able to request and assess precision information from the laboratory over the usual clinical range of lipid values.

The Lipid Standardization Panel of the National Cholesterol Education Program has also defined national guidelines and has set targets similar to those for accuracy. The goal for 1988 for precision as the CV was 5% at maximum with a goal of achieving 3% or less by 1992.

To assess the current state of affairs in the United States in terms of accuracy and precision, it appears from the College of American Pathologists (CAP) Survey of approximately 5000 laboratories that precision goals of 3% are already probably being achieved or close to being achieved. This figure almost certainly reflects advances in methodology for cholesterol and triglyceride analysis, which has been fueled by a switchover from purely chemical and primarily manual procedures to techniques using automated, enzymatic processes; it also reflects improvements in automated instrumentation.

The major problem, however, appears to be accuracy (bias) among laboratories' instrument/reagent systems. Significant strides are being made by individual laboratories and especially by manufacturers to achieve more accurate analyses by adopting common calibration systems that are traceable back to the CDC reference method. This single modification can in many situations significantly reduce bias among methods. It is, however, recommended that individual laboratories not only request from manufacturers their studies on calibration but also conduct their own studies using one of the reference network laboratories set up by the CDC to ensure that they are providing accurate results.

Although total cholesterol measurements have been addressed in great detail by the NCEP Lipid Standardization Panel, triglycerides, HDL cholesterol isolation and quantitation, and LDL cholesterol have still to be addressed. It is anticipated that the NCEP Working Group on Lipoprotein Measurements will provide specific recommendations for laboratories measuring these parameters (by 1991). In the interim, it would be reasonable to expect laboratories to be achieving coefficients of variations of less than 5% for the two measured parameters (triglycerides and HDL cholesterol). Accuracy is more difficult to assess for triglycerides, as no current definitive method exists; although the CDC does have a reference method, it has not been widely used to provide calibrating material. HDL cholesterol accuracy is still more difficult, as it involves isolation of HDL as well as quantitation of relatively small amounts of cholesterol. Again, the CDC has a recommended reference procedure that is currently being implemented along with triglyceride measurements in the lipid reference laboratory network.[7]

HDL cholesterol is important not only for lipid assessment as a component of the Friedewald formula used to calculate LDL cholesterol, but it has additional significance in its own right as a potential risk factor. The adult treatment panel has recognized this fact by incorporating HDL as an additional parameter assess when diet or drug therapy for lowering LDL is indicated. The selected cutoff point for HDL is 35 mg/dl. Given the rather narrow physiological range of HDL and the fact that a value of 35 mg/dl is just below the 10th percentile in women and 25th percentile for men, whereas the 50th percentiles are 55 and 45 mg/dl for women and men, respectively, it is essential that HDL cholesterol measurements be both accurate and precise. The 35 mg/dl cutoff point was established based on epidemiological data gathered through the Lipid Research Clinic's Programs as well as other epidemiological studies, which used a common method for HDL isolation and a standardized method for its cholesterol measurement. This original isolation procedure utilized heparin and manganese chloride and was shown to be consistent with the reference (laborious and expensive) technique of preparative ultracentrifugation. For a variety of reasons, mainly convenience and reagent stability, few commercial procedures, if any, have adopted the heparin/manganese HDL isolation procedure. Instead, the most common procedures involve dextran sulfate or sodium phosphotungstate.[8] Furthermore, dextran sulfate procedures can be subdivided into those using dextran sulfate 50,000 and 500,000 molecular weight (MW) solutions. All of these reagent systems produce negative bias compared to the CDC reference technique.[8] It can be seen that if a technique is 10 to 12% biased (i.e., reads 4–6 mg/dl below the true value), subjects with HDL cholesterols levels close to the 50th percentile could be assigned to the high risk category based on an HDL level below 35 mg/dl. The most negatively biased of all the isolation techniques is dextran sulfate 500,000 MW followed by the sodium phosphotungstate procedure. With certain manipulations, the dextran sulfate 50,000 MW procedure can be made comparable to that of heparin manganese. The clinician should be aware of these potential differences, as low HDL cholesterol errors have two significant implications for patients. First, they result in overestimation of LDL cholesterol by the Friedewald formula; and second, they can result in placing subjects on therapy owing to the presence of an additional risk factor by NCEP guidelines. It is anticipated because of the development of national guidelines produced by the NCEP Working Group on Lipoprotein Measurement, laboratory performance and standardization for HDL together with triglycerides and LDL evaluation will improve.

References

1. Lanfant C. A new challenge for America: the National Cholesterol Education Program. Circulation 1986;265:2839–2842.
2. Report of the National Cholesterol Education Program Expert Panel on detection, evaluation and treatment of high blood cholesterol in adults. Arch Intern Med 1988;148:36–69.
3. Naito HK. Current status of blood cholesterol measurement in clinical laboratories in the United States: a report from the Laboratory Standardization Panel of the National Cholesterol Education Program. Clin Chem 1988;34:193–201.
4. Friedewald WT, Levy RI, Frederickson DS. Estimation of concentration of low-density lipoprotein cholesterol in plasma without use of the preparative ultracentrifuge. Clin Chem 1972;18:499–502.
5. Naito HK. The cholesterol challenge: from laboratory to clinician. Clin Chem 1988;34:3–7.
6. Abell LL, Levy BB, et al. Simplified methods for estimation of total cholesterol in serum and demonstration of its specificity. J Biol Chem 1952;195:357–366.
7. National Reference System for Cholesterol: A National Reference Method Laboratory Network. US Department of Health and Human Services, Public Health Service, Centers for Disease Control, Atlanta. 1989;1–10.
8. Warnick GR, Cheung MC, Albers JJ. Comparison of current methods for high-density lipoprotein quantitation. Clin Chem 1979;25:596–601.

5
Sex Steroids and Lipoproteins

VALERY T. MILLER and JOHN C. LA ROSA

For women the use of exogenous sex steroids is taking on an importance beyond the areas of sexual development, contraception, fertility, and menopausal symptom relief. Appropriate use of estrogens and progestogens at different times in a woman's life may have the potential to either accelerate or prevent atherosclerotic heart disease.[1,2] Because in women, as in men, heart disease is the number one cause of death, physicians caring for women must understand how sex steroids influence death and disability due to heart disease.[3]

Estrogens

Potency

Some comprehension of the relative potencies among estrogens is necessary to understand and compare their effects. Estrogens can be divided into three groups: synthetic, equine, and natural (Table 5–1). Although a natural estrogen, equine estrogens contain equilin, which is not natural to humans.

Synthetic estrogens are more potent on a weight basis when measured by most end-organ assays, i.e., hepatic induction of proteins (including lipoproteins), suppression of pituitary gonadotropins, and vaginal cornification and endometrial stimulation.[4–8] Conjugated equine estrogens (CEE) are next in potency, followed by micronized estradiol and the various estrone conjugates. Table 5–2 demonstrates the relative potencies of various estrogens according to three hepatic protein parameters.[6] The chemical structures of both ethinyl estradiol and CEE influence hepatic induction.[9] On a milligram to milligram basis, oral ethinyl estradiol is 75 to 200 times more potent than CEE in terms of affecting hepatic globulins.[6] Equilin sulfate, the equine estrogen, which makes up 25% of conjugated equine estrogen, is two to four times more potent in the liver than native estrogens (estrone and estradiol) and at least twofold more potent than CEE itself.[10]

TABLE 5–1. Estrogen compounds

Synthetic estrogens
  Diethylstilbestrol
  17α-ethinyl estradiol
  Mestranol

Equine estrogen
  Conjugated equine estrogen

Natural estrogens
  Micronized estradiol
  Piperazine estrone sulfate
  Estradiol valerate

TABLE 5–2. Relative potency according to three parameters of estrogenicity

Estrogen	Serum FSH	Serum SHBG-BC	Serum angiotensinogen
Piperazine estrone sulfate	1.1	1.0	1.0
Micronized estradiol	1.3	1.0	0.7
Conjugated estrogens	1.4	3.2	3.5
Diethylstilbestrol	3.8	28	13
Ethinyl estradiol	80–200	614	232

Modified from Maschak CA et al.,[6] with permission.
SHBG-BC = sex hormone-binding globulin-binding capacity.

Routes of Administration

All estrogens induce predictable dose-related hepatic protein changes, including lipoprotein changes, when administered orally. This phenomenon is due to the high concentrations delivered to the liver after intestinal absorption via the portal system, the "first pass."

Hepatic induction of lipoproteins by nonoral routes of administration depends on the particular estrogen and its dose and the vehicle (cream, gel, pellet, or patch). CEE, a potent lipoprotein inducer orally, does not have an effect on lipoproteins when administered vaginally.[5] Ethinyl estradiol is so potent, however, that a vaginally administered dose can induce hepatic protein levels equal to those produced by oral administration.[9] In general, data are accumulating to suggest that a system that can induce a sustained level of circulating estradiol over a period of time induces lipoprotein changes. Estradiol in subcutaneous pellet and estradiol gel applied to the abdomen has been shown to change lipoproteins.[11,12] To date, the estradiol patch (0.1 mg) available in the United States has been shown to alter lipoprotein levels after 24 weeks in only one study.[13]

TABLE 5–3. Effects of estrogens versus synthetic progestogens on lipids and lipoproteins[a]

Lipid effect	Estrogen effect	Progestogen
HDL-C	Increased	Decreased
HDL$_2$	Increased	Decreased
HDL$_3$	Increased	Decreased
Apo A-I	Increased	Decreased
Apo A-II	Increased	Variable
LDL-C	Decreased	Increased
Apo B	Decreased	Increased
VLDL-C	Increased	Decreased
Total triglycerides	Increased	Decreased

[a]The newer gonanes do not follow this progestogen pattern of effect.

Lipid and Lipoprotein Effects of Estrogens

Basic lipoprotein metabolism is reviewed elsewhere in this text. Some specific effects of lipoprotein metabolism as it relates to estrogen and progestogen administration are discussed here.

Table 5–3 shows the effects of estrogen on lipids and lipoproteins.[14,15] These effects are both dose- and structure-related. Many of the effects, such as increases in high density lipoprotein cholesterol (HDL-C) and HDL$_2$ and decreases in low density lipoprotein cholesterol (LDL-C), are antiatherogenic.[16–18] Increases in very low density lipoprotein cholesterol (VLDL-C) and triglycerides, however, may not be. There is disagreement in the literature as to whether, in women, hypertriglyceridemia is an independent risk factor for coronary artery disease.[19,20]

In addition to increasing triglyceride levels, estrogen enhances the secretion and metabolism of VLDL-C, the major lipoprotein carrier of triglyceride in fasting plasma.[21] This increased turnover may be associated with increased transfer of lipoprotein surface remnants, including cholesterol, to HDL, reflecting reverse cholesterol transport, i.e., the process of moving cholesterol from cells to catabolic sites, a phenomenon thought to be antiatherogenic. Moreover, oral estrogen raises levels of HDL-C, HDL$_2$ and apoprotein A-I (apo A-I), all of which have been inversely associated with coronary risk.[14,22] The mechanisms by which these changes in HDL fractions and apoproteins occur are not entirely clear but are probably related to estrogen's effect of reducing hepatic triglyceride lipase activity and inhibiting hepatic HDL catabolism.[23] Increased turnover of VLDL, with enhanced HDL production, may also play a role. Measurements of HDL-C and its associated subfractions, of course, may not accurately reflect HDL function. Estimates of HDL function must await simpler, more reliable methods for measuring reverse cholesterol transport.

TABLE 5–4. Progestogens and progestins

19-Nortestosterone-related progestogens
Gonanes
Levonorgestrel
Desogestrel
Gestodene
Norgestimate
Estranes
Norethindrone
Norethindrone acetate
Ethynodiol diacetate
Lynestranol
Norethynodrel
17-α-Hydroxyprogesterone-related progestins
Pregnanes
Medroxyprogesterone
Chlormadinone acetate
Megestrol acetate
Cyproterone acetate
Natural progesterone

In addition to the effect on VLDL-C and HDL-C, estrogen decreases LDL-C.[14,24] The exact mechanisms are unclear, but it is known that LDL-C reduction is associated with enhanced synthesis of LDL receptors.[25]

Progestogens

Potency

Interest in the United States has concentrated on progesterone (the only natural progestogen), its synthetic derivative medroxyprogesterone acetate (MPA), and the synthetic progestogens derived from 19-nortestosterone, i.e., norgestrel, norethindrone, and ethynodiol diacetate. Progestogen potency can be estimated in terms of androgenicity, estrogenicity, and antiestrogenicity.[26] Androgenicity is the progestogen characteristic most closely related to lipoprotein effect. Unfortunately, there is no measurement comparable to hepatic proteins with which to compare progestogen potency. Table 5–4 lists the progestogens by conventional chemical group, i.e., gonanes, estranes, and pregnanes. Prior to the introduction of the newer gonanes, e.g., desogestrel and gestodene, it could be said that gonanes were the most androgenic and had the greatest adverse effect on the lipoprotein profile. Newer gonanes, however, are less androgenic than the norethindrones and demonstrate a beneficial effect on lipoproteins.[27] Estranes have a more adverse effect on lipoproteins than do the pregnanes.

Route of Administration

As in the case of natural estrogens, the first pass is apparently necessary for MPA and for the norethindrones to induce lipoprotein effects in the liver. Levonorgestrel, however, like ethinyl estradiol, is less dependent on the first pass phenomenon.[28] Progesterone, the only natural progestogen, has no apparent effect on circulating lipoproteins, although this question has not been thoroughly researched.[29]

Lipid and Lipoprotein Effects of Progestogens

Table 5–3 summarizes the effects of progestogens on lipids and lipoproteins. The mechanisms by which progestogens affect cholesterol and lipoproteins are still basically unknown. Progestogens increase the activity of lipoprotein lipase, an enzyme bound to capillary endothelium in muscle and adipose tissue, which clears the blood of chylomicrons and VLDL.[30] Progestogens inhibit VLDL secretion by the liver, thus reducing serum total triglyceride.[31] This effect may be beneficial if triglyceride levels are valid predictors of coronary risk in women. HDL-C levels are also reduced, however, perhaps because hepatic triglyceride lipase activity increases with progestogen activity.[32] Diminished synthesis of LDL receptors appears to be one reason for increased levels of LDL-C in the presence of progestogens.[33]

In general, all synthetic progestogens, except for the newer gonanes, have an effect opposite to that of estrogen on lipids and lipoproteins, and their effects are drug- and dose-related. Theoretically, then, most progestogens have the potential for increasing the risk of coronary artery disease.

Oral Contraceptives

Oral contraceptives (OCs) are a combination of two sex steroids that have opposite effects on lipoproteins. The administration of such potent agents to millions of women has focused attention on the possible long-term effects of these agents. Recognition that lipoprotein changes associated with an increased risk of atherosclerosis may result from the progestogen component in OCs has led to both a reduction in dose and a search for new, less androgenic progestogens.

Contraceptive Formulation

Oral contraceptive formulation is based on a balance between two essential considerations: contraceptive efficacy versus adverse changes in lipoprotein and carbohydrate metabolism. As discussed previously, the ability of

TABLE 5–5. Estrogen and progestogen content of commonly used oral contraceptives and their total estrogen and progestogen (dose/cycle)

Oral contraceptive	Ethinyl estradiol (μg/cycle)	Progestogen (mg/cycle)	
Nordette	630	levonorgestrel	3.15
Triphasil	680	levonorgestrel	1.925
Lo/Ovral	630	dl-norgestrel	6.3
Ovral	1050	dl-norgestrel	10.5
Loestrin	420	norethindrone acetate	21.0
Norlestrin	1050	norethindrone acetate	21.0
Norlestrin 2.5	1050	norethindrone acetate	52.5
Brevicon	735	norethindrone	10.5
Norinyl	735	norethindrone	21.0
Ortho-Novum 7/7/7	735	norethindrone	15.75
Ovcon	735	norethindrone	8.4
Ovcon-50	1050	norethindrone	21.0

a progestogen to change lipoproteins appears closely related to its androgenicity. The more androgenic the agent, the greater the decrease in HDL-C and the increase in LDL-C levels. However, the third generation gonane desogestrel is less androgenic than is norethindrone, an estrane, and has a more favorable effect on lipoproteins when combined with estrogen in oral contraceptives.[27]

Pitfalls Comparing Contraceptives

Comparisons between OCs are fraught with difficulty because of differences in estrogen dosage and in progestogen type and dose. Even though ethinyl estradiol is used in all but 4 of 35 OC formulations in the United States, comparisons must be made between formulations containing 20-, 30-, and 50-μg doses.

Phased-dosage OCs add another dimension to the problem. Tri- and biphasic OCs contain varying amounts of estrogen as well as progestogen per cycle. It is helpful in these instances to identify the total cycle dose of each hormone when comparing these formulations.[34] Table 5–5 demonstrates the differences between both estrogen and progestogen doses per cycle of 12 commonly used OCs.

Because gonanes such as norgestrel are five- to tenfold more androgenically potent per equivalent weight than estranes, the same doses cannot be compared. It is also important to note that "norgestrel" indicates dl-norgestrel, the racemic mixture of d-norgestrel (levonorgestrel) and l-norgestrel. Milligram per milligram, levonorgestrel, the active form, is twice as potent as dl-norgestrel.[26]

Although the literature is replete with studies of the effect of OCs on

TABLE 5–6. Percent change of lipids and lipoproteins due to oral contraceptives

| Reference (1st author) | Progestogen | | | | HDL-C | HDL$_2$ | HDL$_3$ | Apo A-I | LDL-C | Apo B | Total trig. |
	Ethinyl estradiol (µg)	Name	mg	Total cycle dose (mg)							
Lipson[36]	50	Norgestrel	0.5	10.5	-13	-27	5	-9	18	—	32
Powell[37]	30	Levonorgestrel	0.15	3.15	-12.2	—	—	—	11.8	—	26.0
Burkman[38]	30	Levonorgestrel	0.15	3.15	-8.7	—	—	3.2	15.6	28.9	17.5
Krauss[39]	30	Levonorgestrel	0.15[a]	3.15	-4.3	—	—	—	4.2	—	18.2
Powell[37]	30	Ethynodiol acetate	2.0	42	-6.3	—	—	—	8.8	—	25
Burkman[38]	35	Ethynodiol acetate	1.0	21	2.4	—	—	19.3	10.0	28.8	38
Lipson[36]	50	Ethynodiol acetate	1.0	21	1	4	5	11	10	—	57
Powell[37]	50	Ethynodiol acetate	1.0	21	-0.5	—	—	—	12.5	—	—
Lipson[36]	50	Norethindrone acetate	1.0	21	3	-3	11	9	6	—	45
Burkman[38]	35	Norethindrone	1.0	21	-2.6	—	—	12.3	14.9	30.0	24.4
Burkman[38]	35	Norethindrone (biphasic)	0.5, 1.0	16	-4.5	—	—	12.2	10.0	24.8	45.3
Krauss[39]	35	Norethindrone	0.4	8.4	10.9	—	—	—	11.9	—	11.7
Percival-Smith[40]	Triphasics (30, 40, 30)	Levonorgestrel	0.05, 0.075, 0.125	1.925	-1.7	—	—	—	18.5	—	50.0
Havengt[41]	Triphasics (30, 40, 30)	Levonorgestrel	0.05, 0.075, 0.125	1.925	-1.6	-51.5	—	0.0	8.7	3.3	14.6
Kloosterboer[42]	Triphasics (30, 40, 30)	Levonorgestrel	0.05, 0.075, 0.125	1.925	0.0	-22.0	1.6	2.7	-6.3	22.5	—
Gaspard[43]	Triphasics (30, 40, 30)	Levonorgestrel	0.05, 0.075, 0.125	1.925	0.0	—	—	13.2	0.9	2.3	29.7
März[44]	30	Desogestrel	0.15	3.15	8.3	-1.3	14.2	21.1	2.1	0.1	35.1
Havengt[41]	30	Desogestrel	0.15	3.15	13.0	-4.5	—	22.6	-1.9	0.0	46.3
Kloosterboer[42]	30	Desogestrel	0.15	3.15	11.8	-4.4	9.8	18.1	-8.1	19.4	35.0
Gaspard[43]	30	Desogestrel	0.15	3.15	5.4	—	—	14.5	-3.2	-19.2	21.4

Trig. = triglycerides.
[a] Actually dl-norgestrel 0.3 mg.

circulating lipoproteins, making sense of them is sometimes difficult. When comparing such studies it should be remembered that not all laboratories reporting lipids and lipoproteins are standardized through the Centers for Disease Control or other standardizing agencies. The measurement of HDL-C and HDL subfractions in particular is prone to laboratory error.[35] Moreover, there is no agreement in standardization of apoprotein measurements. Study duration may also be critical.

Lipoprotein Effects of OCs

The result of 11 clinical trials of OCs and their effects on lipids and lipoproteins are summarized in Table 5–6. The formulations have been arranged in descending order of progestogen androgenicity. It is readily apparent that the adverse effects on lipoproteins are directly related to androgenicity.

The most easily recognized patterns appear with HDL-C and related measurements. HDL-C, HDL_2, and apo A-I levels are inversely related to androgenicity. Norgestrel in particular, although reducing the HDL-C and apo A-I less as total monthly dose is reduced, remains (even in the triphasic preparations) potent in terms of its adverse effects on HDL_2. Desogestrel actually has a positive effect on HDL-C. Apo A-I is decreased by only one formulation, the most androgenic; its levels are increased by all other formulations.

LDL-C, the lipoprotein most clearly associated with risk of atherosclerosis, appears to be similarly increased by all formulations apparently without correlation to dose or androgenicity. Preparations containing desogestrel, the new gonane, however, decrease LDL-C levels below baseline. Triglyceride levels are increased by every contraceptive and demonstrate no recognizable pattern related to formulation.

The results of an elevated LDL-C level or a reduced HDL-C level may not be apparent for many years. Therefore it seems prudent to use the OC formulation that has the least adverse effect on lipids and lipoproteins. OCs containing the newer gonanes, such as desogestrel, are not currently available in the United States.

Hormone Replacement During Menopause

Postmenopausal use of estrogen is on the increase again in the United States for three reasons: (1) progestogen use has proved protective of the endometrium; (2) osteoporosis can be prevented by early estrogen replacement; and (3) a growing body of evidence supports the theory that postmenopausal estrogen use protects women from heart disease.[2,45,46]

Table 5–7 demonstrates the lipoprotein effects of various unopposed estrogens administered orally to postmenopausal women. Even low doses

TABLE 5–7. Effects of unopposed oral estrogen on lipoproteins (percent change)

Study (1st author)	(n)	Duration	Estrogen	mg/day	LDL-C	HDL-C	HDL$_2$	HDL$_3$
Miller[47]	27	3 months	CEE	0.625	−15.7	11.3	19.4	5.3
Hart[48]	20	10 years	Mestranol	0.026	−13.0	38	97	17
Bradley[49]	32	—	EE	0.02	—	26	—	—
Wallentin[50]	20	6 months	EE	0.05	−27.0	33	—	—
Blumenfeld[51]	11	—	EE	0.05	—	30	29	76
Farish[52]	21	6 months	CEE	0.625	−5.0	16	23	—
Cauley[53]	48	—	CEE	0.370	—	24	60	2
Fahraeus[54]	19	—	Estradiol	2–4	—	19	21	14

EE = ethinyl estradiol; CEE = conjugated equine estrogen.

of synthetic estrogens raise HDL-C levels 26 to 38%, increasing mainly the HDL$_2$ subfraction. Oral CEE and 17β-estradiol increase HDL-C levels to 11 to 24%, again mainly in the HDL$_2$ subfraction. LDL-C levels are lowered by all oral estrogens. Data not shown in the table indicate that oral estrogens increase apo A-I and decrease apo B levels.[47]

Table 5–8 demonstrates the lipoprotein effects of nonoral administration of estrogen. Vaginally administered ethinyl estradiol (EE) significantly alters HDL-C and LDL-C, in contrast to even the highest dose of CEE, which has no effect when administered vaginally.

Subdermal pellets of 17β-estradiol also show substantially beneficial effects on HDL-C and LDL-C at 3 months. However, there may be little or no effect after 6 months, which is the limit of estradiol delivery for most pellets and implants.

Transdermal administration of estrogen has not been shown to affect lipoproteins to the extent that oral estrogens do. Only minor lipoprotein changes are reported with estradiol creams and gels even after 6 to 12 months of therapy.[11,57] To date, a significant HDL-C elevation ($p > 0.03$) has been reported by only one group of investigators.[13] They used a 0.1 mg estradiol transdermal patch for 24 weeks.

Combined Estrogen / Progestogen Replacement

The experience with combination estrogen/progestogen therapy during menopause is reminiscent of that with OCs. Progestogens are accepted as a necessary part of postmenopausal hormone replacement for women with an intact uterus to prevent estrogen-induced endometrial hyperplasia. On the other hand, there is concern about the possible long-term effects on cardiovascular risk when progestogens are used. The epidemiological data that relate decreased coronary disease risk to postmenopausal estrogen use is almost entirely based on cohorts of women who used estrogen without a progestogen.

TABLE 5–8. Effects of nonoral estrogens on lipoproteins (percent change)

Study (1st author)	(n)	Duration (months)	Estrogen	Dose/day (mg)	Route	LDL-C	HDL-C
Mandel[5]	20	1	CEE	0.3	Vaginal cream	0	0
Goebelsmann[a]	3	25 days	EE	50 μg	Vaginal suppository	−20	25
Lobo[12]	22	3	Estradiol	25	Pellet	3	48
Farish[55]	14	6	Estradiol	50	Pellet	−6	7
Sharf[56]	8	3	Estradiol	100	Pellet	−31	32
Jensen[11]	20	12	Estradiol	5	Abdominal cream	10	6[a]
Fahraeus[57]	17	6	Estradiol	3	Abdominal gel	—	4
Chetkowski[58]	23	4	Estradiol	0.2	Patch	0	0

EE = ethinyl estradiol; CEE = conjugated equine estrogen.
[a]Percent change from placebo group.

TABLE 5–9. Change of lipoproteins with conjugated equine estrogen 0.625 mg (days 1–25) and low dose progestogens (days 13–25) (percent change)

Lipoprotein	Medroxyprogesterone (10 mg)	Norethindrone acetate (1 mg)	dl-Norgestrel (0.15 mg)
LDL-C	−12	−10	−7
Apo B	−13	−5	−8
HDL-C	−6	−10	−2
HDL_2	0	−27	−17
HDL_3	−9	−1	+4
Apo A-I	−4	+4	−5

Raw data from Miller et al.[61]

Studies showed that when added to natural estrogens the 19-nortestosterones, in doses available during the late 1970s, could reduce HDL-C by as much as 27% below baseline.[59] Subsequently, investigations were undertaken to identify lower progestogen doses that could still protect the endometrium and have fewer adverse lipoprotein effects. Whitehead et al. reported the lowest doses of several progestogens that in the presence of variable absorption would protect the endometrium.[60] Using those progestogen doses, Miller et al. compared the lipoprotein effects of CEE 0.625 mg (days 1–25) unopposed for 3 months and opposed by the three progestogens (days 13–25) for an additional 3 months. Table 5–9 shows the lipid and lipoprotein results of that study.[61] In general, even at these lower doses for the 19-nortestosterone, there was little difference between the lipoprotein effects of these three regimens, except HDL_2 levels. Both 19-nortestosterones decreased HDL_2 levels significantly, whereas MPA did not, after 3 months.

Table 5–10 describes lipoprotein changes reported in prospective studies on combined regimens, both cyclic (13 days) and continuous (daily) use of progestogen. These studies indicate that there is little difference between these regimens and their effect on LDL-C. Adjusting for differences in size between the studies and not considering lengths of study, the mean LDL-C lowering for the studies combined is 15.3 mg/dl.

Unfortunately, even at low doses, the more potent 19-nortestosterones adversely affect HDL-C and HDL_2. The monthly dose of MPA, however, can be reduced to give improved lipoprotein values even resulting in some studies in increased HDL-C. As with OCs, decreasing androgenic potency increases HDL-C and HDL_2 levels. Monthly doses of 65 to 75 mg, regardless of the number of days administered, appear to provide more beneficial lipoprotein effects than do higher doses.

Apoproteins A-I and B, which some have suggested are better markers for coronary disease risk, tend to follow HDL-C and LDL-C levels, respectively.[61,66,67] As more sophisticated studies become available, subtle

TABLE 5–10. Lipoprotein changes with differing progestogens and doses (plus 0.625 mg conjugated equine estrogen)

Study (1st author)	(n)	Duration (months)	Progestogen & dose (mg)		Regimen	Dose (mg)/month	Lipoprotein change (percent change)		
							LDL-C	HDL-C	HDL$_2$
Farish[62]	21	6	NE	0.15	Cyclic	1.95	−13	−5	−10
Miller[61]	10	3	NE	0.15	Cyclic	1.95	−7	−2	−17
Jensen[63]	21	12	NE	1	Continuous	30	−20	−5	—
Miller[61]	10	3	NE	1	Cyclic	13	−10	−10	−27
Weinstein[64]	12	3	MPA	5	Continuous	150	−19	4	—
Miller[61]	7	3	MPA	10	Cyclic	130	−11.6	−6	0.0
Prough[65]	10	9	MPA	10	Cyclic	130	−11.8	25	—
Weinstein[64]	12	3	MPA	2.5	Continuous	75	−21	4	—
Prough[65]	16	9	MPA	2.5	Continuous	75	2	12	—
Weinstein[64]	12	3	MPA	5	Cyclic	65	−18	11	—

NG = dl-norgestrel; NE = norethindrone acetate; MPA = medroxyprogesterone acetate.

but significant differences between apoproteins A-I and A-II as well as HDL subfractions may provide a better understanding of the true differences in postmenopausal replacement between these progestogens.

Summary

Long-term use of sex steroids, whether OCs or postmenopausal hormone replacement, has the potential to powerfully influence circulating lipoprotein levels. Whether these changes result in altered risk of atherosclerosis is less clear. Although much remains to be clarified, enough information is currently known to guide physicians to safe, more beneficial use of these drugs.

Combinations of estrogen and progestogen that decrease HDL-C and HDL$_2$ levels the least should be used. The Framingham Study has provided evidence that HDL-C is inversely related to the development of a myocardial infarction in both men and women. Even in the presence of normal total cholesterol levels, moreover, low HDL-C increases risk.[19] Furthermore, there are now two studies that appear to show that at least in men pharmacologically increased HDL-C reduces cardiovascular risk.[68,69]

Atherosclerosis is a long-term process enhanced by many risk factors. Circulating total cholesterol and LDL-C levels are some of the most important. Early atherosclerotic changes can be found in the arterial intima of children, and the degree of the change correlates with the level of plasma cholesterol in those children.[70] It is possible that the association between OCs and heart disease is mediated through long-term elevations of LDL-C and reductions in HDL-C levels produced by high-dose progestogen OCs in the past. The more immediate thrombotic effects of higher-dose estrogen formulations of the past are also implicated.[1,71] With the newer low-dose formulations of OCs, the baseline risk, particularly in younger women, is low.[72] However, with increasing age and in smokers, the baseline risk increases in current users. The literature is unclear as to whether past use of OCs predicts cardiovascular risk.[73,74] In general, until these relations are clarified, formulations that increase LDL-C and decrease HDL-C the least should be used.

Unopposed estrogen induces beneficial lipoprotein changes in postmenopausal women. The data from cross-sectional and cohort studies that support decreased cardiovascular risk with unopposed estrogen, moreover, are extensive.[2,75,76] When possible, then, as in the case of hysterectomized women, unopposed estrogen should be used. The authors do not believe that current data support the notion that unopposed estrogen is associated with breast cancer or that the use of a progestogen protects the breast from cancer.

Although there are no clinical trial data to support the notion that combined hormone replacement during menopause has an adverse impact on cardiovascular risk, the lipoprotein effects suggest reason for concern. It is true that LDL-C is decreased by current combination regimens. Unfortunately, it is also true that HDL-C and its subfractions may be lowered in the short term. More studies are needed to detail the lowest doses of the various progestogens that still protect the endometrium. Until more data are available, the use of the lowest dose of MPA that can protect the endometrium appears to be the best choice.

References

1. Stadel BV. Oral contraceptives and cardiovascular disease. N Engl J Med 1981;305:612–18.
2. Bush TL, Barrett-Connor E, Cowan LD, et al. Cardiovascular mortality and noncontraceptive use of estrogen in women: results from the Lipid Research Clinic Program's Follow-up Study. Circulation 1967;75:1102–1109.
3. Vital Statistics of the United States, 1981. Mortality Part A, 1986. Hyattsville, MD: National Center for Health Statistics, 1986.
4. Mandel FP, Geola FL, Lu JKH, et al. Biologic effects of various doses of ethinyl estradiol in postmenopausal women. Obstet Gynecol 1982;59:673–678.
5. Mandel FP, Geola FL, Medrum DR, et al. Biological effects of various doses of vaginally administered conjugated equine estrogens in postmenopausal estrogen. J Clin Endocrinol Metab 1983;57:133–137.
6. Maschak CA, Lobo RA, Dozono-Takano R, et al. Comparison of pharmacodynamic properties of various estrogen formulations. Am J Obstet Gynecol 1982;144:511–518.
7. Frumar AM, Geola F, Tataryn IV, et al. Biological effects of estrogen at different sites of action in postmenopausal women. In: Scientific Abstracts, Twenty-sixth Annual Meeting of the Society for Gynecological Investigation, San Diego, 1979:66.
8. Geola FL, Frumar AM, Tataryn IV, et al. Biological effects of various doses of conjugated equine estrogens in postmenopausal women. J Clin Endocrinol Metab 1980;51:620–625.
9. Goebelsmann U, Maschak CA, Mishell DR. Comparison of hepatic impact of oral and vaginal administration of ethinyl estradiol. Am J Obstet Gynecol 1985;151:868–877.
10. Lobo RA. Absorption and metabolic effects of different types of estrogens and progestogen. Obstet Gynecol Clin North Am 1987;14:143–165.
11. Jensen J, Riis BJ, Strøm V, et al. Longterm effects of percutaneous estrogen and oral progesterone on serum lipoproteins in menopausal women. Am J Obstet Gynecol 1987;156:66–71.
12. Lobo RA, March CM, Goebelsmann UT, et al. Subdermal estradiol pellets following hysterectomy and oophorectomy. Am J Obstet Gynecol 1980;138:714–719.
13. Stanczyk FZ, Shoupe D, Nunez V, et al. A randomized comparison of ethinyl estradiol delivery in postmenopausal women. Am J Obstet Gynecol 1988;159:1540–1546.

14. Bush TL, Miller VT. Effects of pharmocologic agents used during the meno-pause, In: Mishell DR Jr, ed. Menopause: Physiology and Pharmacology. Chicago: Year Book Medical Publishers, 1987:187–208.
15. Cheung MD, Albers JJ. The measurement of apolipoprotein A-I and A-II levels in men and women by immunoassay. J Clin Invest 1977;60:43–50.
16. Gordon T, Castelli WP, Hjortland MC, et al. High density apoprotein as a protective factor against coronary heart disease. Am J Med 1977;62:707–714.
17. Kannel WB, Castelli WP, Gordon T, et al. Serum cholesterol, lipoproteins and the risk of coronary diseases: the Framingham Study . Ann Intern Med 1971; 74:1–12.
18. Abbot RD, Wilson PWF, Kannel WP, et al. High density lipoprotein cholesterol, total cholesterol screening, and myocardial infarction: the Framingham Study. Arteriosclerosis 1988;8:207–211.
19. Kannel WB, D'Agostino RB, Belanger AJ. New insights on cholesterol-lipoprotein profiles: the Framingham Study. Presented at the 61st Scientific Sessions of the AHA, November 1988.
20. Freedman DS, Gruchow HW, Anderson AJ, et al. Relation of triglyceride levels to coronary artery disease: the Milwaukee cardiovascular data registry. Am J Epidemiol 1988;127:1118–1130.
21. Schaefer EJ, Foster DM, Zech LA, et al. The effects of estrogen administration on plasma lipoprotein metabolism in premenopausal females . J Clin Endocrinol Metab 1983;57:262–267.
22. Bradley DD, Wingerd J, Petitti DB, et al. Serum high density lipoprotein cholesterol in women using oral contraceptives, estrogen and progestin. N Engl J Med 1978;299:17–20.
23. Applebaum DM, Goldberg AP, Pykalisto OJ, et al. Effect of estrogen on post-heparin lipolytic activity; selective decline in hepatic triglyceride lipase. J Clin Invest 1977;59:601–608.
24. Wahl P, Walden C, Knopp R, et al. Effect of estrogen/progestin potency on lipid and lipoprotein cholesterol. N Engl J Med 1983;308:862–867.
25. Kovanen PT, Brown MS, Goldstein JL. Increased binding of low-density lipoprotein to liver membrane from rats treated with 17 alpha-ethinyl estradiol. J Biol Chem 1979;254:1367–1373.
26. Brenner PF. The pharmacology of progestogens. J Reprod Med 1982;27:490–497.
27. Runnebaum B, Rabe TR. New progestogens in oral contraceptives. Am J Obstet Gynecol 1987;157:1059–1063.
28. Humpel M, Wendt H, Pommerenke G, et al. Investigations of pharmacokinetics of levonorgestrel to specific considerations of a possible first pass effect in women. Contraception 1978;17:207–212.
29. Ottosson UB, Johansson BG, Von Schoultz B. Subfractions of high density lipoprotein cholesterol during estrogen replacement: a comparison between progestogens and natural progesterone. Am J Obstet Gynecol 1985;151:746–750.
30. Glueck CJ, Levy RI, Fredrickson DS. Norethindrone acetate, post-heparin lipolytic activity and plasma triglycerides in types I, III, IV and V: studies in 20 patients and 5 normal persons. Ann Intern Med 1971;75:345–352.
31. Kim H, Kalkhoff RK. Sex steroid influence on triglyceride metabolism. J Clin Invest 1975; 56: 888–896.

32. Tikkanen MJ, Nikkila EA. Regulation of hepatic lipase and serum lipoproteins by sex steroids. Am Heart J 1987;113:562–567.
33. Khokha R, Huff MW, Wolfe BM. Divergent effects of d-norgestrel on the metabolism of rat very low density and low density apoliproteins. J Lipid Res 1986;27:699–705.
34. Oral Contraceptives. Med Lett 1988;30:106.
35. Albers JJ, Warnick GR, Nichols AV. Laboratory measurement of HDL. In: Miller NE, Miller GJ, eds. Clinical and Metabolic Aspects of High-Density Lipoproteins. Amsterdam: Elsevier, 1984:381–387.
36. Lipson A, Stoy DB, LaRosa JC, et al. Progestins and oral contraceptive-induced lipoprotein changes: a prospective study. Contraception 1986;34:121–134.
37. Powell MC, Hedlin AM, Cerskus I, et al. Effects of oral contraceptives on lipoprotein lipids: a prospective study. Obstet Gynecol 1947;63:764–770.
38. Burkman RT, Robinson JC, Kruszon-Moran D, et al . Lipid and lipoprotein changes associated with oral contraceptive use; a randomized clinical trial. Obstet Gynecol 1988;71:33–38.
39. Krauss RM, Roy S, Mishell DR Jr, et al. Effects of two low-dose oral contraceptives on serum lipids and lipoproteins: different changes in high-density lipoprotein subclasses. Am J Obstet Gynecol 1183;145:446–452.
40. Percival-Smith RKL, Morrison BJ, Sizto R, et al. The effects of triphasic and biphasic oral contraceptive preparations on HDL cholesterol and LDL cholesterol in young women. Contraception 1987;35:179–187.
41. Harvengt C, Desager JP, Gaspard U, et al. Changes in lipoprotein composition in women receiving two low-dose oral contraceptives containing ethinyl estradiol and gonane progestins. Contraception 1988;37:565–575.
42. Kloosterboer HJ, van Wayjen RGA, van den Ende A. Comparative effects of monophasic desogestrel plus ethinyloestradiol and triphasic levonorgestrel plus ethinyloestradiol on lipid metabolism. Contraception 1986;34:135–144.
43. Gaspard UJ, Buret J, Gillian D, et al. Serum lipid and lipoprotein changes induced by new oral contraceptives containing ethinyl estradiol plus levonorgestrel or desogestrel. Contraception 1984;31:395–408.
44. März W, Gross W, Gahn G, et al. A randomized crossover comparison of two low-dose contraceptives: effects on serum lipids and lipoproteins. Am J Obstet Gynecol 1985;153:287–293.
45. Whitehead MI, King RJB, McQueen J, et al. Endometrial histology and biochemistry in climacteric women during oestrogen and oestrogen/progestin therapy. J R Soc Med 1979;73:322–327.
46. Lindsay R, Hart DM, Forrest C, et al. Prevention of spinal osteoporosis in oophorectomized women. Lancet 1980;2:1151–1154.
47. Muesing RA, Miller VT, LaRosa JC. Quantitative and qualitative effects of unopposed estrogen on HDL subproteins and apoproteins in 30 postmenopausal women. In preparation, 1990.
48. Hart DM, Farish E, Fletcher CD, et al. Ten years postmenopause hormone replacement therapy—effect on lipoproteins. Maturitas 1984;5:271–276.
49. Bradley DD, Wingerd J, Petitti DB, et al. Serum high-density-lipoprotein cholesterol in women using oral contraceptives, estrogen and progestins. N Engl J Med 1978;299:17–20.
50. Wallentin L, Larsson-Cohn V. Metabolic and hormonal effects of postmeno-

pausal oestrogen replacement therapy treatment. II. Plasma lipids. Acta Endocrinol (Copenh) 1977;86:597–607.
51. Blumenfeld Z, Aviram B, Brook GJ, et al. Changes in lipoproteins and subfractions following oophorectomy and estrogen replacement in perimenopausal women. Maturitas 1983;5:77–83.
52. Farish E, Fletcher CD, Hart DM, et al. The effects of conjugated equine estrogens with and without a cyclical progestogen on lipoproteins and HDL subfractions in postmenopausal women. Acta Endocrinol (Copenh) 1986; 113:123–127.
53. Cauley JA, LePorte RE, Kuller LH, et al. Menopausal estrogen use, high-density lipoprotein cholesterol subfractions and liver function. Atherosclerosis 1983;49:31–39.
54. Fahraeus L, Wallentin L. High density lipoprotein subfraction during oral and cutaneous administration of 17 beta-estradiol to menopausal women. J Clin Endocrinol Metab 1983;56:797–801.
55. Farish E, Fletcher CD, Hart R, et al. The effects of hormone implants on serum lipoproteins and steroid hormones in bilaterally oophorectomized women. Acta Endocrinol (Copenh) 1984;106:116–120.
56. Sharf M, Oettinger M, Lanir A, et al. Lipid and lipoprotein levels following pure estradiol implantation in postmenopausal women. Gynecol Obstet Invest 1985;19:207–212.
57. Fahraeus L, Larsson-Cohn U, Wallentin L. Lipoproteins during oral and cutaneous administration of estradiol-17 beta to menopausal women. Acta Endocrinol (Kbl) 1982;101:597–602.
58. Chetkowski RJ, Meldrum DR, Steingold KA, et al. Biological effects of transdermal estradiol. N Engl J Med 1986;314:1615–1620.
59. Hirvonen E, Mälkönen M, Manninen V. Effects of different progestogens on lipoproteins during postmenopausal replacement therapy. N Engl J Med 1981;304:560–563.
60. Whitehead MI, Townsend PT, Pryse-Davies J, et al. Effects of various type and dosages of progestogens on the postmenopausal endometrium. J Reprod Med 1982;27:539–548.
61. Miller VT, Muesing RA, LaRosa JC, et al. Effects in postmenopausal women of conjugated equine estrogen with and without three different progestogens on circulating lipoproteins and apoproteins. Submitted, 1990.
62. Farish E, Fletcher CD, Hart DM, et al. A long-term study of the effects of norethisterone on lipoprotein metabolism in menopausal women. Clin Chim Acta 1983;123:193–198.
63. Jensen J, Riis BJ, Strøm V, et al. Continuous estrogen-progestogen treatment and serum lipoprotein in postmenopausal women. Br J Obstet Gynaecol 1987;94:130–135.
64. Weinstein L. Efficacy of a continuous estrogen-progestin regimen in the menopausal patient. Obstet Gynecol 1987;69:929–932.
65. Prough SG, Aksel S, Wiebe RH, et al. Continuous estrogen/progestin therapy in the menopause. Am J Obstet Gynecol 1987;157:1449–1453.
66. Miller NE, Hammet F, Saltissi S, et al. Relationship of angiographically defined coronary artery disease to plasma lipoprotein subfractions and lipoproteins. Br Med J 1981;282:1741–1744.

67. Avogero P, Bittolo BG, Cazzolato GE, et al. Are apolipoproteins better discriminators than lipids for atherosclerosis? Lancet 1979;1:901–903.
68. Manninen V, Elo MO, Frick MH, et al. Lipid alterations and decline in the incidence of coronary heart disease in the Helsinki Heart Study. JAMA 1988;260:641–651.
69. Tyroler HA, Levy RI, Thorn MD, et al. High density lipoprotein cholesterol and coronary heart disease mortality: experience of white men aged 40–59 years in the U.S. Lipid Research Clinics mortality follow-up study. In: Levy RI, et al, eds. Atherosclerosis Reviews. New York: Raven Press, 1988:277–286.
70. Newman WP, Freedman DS, Voors AW, et al. Relation of serum lipoproteins and systolic blood pressure to early atherosclerosis: the Bogalusa Heart Study. N Engl J Med 1986;314:138–144.
71. Kay CR. Progestogens and arterial disease: evidence from the Royal College of General Practitioners' study. Am J Obstet Gynecol 1982;142:762–765.
72. Hennekens CH, Evans D, Peto O. Oral contraceptive use, cigarette smoking and myocardial infarctions. Br J Fam Plann 1979;5:66–67.
73. Slone D, Shapiro S, Kaufman DW, et al. Risk of myocardial infarction in relation to current and discontinued use of oral contraceptives. N Engl J Med 1981;305:420–442.
74. Stampfer MJ, Willett WC, Colditz GA, et al. A prospective study of past use of oral contraceptive agents and risk of cardiovascular disease. N Engl J Med 1988;319:1313–1317.
75. Stampfer MJ, Willett WC, Colditz GA, et al. A prospective study of postmenopausal estrogen therapy and coronary heart disease. N Engl J Med 1985;313:104–109.
76. Knopp RH. Cardiovascular effects of endogenous and exogenous sex hormones over a woman's lifetime. Am J Obstet Gynecol 1988;158:1630–1643.

6
Metabolic Changes of Menopause

LIAN G. ULRICH

The term menopause is defined as the permanent cessation of menstruation resulting from loss of ovarian follicular activity.[1] However, in clinical practice and medical literature, the term menopause is used extensively to describe the years immediately before and after the last menstrual period, viz., the perimenopause or the climacteric. Climacteric is derived from the Latin word climactericus, literally meaning rung of ladder relating to a critical period of life, and this period of a woman's life is indeed characterized by major biological and psychological changes.

Research has emphasized the extensive changes in bone metabolism that take place during the menopausal years. A detailed description of these metabolic changes is outside the scope of the present work, and the interested reader is referred elsewhere for discussion of this issue.[1] Instead, this chapter covers the endocrinological events of menopause in relation to lipid metabolism, a matter of equal importance that has received little attention in the past. The changes in sex hormones during the menopausal years are therefore dealt with briefly; and in relation to this topic, the differences that can be expected between natural and surgical menopause are discussed. Other psychological, physiological, or metabolic factors influenced by menopause or age and that relate to lipid and lipoprotein metabolism and cardiovascular risk are touched on.

Hormonal Changes Associated with Menopause and Aging

The hormonal changes of the peri- and postmenopausal years were once thought to be of little significance because they merely signaled the end of a woman's reproductive function. Now, however, they are recognized to be important determinants of a woman's health in her later years. For this reason, an understanding of the sequence of changes in hypothalamic-pituitary-ovarian function is as important for understanding the particular health problems of mature women as is an understanding of menstrual physiology for women's health at a younger age.

The number of ovarian follicles steadily decline from midfetal life onward, and it is assumed that menopause occurs as a result of depletion of the follicular reserve. There is some evidence of accelerated depletion of primordial follicles just prior to menopause that may be related to increased recruitment caused by increasing levels of follicle-stimulating hormone (FSH) during the premenopausal years.[2] This rise in FSH could in turn be caused by decreased sensitivity to gonadotropins of the remaining follicles or be due to some other alteration in hypothalamic control mechanisms.

Whatever the underlying mechanism, an increase in the gonadotropins is seen during the perimenopausal years. FSH levels start to increase as early as 10 years before menopause and continue to rise for a few years after cessation of menstruation until FSH reaches a level 10 to 20 times higher than the normal premenopausal level.[1,3–6] The increase in luteinizing hormone (LH) starts later than the increase in FSH, and the postmenopausal level of three to six times the premenopausal level is reached about 6 months after menopause. Maximum gonadotropin levels are seen during the early postmenopausal years and subsequently decline slightly with increasing age.[1,3–6]

The high levels of serum progesterone seen during the luteal phase of the normal menstrual cycle are due to secretion by the corpus luteum. There does not appear to be any decrease in the high luteal levels of progesterone with age so long as the menstrual cycle is still regular and ovulation takes place.[7] During the follicular phase a small amount of progesterone is present in the circulation. Some of it may be of ovarian origin, but most is probably derived from extraglandular conversion of adrenal pregnenolone and pregnenolone sulfate, as well as from secretion of small amounts of progesterone from the adrenals.[7,8] The constant postmenopausal level of progesterone equal to or even below the premenopausal follicular level is reached within a few months after cessation of menstruation.[5,7–8] In addition, there is some evidence for an age-related decline in follicular phase serum progesterone taking place during several years prior to the menopause. However, so long as ovulation occurs, luteal phase serum progesterone is unaltered.[7]

The primary sources of estradiol in the fertile women are the ovarian follicle and corpus luteum. Consequently, during the months following menopause a considerable decrease in estradiol is seen, a decrease that continues during the following few years although at a lower rate. Estrone levels also decline but more gradually; as a result, the level of serum estrone is higher than that of serum estradiol in the postmenopausal woman. This finding is opposite to what is the case in the premenopausal woman.[1,4–9] There is as yet no consensus as to whether serum estrogens continue to fall with increasing age after menopause and whether the postmenopausal ovary still secretes small amounts of estrogen. However, it is generally accepted that the major source of estrogens in the postmenopausal women is extraglandular conversion of androgen precursors, notably androstenedione.[1,6,9,10]

The net effect of these changes is a relative excess of estrogen compared to progesterone just prior to menopause. After menopause there is a relative absence of progesterone and diminishing estrogen level. If the lipid profile is influenced by these hormonal changes, an estrogenic profile should be expected prior to menopause, with a rapid decrease in estrogen effect just after menopause and a further decrease over the following years.

Androstenedione, testosterone, and dihydrotestosterone are of mixed adrenocortical and ovarian stromal origin. Dehydroepiandrosterone (DHEA) and dehydroepiandrosterone sulfate (DHEA-S), however, originate mainly from the adrenals.[1,8,9] A continuing decline with age is seen in androstenedione, DHEA, and DHEA-S levels throughout adult life and probably in dihydrotestosterone and testosterone levels as well, although the latter has been questioned.[1,4,6,9–11]

Thus secretion of estradiol, estrone, and progesterone changes rapidly and dramatically in relation to menopause, whereas the decline in androstenedione, testosterone, dihydrotestosterone, DHEA, and DHEA-S is a more gradual one related to age (although more abrupt changes related to menopause may occur). Androgens are discussed in more detail in Chapter 7. In contrast to this sequence of changes observed with natural menopause, oophorectomy during the premenopausal years causes an immediate fall in all of these hormones, resulting in late postmenopausal levels of estradiol, estrone, and androstenedione and even dihydrotestosterone, and DHEA.[1] The abrupt hormonal changes resulting from surgical menopause could result in different effects on serum lipids and other processes modulated by sex steroids.

Estradiol and estrone levels in the postmenopausal woman are related to the extent of body fat, probably reflecting the ability of fat cells to convert androstenedione to estrone.[6,9,10] The rate of conversion of androstenedione to estrone and of estrone to estradiol increases with age counteracting the effect of the decreasing androstenedione concentrations.[9,10] Testosterone secreted by the adrenals and the postmenopausal ovary also can be converted to androstenedione and estradiol in peripheral tissues.[9]

Endogenous Sex Hormones and Lipids

Because women have a decreased risk for arteriosclerotic cardiovascular disease compared with men of the same age,[1] considerable attention has been paid to possible causes for this difference, and much focus has been put on the female sex hormones. During the reproductive years, massive fluctuation in serum estrogen levels are seen during the menstrual cycle, offering the opportunity to study the effect of endogenous hormones on plasma lipids.

It is well known that exogenous estrogens influence the lipid profile in a manner that may be protective against cardiovascular disease. This influence of exogenous estrogens on serum cholesterol and lipoproteins is dose-related and occurs within a few days, depending on the relative content of estrogen and progestogen.[12] However, because the effects of exogenous sex steroids could arise from the pharmacologic doses employed because of the first-pass effect through the liver, the changes observed are not necessarily the same as those that occur during normal, physiologic hormonal fluctuations.

If endogenous estrogens affect the lipid profile in a manner similar to that of exogenous estrogens during the postmenopausal period, one might expect to find cyclic variation in this profile with the menstrual cycle.

Most of the few published studies in this field have reported a decline in low density lipoprotein cholesterol (LDL-C) starting early in the follicular phase and continuing throughout the luteal phase. High density lipoprotein cholesterol (HDL-C), surprisingly, is unchanged.[13] However, most of these studies were not controlled for diet; and two studies that were controlled for diet seemed to show different results.[14,15] Jones et al.[14] reported a significant decrease in total plasma cholesterol during the luteal phase regardless of diet, the magnitude of which (from 0.29 mmol/liter to 0.48 mmol/liter) was stated to be similar to that in other previous reports. An increase in HDL-C was significant only in patients on a high fat diet (0.10 mmol/liter), and a luteal decrease in triglycerides was significant in patients on a low fat diet (0.08 mmol/liter). In patients on a normal diet no changes at all were seen in triglycerides or HDL-C (≤ 0.01 mmol/liter). However, Woods et al.[15] found a significant ovulatory increase in total triglyceride compared to that during the follicular phase (0.23 mmol/liter), primarily because of an increase in very low density lipoprotein in (VLDL) triglycerides (of 0.19 mmol/liter). There was no significant change in plasma VLDL-C, LDL, or total cholesterol. These studies did not take cycle-related hydration changes into account; data have now been presented showing no significant difference in plasma lipid fractions when changes in plasma volume during the menstrual cycle were taken into account.[16] Thus no firm conclusions can be drawn at this time as to the extent to which cyclic changes in endogenous estrogens and progesterone influence the lipid profile during fertile life.

Lipid Profile as Influenced by Age and Sex

Epidemiological studies, cross-sectional as well as cohort, British as well as American, have shown a rise in total serum cholesterol with age throughout adult life in women as well as in men.[17–20] The pattern of cholesterol rise, however, is sexually dimorphic. Cholesterol levels are similar in the sexes at the age of 20; but in women total cholesterol then increases slowly until midlife, after which a steeper increase is seen. In men a steep increase is seen during the twenties, thirties, and early forties, leveling off by mid-life. Thus whereas men in their second, third, and fourth decades have higher total cholesterol levels than women, the opposite is true after the age of 50. These total cholesterol changes are mostly due to changes in LDL-C. This subfraction shows the same pattern of age-related increases and differences between the two sexes.[17,18,20,21]

Age-related changes are also seen in serum triglycerides. Women start out with lower levels of triglycerides after puberty and throughout fertile life. The difference between the sexes decreases with age, and serum levels become similar in men and women around age 70, but there is no actual crossover.[17,18,20,21] Interestingly, the higher levels of HDL-C and HDL triglycerides that appear at puberty seem to remain more or less constant throughout life, although at different levels in the two sexes without change after menopause.[13,17]

These lipid patterns are even more interesting when considering the difference between coronary heart disease and age-specific mortality rate for ischemic heart disease between the sexes. Contrary to popular belief, the number of myocardial infarctions in men and women is similar, but myocardial infarction occurs an average of 10 years later in women than in men.[22] The differences between the two sexes in coronary mortality decreases after menopause, but there is evidence that this declining difference between the two sexes could stem from a slowing down of the rate at which coronary heart disease risk increases in men rather than from an accelerated increase in the rate of risk in women.[23,24] Thus although the risk of coronary heart disease continues to rise with age in men as well as in women, if looked at on a logarithmic scale the increase in risk for women is linear whereas it seems to decline for men after age 45. This finding has led to speculation as to whether some young men, owing to an unknown factor, have an increased risk for cardiovascular disease leading to death before age 55 with the remaining male population having no greater risk of coronary heart disease than women. However, it is also possible that without menopause the curve for women would level off as well and that menopause is an independent risk factor.

Clearly, age itself seems to be one of the most important risk factors with regard to coronary heart disease in men as well as in women. In addition, high total cholesterol, LDL-C and triglycerides, as well as low HDL-C are independent risk factors for coronary heart disease in women.[24,25] Aging is associated with many metabolic changes, and sex steroid changes probably account for only some of them. The increase in LDL-C and total cholesterol seen from the age of 20 in both sexes cannot be explained on the basis of endogenous sex hormone changes. This point must be kept in mind during the following discussion of changes seen during the menopausal years even though it is tempting to relate such changes to declining estrogen levels.

Menopause, Surgical or Natural, and Cardiovascular Risk

Although total cholesterol, LDL-C and triglycerides increase steadily throughout adult life, and though the risk curve for cardiovascular death continues exponentially with no change as a result of menopause, it is possible that if there were no menopause the increases in the deleterious lipoproteins would level off with age and the curve of cardiovascular death would flatten as for men. Major epidemiological studies, among which are the Framingham Study, the Nurse Health Care Study, and the Göthenburg Study from Sweden,[1,26–28] have linked cardiovascular risk to menopause, whether natural or surgical. The association between increased cardiovascular risk and menopause is stronger for surgical than for natural menopause. This fact has been confirmed in pathologic studies using autopsy material, case-control studies, and cohort studies.[1] Thus in the Framingham Study the risk of coronary heart disease was tripled after surgical menopause compared to premenopausal women in the same age group.[26] Interestingly, however, there was no difference as to whether the ovaries were removed in addition to the uterus or not. This point could be explained if a factor associated with monthly bleeding had an impact on cardiovascular risk or if blood supply to the ovaries was impaired by surgery. It seems likely that the function of remaining ovaries after hysterectomy is frequently severely impaired.[29] In contrast, in the Nurse Health Care Study, where removal of one ovary or hysterectomy alone was performed, there was no appreciable association between menopause and risk of coronary heart disease in non-estrogen treated women, whereas the risk with bilateral oophorectomy was doubled.[27] The number of women who had undergone surgical menopause in the Framingham Study, however, was only 419 compared with 22,854 in the Nurse Health Care study. The former study is thus less likely to find differences between subgroups and is more vulnerable to variations due to surgical impairment to remaining ovaries.

In contrast to the uniform findings that surgical menopause with bilateral oophorectomy increases cardiovascular risk, not all studies agree that there is an association between natural menopause and cardiovascular risk. In the Framingham Study, coronary heart disease was increased almost threefold in the age groups 40 to 44 and 45 to 49, and this increased risk could not be explained completely by such factors as increased lipids or excessive cigarette smoking. These two factors were stated to account for the increased incidence of coronary heart disease in the Göthenburg Study, but a change in the lipids may of course be caused by the changing hormone levels of menopause. In the Nurse Health Care Study, controlling for age and cigarette smoking did reduce the relative risk of coronary heart disease for naturally postmenopausal women, compared to premenopausal women, to 1.0. Hence in this study there was no increased risk.

Despite conflicting evidence, some conclusions may be drawn from these studies. Aging and smoking are major risk factors for cardiovascular disease and outweigh the influence of menopause, whether natural or surgical. The effect of aging on cardiovascular disease is likely to be at least partly due to increasing levels of total and LDL cholesterol. Total hysterectomy with bilateral oophorectomy before the normal age of menopause is definitely associated with increased cardiovascular risk if the patient is not treated with exogenous estrogens. Data on cardiovascular risk as sociated with hysterectomy without oophorectomy or natural menopause are conflicting, with an association likely but not yet proved.

Smoking is an independent risk factor for cardiovascular disease,[30] and studies should therefore be controlled for smoking, especially as smoking itself may hasten the onset of menopause even though the mechanism is not clear.[31,32] An antiestrogenic effect of smoking has been suggested that might be due to higher levels of dehydroepiandrosterone and androstenedione, a small rise in sex hormone binding globulin (SHBG) resulting in increased protein binding of estrogens, or altered estrogen clearance. Alternatively, the mechanism could be lower body fat in smokers.

The discrepancy between surgical and natural menopause with respect to an increase in cardiovascular risk is puzzling. One explanation could be that although there is an abrupt decrease in serum estradiol by the time of menopause, the decline in estrogen levels takes place over several years and may mask the effect of a few years' difference in menopausal age. Furthermore, it is possible that the level of estrogen necessary to render some protection against coronary heart disease is lower than the level necessary to stimulate the endometrium. Finally, possible differences could be masked by a strong effect of age itself. Regardless of whether there actually is an increased cardiovascular risk associated with natural menopause, treatment with exogenous estrogens, in most epidemiological studies, is definitely associated with a decreased relative cardiovascular risk. This matter is discussed in detail in Chapters 2 and 5.

Lipid Profile in Relation to Menopausal Status

With all the above-mentioned reservations, it is still relevant to review the lipid profile in relation to menopausal status in itself. To study this area, different approaches have been taken to try to overcome the confounding age factor. One approach is to compare the lipid profile after surgical menopause with that obtained before oophorectomy or in a control group (or, preferably, both). In such studies, however, one cannot eliminate the effect of removing the ovaries on the testosterone, dihydrotestosterone, and dehydroepiandrosterone levels. As mentioned previously, these hormones reach lower levels after oophorectomy than after natural menopause, so that the endocrine milieu is not identical in the two forms of menopause. Another approach is to study lipid levels in women of similar age but different menopausal status. Such studies, however, need to consider bias, which may be introduced by factors such as obesity, smoking habits, and other biological variables capable of influencing the age of menopause, the cardiovascular risk, or both. Finally, one might follow large groups of women in longitudinal studies covering the years before and after menopause. However, even such long-term studies are vulnerable to methodological flaws, e.g., changes of laboratory procedures over the years, effects of storage of samples, the effect of age, and often the lack of control except for baseline values.

As early as 1959, women subjected to oophorectomy bilaterally before the age of 35 were shown to have higher levels of serum cholesterol than did women who had undergone unilateral surgery.[33] Furthermore, in 1959 Robinson et al. reported a large study of women aged 40 to 59 years.[34] A total of 112 women oophorectomized before the age of 45 were compared with 104 age-matched controls who had had a hysterectomy but not oophorectomy. The oophorectomized women showed higher serum cholesterol, phospholipids, and β-lipoprotein cholesterol levels (LDL) than the controls. There was no statistically significant difference between the two groups with respect to α-cholesterol (HDL).[34] More recently, Notelovitz et al. compared 19 oophorectomized young women with 21 nonmenopausal age-matched controls and found cholesterol and triglyceride levels were significantly higher and HDL significantly lower in cases compared to the controls. There was no difference between the groups with regard to LDL and VLDL.[35] Finally, Johansson et al. reviewed young females aged 15 to 30 years at the time of bilateral salpingo-oophorectomy done between 1910 and 1940.[36] Of 146 patients, 42 had died; information was obtained on 68 of the women, 11 of whom, however, were found to have menstruated again after the operation. Thus the estrogen status of the subjects was uncertain, which might explain why no overall changes in serum cholesterol or serum triglycerides could be demonstrated with certainty after oophorectomy. However, serum cholesterol in the age group under 60 and serum triglycerides in the age group under 65 were significantly higher in oophorectomized women than in controls, which indicates that increasing age could have effects similar to those of oophorectomy.[36]

Thus studies on surgical menopause seem to agree that bilateral oophorectomy results in an increase in total cholesterol and, less consistently, in triglycerides. The rise in total cholesterol may be due to a rise in LDL, but additional data on this point as well as on the effect of oophorectomy on HDL are clearly needed.

The age-related rise in levels of total cholesterol, LDL-C, and triglycerides becomes steeper in women between 40 and 60 years compared to younger women and men.[18,20] More than two decades ago two Swedish groups in Göthenburg tried to link menopausal status to plasma lipids by studying premenopausal and postmenopausal 50-year-old women.

Hallberg and Svanborg in 1967 published data on 71 fifty-year-old women grouped as premenopausal, less than 8 weeks' postmenopausal, 8 weeks' to 3 years' postmenopausal, and more than 3 years' postmenopausal. Serum cholesterol, phospholipids, and triglycerides were found to be lowest in the less than 8 weeks' postmenopausal group, but it was not statistically significant. If this difference is real, however, it could be related to the relatively higher level of estradiol compared with progesterone during the perimenopausal years. Significant increases in serum cholesterol, phospholipids, and triglycerides were shown with increasing time after menopause.[37]

Consistent with this observation were the 1973 results of Bengtsson et al., who compared 185 premenopausal women to 148 who were postmenopausal. In these 50-year-old women serum cholesterol and serum triglycerides were significantly higher in the postmenopausal group.[38]

The Lipid Research Clinics Program Prevalence Study finding a steep increase in the level of LDL-C in women around age 50 also could be reflecting metabolic changes due to menopause.[21] Data from the Framingham Study examined differences in LDL subfractions and apolipoproteins in premenopausal and postmenopausal women.[39] The study group consisted of 87 premenopausal and 43 postmenopausal women. The postmenopausal women were more likely to have low-molecular-weight, small, dense LDL compared to the premenopausal women. Adjusting for age and body mass index, postmenopausal women had significantly higher LDL-C levels, lower HDL-C and total cholesterol levels, and lower apolipoprotein (apo) A_1/apo B ratios. Differences in HDL, total cholesterol, apo A_1, and apo B did not reach statistical significance except that HDL-C was found to be significantly lower in postmenopausal women than in age-matched premenopausal women. Adjusting for age and body mass index broadened the differences between the groups with respect to HDL-C and apo A_1. This finding may indicate a relatively greater effect of menopause itself on HDL and apo A_1 compared to a greater age-related effect on total cholesterol and LDL.

Longitudinal data on changes in lipids during the menopausal transition are few. Bengtsson et al. found decreasing levels of cholesterol and triglycerides during the 5 years before menopause. By the time of menopause the trend had changed to an upward on.[28] More recently, Matthews et al. published prospective data on 69 women evaluated when premenopausal at study entry and again after 12 months without menses. They were compared with 69 age-matched premenopausal controls. Cases showed greater increases in LDL-C, whereas controls showed greater increase in HDL-C from the first to the second evaluation.[40]

In summary, studies on surgical and natural menopause seem to agree that menopause is associated with an increase in total cholesterol and probably triglycerides, exceeding the increase caused by age. This increase at menopause is probably related to an increase in LDL-C. The decrease in relative HDL-C/total cholesterol levels is due primarily to the increase in total cholesterol. In addition, some investigators have found decreasing levels of HDL-C associated with menopausal status, whereas others have not. However, the relative importance of age and menopause in producing these changes is far from settled. Likewise, the relative importance of changes in the various lipid fractions is not resolved. Apart from an urgent need of major epidemiologic studies assessing cardiovascular risk in connection with estrogen therapy opposed by different progestogens, further studies on the changes in lipid metabolism with natural as well as surgical menopause may be of help. Controlling for possible differences in plasma volume would also be relevant, keeping in mind the differences seen during the menstrual cycle.

Other Factors Relating to Cardiovascular Risk, Menopause, and Metabolism

No matter how obvious the relation between menopause, changes in lipid profile, and cardiovascular risk seems to be, cardiovascular diseases are nevertheless influenced by multiple factors, some of which are intimately linked with lipid metabolism. Thus changes in blood coagulation, blood pressure, weight, glucose tolerance, psychology, and dietary habits could influence cardiovascular risk around the menopause. Weight changes, dietary habits, and physical training also influence lipid metabolism. Therefore these factors are briefly touched on here, although with no attempt to offer a complete overview.

Regardless of age or type of menopause, the estrogen-deficient postmenopausal woman shows increases in antithrombin III, plasminogen, and α-antitrypsinantigen, all of which favor clot inhibition and fibrinolysis. This fact was shown by Notelovitz et al. in 1981, comparing normal, young premenopausal women with both young and older surgically menopausal women and naturally postmenopausal women.[41] These changes favor clot inhibition and fibrinolysis and should thus be favorable in relation to cardiovascular risk. In the Framingham Study, fibrinogen levels have been shown to be independent risk factors for cardiovascular disease, and fibrinogen levels were shown to increase with age in both women and men.[42] However, the magnitude of risk diminished with advancing age in women, but not in men with high fibrinogen values. Putting these two studies together, one could speculate whether the increase in fibrinogen as a result of age is a strong cardiovascular risk factor that is actually favorably opposed by coagulatory changes induced by menopause.

Blood pressure is known to increase with age and to be an independent risk factor for cardiovascular disease. However, interesting data from the Framingham Study have shown different results comparing blood pressure in cross-sectional and cohort examination.[19] In the Framingham Study, women were shown to have a lower mean systolic blood pressure than men up to the age of around 50, after which, when examining the cohort, women had higher systolic blood pressure levels than men in cross-sectional data. However, in the longitudinal study, blood pressure increased in women as well as in men, but with no sex difference. It was speculated that these differences were due to a selectively high mortality among young men with high blood pressure.[19] Whatever the cause, these data do not support an influence of menopause itself on blood pressure, whereas such a relation does exist between blood pressure and age.

The prevalence of manifest diabetes increases with age, and some 80% of diabetic women are in the 45+ age group.[24,43] This increase in the prevalence of manifest diabetes mellitus with age, however, is similar in men and women. An association between cardiovascular disease and diabetes is established. Although estrogens and progestogens can influence glucose levels and insulin secretion, menopause does not seem to play a major role with respect to carbohydrate metabolism.[19]

Both lipid metabolism and glucose metabolism could be influenced by weight changes seen with age. Average body weight increases steadily from the early twenties to the end of the fifties, after which it is more stable.[43] Different results have been obtained regarding the association between obesity and coronary heart disease; these topics are reviewed in Chapter 2. There is, however, a correlation between the mass of adipose tissue and the plasma levels of estrogens. Some authors have suggested that overweight women menstruate up to a later age.[24,43] In addition, obesity is positively associated with hyperlipidemia and arterial hypertension.[24] Thus it appears that the body weight increase with age is related to important cardiovascular risk factors such as hyperlipidemia, hypertension, and diabetes and may or may not be independently linked to cardiovascular risk. A large-scale study of 2481 Italian climacteric women was reported in which the relation of body mass index to age and menopausal status was evaluated.[44] These women were divided into five groups according to menopausal status: a late fertile group,* a premenopausal group,† and

---

*Cycling (regular or irregular) women aged 40–50 years and women aged 46–50 years with regular cycles.
†Women aged 40–45 years with amenorrhea but premenopausal levels of estradiol and gonadotropins, women aged 46–50 years with irregular cycles, and cycling women over 50 years of age.

three postmenopausal groups a duration, e.g., 6 to 36 months, 37 to 96 months, and more than 96 months. Comparing women of the same age, the mean body mass index (weight/height squared) was significantly higher in the premenopausal group than in the late fertile age group. No difference was found between recent naturally postmenopausal and premenopausal women. Comparing women of the same age, surgically postmenopausal women did not differ significantly in weight from late fertile women. When women with the same menopausal status were compared, a mild increase with age was seen in body mass index.[2] It was concluded that premenopause is a weight-gain-inducing state.

That physical training and body weight are not independent factors is not surprising. Rainville and Vaccaro[45] compared premenopausal and post-menopausal trained and untrained women; they found significantly higher weight among postmenopausal, untrained women than among postmeno-pausal, trained women, the latter not differing from premenopausal women. LDL-C was significantly higher in the postmenopausal, untrained women than in the trained women, and in the postmenopausal women than in the premenopausal women. HDL-C was significantly lower in the post-menopausal, untrained women than in with the trained women, and tri-glycerides were significantly higher in the postmenopausal, untrained women than in the premenopausal, untrained.[45] It was concluded that menopause adversely alters the cholesterol lipid profile by elevating LDL-C levels, whereas HDL-C was not significantly affected. It was also con-cluded that postmenopausal women may offset the deleterious effect of menopause on lipid risk factors through a regular, physical conditioning program because training seems to increase HDL-C and lower LDL-C. The relation between exercise and lipid levels in women is discussed in Chapter 11.

Thus it can be seen that the relation between cardiovascular risk, meno-pause, and metabolic factors is multifactorial and complex. In addition to the above-mentioned factors, one could speculate that psychological changes at the time of menopause, such as depression, could influence dietary habits, which could further influence the lipid profile. Likewise, psychological changes might influence smoking habits. Vasomotor symp-toms with excessive sweating could be even worse during physical training and thus influence training habits. Diet also could be linked to age and menopausal status.

Conclusion

Compared to the amount of research done regarding the effect of estrogen on metabolic parameters and cardiovascular risk, surprisingly little is found on the relation between natural and surgical menopause, cardiovascular risk, and metabolic changes. From the evidence we have, however, it seems that surgical menopause and possibly natural menopause are independently linked to metabolic changes in the lipid profile thought to be related to increased cardiovascular risk. Thus menopause seems to increase total cholesterol, triglycerides, and LDL-C in excess of changes in these parameters caused by age. Menopause may also be related to decreases in HDL-C and apo A_1 and increases in apo B. Coagulation seems to be favorably influenced by menopause, whereas blood pressure seems related mainly to age. Menopause, in contrast to age, seems to have no effect on glucose intolerance. Weight increases steadily with age, but the premenopausal state may be associated with additional weight increase.

Surgical menopause increases the relative risk for coronary heart disease. Natural menopause has been linked with increased cardiovascular risk, although less strongly. Without doubt, however, lower relative cardiovascular risk and overall mortality have been found with postmenopausal estrogen-treated women compared to untreated women.

References

1. World Health Organization. Research on the Menopause. Report of a WHO Scientific Group. WHO Technical Report Series 670. Geneva: WHO, 1981.
2. Richardsson SJ, Senikas V, Nelson JF. Follicular depletion during the menopausal transition: evidence for accelerated loss and ultimate exhaustion. J Clin Endocrinol Metab 1987;65:1231–1237.
3. Lenton EA, Sexton L, Lee S, et al. Progressive changes in LH and FSH and LH:FSH ratio in women throughout reproductive life. Maturitas 1988;10:35–43.
4. Rannevik G, Carlström K, Jeppsson S, et al. A prospective long-term study in women from premenopause to postmenopause: changing profiles of gonadotrophins, oestrogens and androgens. Maturitas 1986;8:297–307.
5. Longcope C, Franz C, Morello C, et al. Steroid and gonadotropin levels in women during the premenopausal years. Maturitas 1986;8:1989–1996.
6. Kase NG. The management of the postmenopausal woman. In: Fioretti P, Flamigni C, Jasonni VM, Melis GB, eds. Postmenopausal Hormonal Therapy, Benefits and Risks. New York: Raven Press, 1987:35–54.
7. Metcalf MG, Livesey JH. Pregnanediol excretion in fertile women: age-related changes. J Endocrinol 1988;119:153–157.
8. Ross GT, Van de Wiele RL. The ovaries and the breasts. Part I. The ovaries. In: Williams RH, ed. Textbook of Endocrinology. 6th Ed. Philadelphia: Saunders, 1981:355–399.
9. Nocke W. Some aspects of oogenesis, follicular growth, and endocrine involution. In: Greenblatt RB, ed. A Modern Approach to the Perimenopausal Years. New York: de Gruyter, 1986:11–38.
10. Jensen J, Riis BJ, Hummer L, et al. The effects of age and body composition on circulating serum oestrogens and androstenedione after the menopause. Br J Obstet Gynaecol 1985;92:260–265.
11. Carlström K, Brody S, Lunell N-O, et al. Dehydroepiandrosterone sulphate and dehydroepiandrosterone in serum: differences related to age and sex. Maturitas 1988;10:297–306.

12. Jensen J, Nilas L, Christiansen C. Cyclic changes in serum cholesterol and lipoproteins following different doses of combined postmenopausal hormone replacement therapy. Br J Obstet Gynaecol 1986;93:613–618.
13. Knopp RH. Cardiovascular effects of endogenous and exogenous sex hormones over a woman's lifetime. Am J Obstet Gynaecol 1988;158:1630–1643.
14. Jones DY, Judd T, Taylor PR, et al. Menstrual cycle effect on plasma lipids. Metabolism 1988;37:1–2.
15. Woods M, Schaefer E, Morrill A, et al. Effect of menstrual cycle phase on plasma lipids. J Clin Endocrinol Metab 1987;65:321–323.
16. Cullinane EM, Sody M, Mitcheson S, et al. Variations in plasma volume alter total and LDL-cholesterol concentration during the menstrual cycle. Abstract 1535. Circulation 1988;78(Suppl):II–385.
17. Lewis B, Chait A, Wooton IDP, et al. Frequency of risk factors for ischaemic heart disease in a healthy British population. Lancet 1974;1:141–146.
18. Mann JI, Lewis B, Shepherd J, et al. Blood lipid concentrations and other cardiovascular risk factors: distribution, prevalence and detection in Britain. Br Med J 1988;296:1702–1706.
19. Kannel WB, Gordon T. Cardiovascular effects of the menopause. In: Mishell DR, Jr, ed. Menopause: Physiology and Pharmacology. Chicago: Year Book Medical Pulishers, 1987:91–102.
20. Lipid Research Clinics Program Epidemiology Committee. Plasma lipid distributions in selected North American populations. The Lipid Research Clinics Program Prevalence Study. Circulation 1979;60:427–439.
21. Heiss G, Tannis I, Davies CE, et al. Lipoprotein cholesterol distributions in selected North American populations: The Lipid Research Clinics Program Prevalence Study. Circulation 1980;61:302–315.
22. Castelli WP. Cardiovascular disease in women. Am J Obstet Gynecol 1988;158:1553–1560.
23. Wentz AC. Management of the menopause. In: Jones HW, Wentz AC, Burnett LS, eds. Novak's Textbook of Gynecology. 11th Edition. Baltimore: Williams & Wilkins.
24. Johansson S, Vedin A, Wilhelmsson C. Myocardial infarction in women. Epidemiol Rev 1983;5:67–95.
25. Report of the National Cholesterol Education Program Expert Panel on detection, evaluation and treatment of high blood cholesterol in adults. Arch Intern Med 1988;148:36–69.
26. Gordon T, Kannel WB, Hjortland ML, et al. Menopause and coronary heart disease. Ann Intern Med 1978;89:157–161
27. Colditz GA, Willett WC, Stampfer MJ, et al. Menopause and the risk of coronary heart disease in women. N Engl J Med 1987;316:1105–1110.
28. Bengtsson, Lundquist O. Coronary heart disease during the menopause. In: Oliver MF, ed. Coronary Heart disease in Young Women. New York: Churchill Livingstone, 1978;234–239.
29. Aranvantinos DJ. Keeping or removing the ovaries at the time of hysterectomy. Eur J Obstet & Gynecol Reproduct Biol 1988;28:140–146.
30. Goldbaum, GM Kendrick JS, Hogelin GC, et al. The behavioural risk factor surveys group: the relative impact of smoking on oral contraceptive use on women in the United Stats. JAMA 1987;258:1339–1342.
31. Andersen FJ, Transbol I, Christiansen C. Is smoking a promoter of the meno-

pause? Acta Med Scand 1982;212:137–139.

32. Khaw K-T, Tazuke S, Barret-Connor E. Cigarette smoking and levels of adrenal androgens in postmenopausal women. N Engl J Med 1988;318:1705–1709.
33. Oliver MF, Boyd GS. Effect of bilateral ovariectomy on coronary artery disease and serum lipid levels. Lancet 1959;2:690–694.
34. Robinson RW, Higano N, Cohen WD. Increased incidence of coronary heart disease in women castrated prior to menopause. Arch Intern Med 1959; 104:908–913.
35. Notelovitz M, Gudat JC, Ware MD, et al. Lipids and lipoproteins in women after oophorectomy and the response to estrogen therapy. Br J Obstet Gynaecol 1983;90:171–177.
36. Johansson BW, Kaij L, Kullander S, et al. On some late effects of bilateral oophorectomy in the age range 15–30 years. Acta Obstet Gynecol Scand 1975;54:449–461.
37. Hallberg L, Svanborg A. Cholesterol, phospholipids and triglycerides in plasma in 50 year-old women. Acta Med Scand 1967;181:185–194.
38. Bengtsson C, Rybo G, Westerberg H. Ischaemic heart disease in women. Acta Med Scand [Suppl] 1973;549:75–81.
39. Campos H, McNamara JR, Wilson PWF, et al. Differences in low density lipoprotein subfractions and apolipoproteins in premenopausal and postmenopausal women. J Clin Endocrinol Metab 1988;67:30–35.
40. Matthews KA, Wing RR, Meilahn EN, et al. Menopause influences risk factors for coronary heart disease. Abstract 2325. Circulation 1988;78(Suppl): II–583 (Suppl)II, Vol. 78, no. 4. October 1988.
41. Notelovitz M, Kitchens CS, Rappaport V, et al. Menopausal status associated with increased inhibition of blood coagulation. Am J Obstet Gynecol 1981;141:149–152.
42. Kannel WB, Wolf PA, Castelli WP, et al. Fibrinogen and risk of cardiovascular disease. JAMA 1987;258:1183–1186.
43. Teichmann AT. Age, metabolism and oral contraception. Maturitas 1988; (Suppl I):117–130.
44 De Aloysio D, Villeco AS, Fabiani AG, et al. Body mass index distribution in climacteric women. Maturitas 1988;9:359–366.
45. Rainville S, Vaccaro P. The effects of menopause and training on serum lipids. Int J Sports Med 1984;5:137–141.

7
Androgens in Women: Their Effects on Lipid and Carbohydrate Metabolism

GEOFFREY P. REDMOND

The purpose of this chapter is to present a perspective on androgenic disorders that emphasizes their broad health implications. Even though their exact incidence is not known, androgenic disorders clearly comprise the most common endocrinopathy of premenopausal women. For this reason the impact of androgenic disorders on the health of women merits serious attention. Most concern has been focused on the associated infertility, and treatment for this aspect has reached a considerable degree of refinement. The androgenic disorders are not always taken seriously as health problems, perhaps because their most evident effects are on appearance. Although there is treatment for the effects of androgens on appearance, it is complex and not always readily available to women seeking medical help.

It is the author's hope that this chapter can convince the reader that androgenic disorders are indeed a serious health concern. There is considerable evidence, albeit preliminary, that androgenic disorders constitute a significant public health problem because of associated changes in lipid and carbohydrate metabolism.

Androgen Action in Women

Although androgens are generally thought of as "male hormones," they are present in biologically active amounts in all women between puberty and menopause. Additionally, there may be active levels of these hormones during fetal and neonatal life and after menopause. Androgens are responsible for some of the normal events of female puberty. The androgen-mediated changes are the appearance of pubic and axillary hair, rugation of the labia majora, redundancy of the labia minora, and increased pigmentation of the genital skin. There are also changes in the chemical composition of sweat leading to the development of apocrine odor. Sebum production increases and makes the skin of the face, scalp, and upper trunk more oily. When androgen action is excessive, facial hair and body hair increase beyond normal amounts. Significant acne may appear, often with cyst formation and subsequent scarring. When these cutaneous actions of androgens are excessive, the result is a noticeably less feminine appearance to the face and scalp hair. Androgenic alopecia, a mild form of balding, occurs in many women as a result of androgen action. Mild forms of these androgen-induced changes are usually regarded as normal by physicians, and only the extreme forms are recognized as abnormal. However, there is no precise point of discontinuity between normal and abnormal, and so it is more useful to regard these androgen effects as a continuum from minimal to severe. Visible skin changes are a sign that the patient is experiencing increased androgen action and should alert the clinician to the possibility of other associated abnormalities. The latter may include psychological distress over the changes in appearance, reproductive dysfunction, and alterations in lipid and carbohydrate metabolism. The latter effects are generally less well known than the others and form the main subject of this chapter.

The Androgenic Disorders Concept

Despite extensive research, the pathophysiology of androgenic abnormalities in women remains incompletely understood. Areas of uncertainty include the nature of the regulatory abnormality responsible for the excessive androgen secretion, the relative contributions of adrenal and ovary, and the actual incidence of elevated androgens in women with the skin manifestations. Commonly used clinical terminology is a further source of confusion.

Traditionally, women with signs of excessive androgen action have been divided into two groups termed *idiopathic hirsutism* (IH) and *polycystic ovarian disease* (PCOD). Women are usually labeled as having IH if they have increased hair growth but normal menstruation. PCOD is diagnosed when menstrual abnormalities are present, the ovaries are enlarged with a thickened capsule and multiple cysts, or androgens are clearly elevated above normal. Unfortunately, these terms have not always been applied consistently among studies. At times patients were classified as belonging to one group by some investigators and the other group by others. For this reason it is difficult to combine existing studies into a clear picture of the two disorders. It is generally assumed that IH is relatively benign in effects and involves the adrenal more than the ovary. PCOD is more severe and is thought to involve the ovary in a primary role in its pathogenesis.

A different conceptualization is employed in this chapter. Androgen action may be observed in all women and is the result of a chain of events beginning with the hypothalamic-pituitary unit stimulating the ovary, the adrenal, or both, which in turn secrete androgens. These androgens may be secreted in active form as testosterone or less active forms as androstenedione and dehydroepiandrosterone sulfate (DHEA-S), which can be activated peripherally. Testosterone is converted to dihydrotestosterone (DHT) by the enzyme 5 α-reductase in the end-organ. This enzyme is particularly active in the skin, where much of its activity is concentrated in the sebaceous gland. DHT then binds with the receptor, resulting in altered gene expression. An androgenic disorder can be considered to be present whenever excessive androgen *effect* is observed. However, different point(s) along the pathway may be involved in different patients. For example, excessive facial hair may result from increased androgen secretion by the ovary or the adrenal (or both) or from increased activity of 5 α-reductase or increased postreceptor events (target organ sensitivity). It is likely that most patients with androgenic disorders have several of these factors involved to varying degrees.

The use of the term "androgenic disorder" is useful in a clinical context because it specifically refers to the exaggerated androgen effect observed in the patient and does not imply more than is known about causality. The label PCOD is particularly problematic because the ovaries in some women with the associated physiological aberrations do not have a polycystic appearance. Furthermore, some women whose ovaries appear polycystic on ultrasonography have no signs of an androgenic disorder. Although it is unlikely the term will be abandoned in clinical practice, the clinician would be well advised to be aware of its imprecision.

Androgenic Disorders and Lipoproteins

Although studies have been limited, all those reported suggest that androgenic disorders are associated with unfavorable changes in lipoproteins. Principal work has been that of Wild and collaborators.[1-3] One such study compared 29 patients with PCOD to 30 normal women.[1] The women were approximately matched for age and height, but the PCOD women were somewhat heavier, with a mean weight of 73 ± 3.0 kg compared to 62.0 ± 1.0 kg in the normal group. Mean age was 28 years in the PCOD group and 32 years in the other. This age mean is similar to that seen in our own androgen disorders clinic, and is certainly well below the age at which cardiovascular risk is generally evaluated in women. The investigators found higher levels of serum triglycirides (TG), very low density lipoproteins (VLDL), total cholesterol, (TC), low density lipoproteins (LDL), high density lipoproteins (HDL), and TC/HDL ratio in the PCOD group. Total cholesterol was 209.0 ± 11.0 mg/dl in the PCOD group versus 186.0 ± 5.0 in the normal group. HDL was 43.0 ± 2.0 mg/dl compared to 58.0 ± 2.0 mg/dl in the normal group. TC/HDL was 5.1 ± 0.3 in the PCOD group and 3.2 ± 0.2 in the normal group.

It is evident that these differences are sufficiently large to be of potential clinical importance. Obviously such a study cannot establish the cause of the differences among the groups, but it is plausibly related to androgen action. Another possibility would be hyperinsulinism, although this factor was not specifically measured in the study. Although the PCOD group was more obese than the normals, removing the effect of obesity in the statistical analysis did not alter the results. Interestingly, another study has suggested that PCOD patients are not only heavier but also are less active, have higher blood pressure, and have a higher intake of saturated fat together with lower fiber intake.[4] Because it is implausible that the presence of elevated androgens predisposes to these disadvantageous life style choices, it is possible that the life style is somehow conducive to developing PCOD. PCOD is clearly not the result of obesity alone because many obese women do not have the endocrine abnormalities of this syndrome; furthermore, many women with unequivocal PCOD or androgen excess are slender.

An important study[3] investigated women coming to cardiac catheterization. Those who were found to have significant coronary vessel disease were compared to those who did not. There was a greater prevalence of past acne and hirsutism in those who had vessel disease. Recall bias seems unlikely in a study of this sort but of course cannot be excluded. This study is of major importance because it suggests that androgenic disorders are associated not only with a greater incidence of risk factors but with an actual increase in coronary artery disease.

Another endocrine parameter found to be associated with cardiovascular risk factors in women is sex-hormone binding globulin (SHBG). Levels of this substance are suppressed by androgens and elevated by estrogens. Lapidus et al.[5] studied levels of SHBG in naturally menopausal women in Sweden and found that lower levels of SHBG correlated with the following risk factors: higher serum triglycerides, higher body mass, higher body mass index, and increased waist to hip circumference. They also found that low SHBG concentration was a significant risk factor for mortality; however, it did not correlate with angina pectoris, electrocardiographic changes suggestive of ischemic heart disease, or stroke. Although low SHBG was associated with subsequent myocardial infarction, the relation was not linear.

That low SHBG is a risk factor for myocardial infarction of course does not establish that high levels of androgens are the cause of the lower SHBG. The difference could be due to lower estrogen levels, an altered estrogen/androgen ratio, or other, unknown factors. Obesity per se has been found to be associated with lower levels of SHBG independent of androgen and estrogen levels.[4]

Suggestive as these studies are, there are few of them, and they generally have dealt with fairly small numbers of subjects. However, their findings are so plausible in light of what is known about the action of androgens on lipids and cardiovascular risk in men that they must be taken seriously, especially because the author knows of no contrary findings that have been reported. It is well known that androgens unfavorably alter lipoprotein levels, that men have less favorable patterns than women, and that men have earlier coronary artery disease than women.[6,7] These findings are not subject to dispute. Accordingly, it is plausible that increased androgen action in women would result in partial or complete loss of the usual female protection. It is possible, although yet to be demonstrated, that androgenic disorders are major risk factors early for heart disease in women and perhaps account for a significant proportion of the cases. Despite the preliminary nature of the findings, it seems justified to screen women with androgenic disorders for lipoprotein abnormalities and to treat them in accordance with present national guidelines[8] pending the development of a more complete understanding of these issues in women.

Androgenic Disorders and Carbohydrate Metabolism

The association between hyperandrogenism in women and abnormalities of carbohydrate metabolism first emerged in reports of the threefold association of PCOD, acanthosis nigricans, and insulin-resistant diabetes.[9–15] Initially, this disorder was thought to be a rare condition in which insulin resistance was severe. Subsequently it became apparent that the mutual association of PCOD, acanthosis nigrecans and insulin resistance was a rather common one with a considerable range in severity. Finally, work of several investigators has shown that insulin resistance accompanies PCOD even in the absence of acanthosis nigricans or obesity.[16–20] It appears, then, that insulin resistance is a common feature of androgenic disorders. Unfortunately, it is still unclear under what circumstances the insulin resistance progresses to frank diabetes and its complications. The effectiveness of interventions in correcting this situation remains to be fully investigated. This section discusses what is known about the association of insulin resistance and excessive androgen action in women.

If androgens per se produce insulin resistance, there should be relative insulin resistance in men compared to women, which is not the case. Accordingly, more is involved in the pathogenesis of insulin resistance than the direct action of androgens. One theory has been that the anabolic effect of the elevated androgens results in increased appetite and consequent obesity. Although it is true that most women with acanthosis nigrecans are obese, there are many women with significant hyperandrogenism who are slender. It is difficult therefore to conclude that hyperandrogenism by itself engenders obesity. Suppression of ovarian androgen production[21,22] does not, at least in the short term, produce remission of the hyperinsulinism.[23–25] Accordingly, it appears likely that hyperandrogenism of itself does not cause the impaired glucose metabolism associated with the hyperandrogenic states. Even if it were the case, however, it would be apparent that other factors beyond the hyperandrogenism must be operative. An action of estrogen in combination with androgens to produce insulin resistance is plausible, as estrogen levels are elevated in obese men who often do have insulin resistance.

The alternative hypothesis that the hyperandrogenism results from the hyperinsulinism has some support. A variety of growth factors, some of which have insulin-like activity, can effect an increase in androgen production by the ovary. In the syndrome of leprechaunism, insulin resistance is associated with hirsutism and androgen-induced genital changes.[12] Ovarian enlargement is also present. In a review, Barbieri and Ryan[9] commented on the work of Hultquist and Olding,[26] suggesting that the ovaries of infants of diabetic mothers show increased lutein cells and that male infants of diabetic mothers show increased Leydig cells. However, these infants have generalized overgrowth, and so hypertrophy or hyperplasia of a particular tissue should not be presumed to be a direct insulin effect. Also insulin action in the neonate differs in many respects from that in the adult. Furthermore, hyperinsulinemic infants, e.g., those born to diabetic mothers or those with uncommon hyperinsulinemic disorders such as Beckwith-Wiedemann syndrome or nesidioblastosis, are not masculinized.

Additional evidence that hyperinsulinism may be a factor in hyperandrogenism has resulted from the work of Stuart et al.[27] These investigators infused insulin into normal men, normal women, obese women, and women with the triad of insulin resistance, hirsutism, and acanthosis nigricans (ACN). Plasma glucose levels were maintained at 85 mg/dl by dextrose infusion. Although testosterone levels did not change, plasma androstenedione increased in all subjects, normal as well as those with obesity and ACN. Men, however, had a relatively small rise, whereas women had a substantial one. In all but the ACN groups androstenedione returned toward baseline toward the end of the 10-hour infusion period. The ACN subjects had higher baseline and peak androstenedione levels than the normals, although the increase seemed to be of similar proportion. Baseline and peak androstenedione levels were not especially high; the mean peak in the ACN group was less than 180 ng/dl. The authors appropriately commented that the adrenal might as readily be the source of androstenedione as the ovary. That the latter might be the case is suggested by the rise in cortisol seen in all groups. This point raises the possibility that the increase in adrenal activity was part of the counterregulatory response to the infused insulin.

Tissue and animal studies have provided more direct evidence that insulin can act on the ovary. Poretsky et al.[28] examined ovarian tissue from three obese women with PCOD who had undergone ovarian surgery. Tissue from all three subjects exhibited specific ^{125}I-insulin binding. The authors observed that the insulin may have been binding to receptors for insulin-like growth factor 1 (IGF-1). To some extent this issue is a semantic one. The polycystic human ovary appears to exhibit specific binding for insulin. Veldhuis et al.[29] demonstrated that insulin acts on swine granulosa cells in vitro to increase progesterone secretion. Cytochrome P-450 content rose substantially, as did specific mitochondrial cholesterol side chain cleavage activity. These effects were mimicked by somatomedin but not by certain other growth factors. Although androgens were not measured and only granulosa cells were studied, it is plausible that the increased precursor production could permit an increase in androgen synthesis. Garzo and Dorrington[30] found that granulosa cell aromatase synthesis in response to follicle-stimulating hormone (FSH) is enhanced by insulin, which is further evidence for a role of insulin in the regulation of steroidogenesis. Growth hormone (GH) may potentiate the ovulatory response of the ovary to exogenous FSH.[31] That GH, via IGF-1/somatomedin C, has insulin-like actions is further evidence for a role of insulin-like factors in the regulation of ovarian function. It must be pointed out that although this evidence suggests that insulin or insulin-like factors act on the ovaries they do not establish a pathogenetic role for them. The implication that quantitatively greater action of these substances on the human ovary can induce PCOD or hyperthecosis remains hypothetical. Evidence from clinical experience with type 1 diabetes and from growth hormone therapy would argue otherwise. Patients with type 1 diabetes require substantial amounts of exogenous insulin for satisfactory control. Patients on insulin doses sufficient to produce desirable levels of control are found almost invariably to be hyperinsulinemic when free insulin levels are measured. Despite this fact, there do not seem to be any reports suggesting that PCOD or hyperandrogenism is more common in women with insulin-dependent diabetes mellitus. It is my experience that these conditions are not particularly associated with type 1 diabetes; nor do such patients seem to have an unexpectedly high incidence of anovulation when they are otherwise healthy. Doses of GH sufficient to produce acceleration of growth in female adolescents with intact ovaries do not induce clinically evident androgenization. These considerations do not exclude a role for insulin or GH in hyperandrogenism. However, they do imply that increased levels of insulin on GH alone cannot account for PCOD.

Because those originally reported with the PCOD/ACN/insulin resistance (IR) triad had markedly elevated insulin levels, it has been thought that the hyperinsulinism may have induced the ovarian abnormality. However, more recent reports[32] indicate that this triad is actually rather common and that the degree of insulin resistance as well as the degree of hyperandrogenism is variable. Our experience indicates that some patients with obesity and ACN have normal serum androgen levels just as some have normal glucose tolerance and insulin secretion (Fig. 7–1). A plausible interpretation of this situation is that there is another humoral factor that acts on the skin to produce the ACN and may also act on the ovary to produce PCOD. This substance might also produce insulin resistance, although the presence of ACN in patients without insulin resistance is not explained by this hypothesis. However, conditions such as obesity known

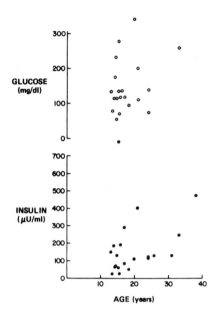

FIGURE 7–1. Glucose and insulin levels 2 hours postprandially in young females with acanthosis nigricans. Levels vary from normal to markedly elevated.

to induce insulin resistance do so gradually. Thus there may be a long period during which the patient has obesity, hyperandrogenism, and ACN before insulin resistance emerges. It is possible, of course, that ACN and insulin resistance are separate effects of obesity and that both are worse with more severe obesity. It seems evident that additional factors not yet clearly identified are involved in this complex situation. The known actions of insulin and androgens cannot by themselves account for the clinical observations.

Range of Insulin Resistance

As mentioned previously, the initial reports of PCO/ACN/IR were cases in which the insulin resistance was extreme. Thus the patient reported by Imperato-McGinley et al.[33] had a fasting insulin level of 425 μU/ml and peak of 2700 μU/ml at 180 minutes. She was only mildly diabetic with a glucose peak of 215 mg/dl at 90 minutes. This 15-year-old girl had presented with primary amenorrhea, hirsutism, and acanthosis nigricans. The patients reported by Tatna et al.[34] also had marked insulin resistance with values in excess of 250 μU/ml. The patients in the original report by Kahn et al. also had extreme insulin resistance. However, Flier et al.[32] published observations of a larger group of patients with acanthosis nigricans and hyperandrogenism. They found that 5% of patients being evaluated for hyperandrogenism had acanthosis nigricans. All of them were obese. All were insulin-resistant, but not all had frank diabetes. Fasting insulin levels ranged from 38 to 70 μU/ml in the group with ACN and 18 to 36 μU/ml in the group of hyperandrogenic women without ACN. These levels, especially those in the ACN group, were abnormal but were well below the extreme values seen in the earlier case report.[35]

Our experience is similar. Figure 7–1 shows glucose and insulin values in a group of young patients with ACN/PCO/IR. It is evident that insulin resistance is present in some but not all. It is equally striking that glucose levels are normal in some patients and clearly diabetic in others. The review by Barbieri and Ryan[9] also indicated that mild insulin resistance is far more commonly seen in this group of patients than the extreme forms. As for many other conditions, the extreme cases of PCOD/ACN/IR are noted and reported first, and the milder end of the disease spectrum becomes apparent only later with closer scrutiny.

The mildest end of the insulin resistance spectrum was shown by Chang et al.[16] in their study of nonobese patients with PCOD. These women did not have ACN and were not diabetic. However, their basal insulin level was 18.7 ± 2.9 μU/ml compared to 11.0 ± 0.8 μU/ml in the normally ovulating (non-PCO) group. Peak insulin levels were 158 ± 23 μU/ml compared to 57 ± 10 μU/ml in normals. This degree of insulin resistance is mild, and glucose-stimulated insulin levels greater than these amounts are frequently seen in mildly or moderately obese women with normal ovarian function.

There is considerable evidence that insulin resistance even without glucose intolerance has adverse effects on health.[37-39] One theory of atherogenesis holds that insulin acts as a growth factor to stimulate cell proliferation in the arterial wall. It is also likely that patients with insulin resistance have an increased risk of developing frank diabetes. However, it is more likely true of obese than nonobese individuals.

Classification of Insulin Resistance States Associated with Androgenic Disorders

There have been a number of attempts to classify or distinguish the various insulin resistance states associated with hyperandrogenism in women. A fundamental difficulty is the confusion regarding classification of the hyperandrogenic states themselves. Several groups have proposed classification schemes based on luteinizing hormone (LH) levels.[39-41] Those who have an elevated LH/FSH ratio are considered to have typical PCOD and the others to have an atypical form. For example, Barbieri and Hornstein distinguished one group with stromal hyperthecosis and a normally or slightly elevated LH level who were thought to have hyperandrogenism due to the hyperinsulinism from another group with more typical PCOD with an elevated LH level. The former are said to have less severe insulin resistance as well. In the present author's view such a scheme is problematic. The LH/FSH ratio may not be nearly so useful a criteria for PCOD as has been generally believed. In our studies patients with adrenal versus ovarian hyperandrogenism did not differ in terms of their LH/FSH ratio.[43] The suggestion that differences in the LH/FSH ratio are associated with different abnormalities of carbohydrate metabolism is speculative and remains to be tested in appropriate clinical studies.

Our experience, which includes many adolescents as well as adults, suggests that the factors involved in this syndrome vary independently in terms of severity. Patients differ in the degree of acanthosis nigricans, insulin resistance, glucose intolerance, hyperandrogenism, and menstrual abnormality. We did not find that patients with more severe acanthosis, for example, clearly had more severe abnormalities of insulin secretion or glucose tolerance. Some patients with ACN and frank diabetes had regular menses and normal androgens. Some with abnormal menses and ACN had normal androgens.

Accordingly, in the absence of a pathophysiological understanding, it may be premature to try to work out an overly neat scheme of these conditions. Rather, it seems clear that the factors of android obesity, acanthosis nigricans, menstrual dysfunction, androgen excess, and ovarian changes are highly associated with each other. However, each parameter can vary in severity independently of the others.

A related issue is which of these factors are prognostic of the development of diabetes. Is the 15-year-old with ACN but as yet normal glucose tolerance more likely to develop diabetes than an equally obese girl without the skin change? It may also be asked whether the glucose intolerance associated with this condition has the same likelihood of evolving into full-blown diabetes mellitus as does glucose tolerance in women without ACN or androgenic changes. In our limited state of knowledge it seems prudent to regard ACN and insulin resistance as risk factors for the development of diabetes.

The PCOD/ACN/IR syndrome has also been classified based on the nature of their insulin resistance and the presence of other abnormalities. Such syndromes include congenital and acquired lipodystrophy,[44] leprechanism,[45] and Kahn types A and B.[35] As originally described by Kahn, the type A syndrome consists of diabetes with marked insulin resistance and a receptor defect. Type B occurs in patients with insulin receptor antibodies.[46] This type has been found to be associated with a variety of autoimmune conditions such as lupus.[47] A case with an as yet incompletely identified circulating inhibitor of insulin action has been reported.[48] An additional form distinct from the type A and B syndromes was described by Flier et al.[32] This report seems to describe women with the milder end of the spectrum as does another series reported by Dunaif et al.[49]

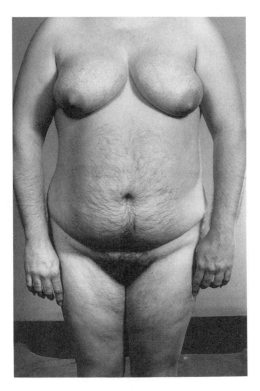

FIGURE 7–2. Hirsutism. Under the influence of androgens, body hair growth on the body of a woman can become as extensive as it is on a man.

Clinical Manifestations of Androgenic Disorders

It is apparent from the foregoing discussion that androgenic disorders affect more than appearance. Accordingly, it is important for the gynecologist, internist, or other physician caring for women to seek signs of increased androgen action as part of the general physical examination because they may be clinical clues to otherwise inapparent metabolic disease.

Increased facial and body hair, generally termed hirsutism, is the most generally known sign of increased androgen action (Fig. 7–2). Androgens transform the delicate, translucent vellous hairs into terminal hairs, which are thicker, darker, and stiffer. The skin areas that are most sensitive to androgens are the pubic and axillary regions, and of course virtually all women have terminal hairs in these regions although the amount varies considerably. Other areas in which terminal hairs commonly appear are the lateral aspect of the upper lip, the chin, the inner aspect of the upper thigh, the linea alba, and the presacral region. Hair frequently is present on the forearms and lower legs, although growth of this hair is not entirely

Hirsutism Rating Scale*

Patient's Name	Address	Date

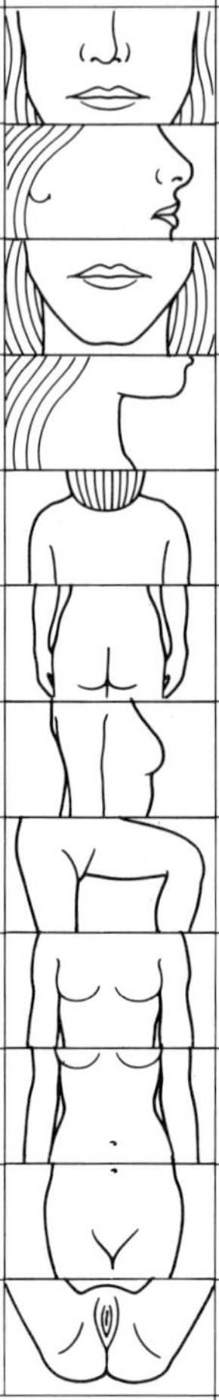

Site		Grade and Definition (Enter numerical grade in box.)			
		1	2	3	4
Upper Lip		A few terminal hairs at outer margin or scattered over upper lip	A small moustache at outer margin or covering less than half of upper lip	A moustache extending halfway from outer margin or halfway up lip	A moustache extending to mid-line and covering most of upper lip
Sideburn Area		A few scattered terminal hairs	Scattered terminal hairs with small concentrations	Light coverage of entire area	Dense coverage of entire area
Chin		A few scattered terminal hairs	Scattered terminal hairs with small concentrations	Complete but light coverage	Complete and heavy coverage
Lower Jaw and Upper Neck		A few scattered hairs	Scattered hairs with small concentrations	Light coverage of entire area	Complete and dense coverage of entire area
Upper Back		A few scattered terminal hairs	More terminal hairs, but still scattered	Complete but light coverage	Complete and dense coverage
Lower Back		Some sacral hair (area of coverage less than 4 cm wide)	With greater lateral extension	Three-quarter coverage	Complete coverage
Upper Arm		Sparse growth affecting not more than a quarter of the limb surface	More than this; coverage still incomplete	Complete but light coverage	Complete and dense coverage
Thigh		Sparse growth affecting not more than a quarter of the limb surface	More than this; coverage still incomplete	Complete but light coverage	Complete and dense coverage
Chest		Terminal circumareolar hairs or midline hairs	Both terminal circumareolar hairs and midline hairs	Three-quarter coverage	Complete coverage
Upper Abdomen		A few midline terminal hairs	More terminal hairs, still midline	Half coverage	Full coverage
Lower Abdomen		A few midline terminal hairs along linea alba	A midline streak of terminal hair	A midline band of terminal hair not more than 1/2 width of pubic hair at base	An inverted V-shaped growth 1/2 width of pubic hair at base
Perineum		Perianal terminal hair	Lateral extension of terminal hair to edge of gluteal cleft	Three-quarter coverage of buttocks	Complete coverage of buttocks
	Column Subtotals				

Total Score

FIGURE 7–3. Hirsutism rating scale. (Modified from Ferriman and Gallwey,[36] with permission; and courtesy of Searle and Company, Chicago.)

dependent on androgens. In some patients with hirsutism the terminal hairs are very apparent on physical examination, whereas in others, because of either fair color or the use of bleaching or other local removal methods the hirsutism may be less obvious. It may be helpful to run the tip of the finger gently along the skin or to ask the patient about the quantity of hair she has. Tact and discretion is required when inspecting for hirsutism because many women are embarrassed by the presence of facial and body hair. Hair growth can be quantitated using the rating scheme devised by Ferriman and Gallwey.[36] Based on discussion with other endocrinologists interested in hirsutism, a modified form of this technique has been developed that considers only hair on androgen-sensitive areas (Fig. 7–3). A limitation of this rating scheme is that it considers area coverage rather than the thickness and darkness of the hairs themselves.

Acne is considered to be a normal developmental event, and so it is when only mild comedones are present. However, when cystic or inflammatory acne occurs in a female, increased androgen action is generally involved (Fig. 7–4). A number of studies have shown an increased incidence of elevated androgens in women with cystic acne,[50] although there is some controversy about it.[51] That androgen action is involved in the pathogenesis of acne is further confirmed by the marked success of therapy with androgen antagonists such as spironolactone[52] and cyproterone acetate.[53] As in the case of hirsutism, there is no clear demarcation between normal and abnormal amounts of acne. The fact that some acne is normal in an adolescent does not mean that any amount is normal at any age.

The entity of androgenic alopecia is less familiar to nondermatologists than hirsutism or acne. In this condition, which affects a large number of women, hair follicles on the scalp become inactive as a result of androgen action.[54] Androgens act on the scalp to cause hair thinning despite their action to increase facial and body hair. The mechanism of this paradoxical action is unknown but its effects are familiar in the normal hair distribution in men. In women the area that has the most thinning is the vertex followed by the crown; some women also have thinning in the temporal area. In contrast to balding men in whom recession of the anterior hair line is a characteristic finding, the anterior hair line is relatively preserved in women with androgenic alopecia. When there is anterior recession, it is to a much lesser extent than is usual in men. Androgenic alopecia in both sexes tends to spare the sides of the scalp compared to the top. A variety of other conditions can cause alopecia in women, and not all alopecia is due to androgen action.

Many women have an acceleration of alopecia in androgenic distribution during the perimenopausal years, which likely involves estrogen deficiency rather than direct androgen action. Whether the falling estrogen levels predispose to alopecia by lowering sex steroid binding globulin levels or by a totally distinct mechanism is unknown.

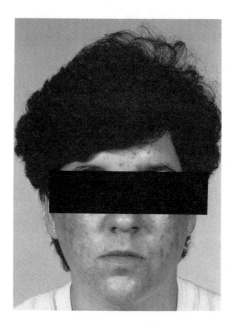

FIGURE 7–4. Cystic-inflammatory acne in a young woman. Although acne is often dismissed as merely cosmetic, more severe forms, as seen here, suggest the presence of an androgenic disorder.

Severe manifestations of androgen excess are termed *virilization*. They include temporal hair recession comparable to that seen in men, severe hirsutism requiring daily shaving, deepening of the voice, and enlargement of the clitoris. These effects are suggestive of a testosterone level of 150 ng/dl or higher, but an occasional virilized woman is found to have lower androgen levels. When virilization is present, thorough investigation is essential including search for a possible ovarian or adrenal tumor. However, the clinician should bear in mind that many women who do not have frank virilization may still be experiencing excessive androgen action with detrimental effects on their health. The absence of classic signs of virilization do not rule out a significant androgenic disorder.

The relation of ACN to androgenic disorders and carbohydrate abnormalities has been discussed earlier in this chapter. It is an important physical sign whose presence should be sought (Figs. 7–5, 7–6, and 7–7). The initial impression that ACN is rare is incorrect; rather, ACN appears on areas that usually are not inspected during physical examination: the back of the neck and axillae. Other intertriginous areas may be affected, including the inferior aspect of the breast, skin folds of obese patients, the belt line, and the groin. The skin becomes hyperpigmented with exaggerated markings and a velvety appearance (Figs. 7–2, 7–4 to 7–7). In more severe

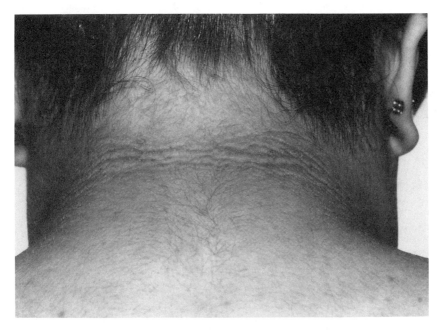

FIGURE 7–5. Acanthosis nigricans on the back of the neck. When the hair is lifted, the hyperpigmentation, increased skin markings, and a velvety appearance are evident.

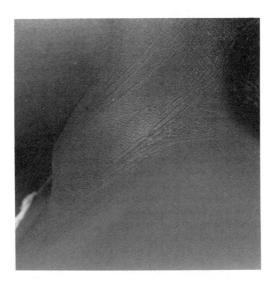

FIGURE 7–6. Acanthosis nigricans on the neck of a black woman. Some degree of increased intertriginous pigmentation is normal in blacks. However, the increased skin markings indicate the presence of acanthosis nigricans.

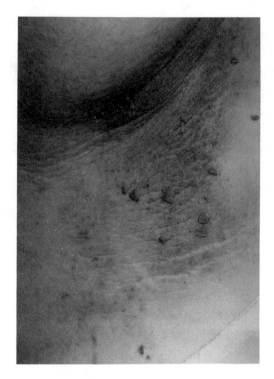

FIGURE 7–7. Acanthosis nigricans on the skin of the axilla. Skin tags are another feature of this skin lesion.

cases skin tags are noted. The appearance of ACN indicates the need to do a glucose tolerance test with simultaneous measurement of insulin levels.

Laboratory Investigation of Androgenic Disorders

When physical signs of androgenic disorders or abnormal menstruation are present, laboratory investigation is warranted. A complete evaluation would include measurement of total and free testosterone, androstenedione, and DHEA-S. Of these assays, that for androstenedione is the least useful, as it is unusual for this substance to be increased when the other androgenic steroids are normal. However, it may be abnormally high when the elevation of testosterone is at the upper limit of the normal range. Free testosterone may be elevated when total testosterone is normal and probably correlates more closely with the skin and metabolic manifestations of androgen excess. The sex steroid-binding globulin (SSBG) assay is useful in some instances. Prolactin should always be measured when there is menstrual abnormality present because galactorrhea is not always evident in women with hyperprolactinemia. Although the LH/FSH ratio is touted as the "gold standard" for PCOD, its relation to androgen excess is uncertain. There is considerable evidence that LH secretion is increased in women who have the manifestations of PCOD; however, a single measurement frequently fails to show an elevation of the ratio.

The author believes that lipid studies should be carried out in any woman who shows signs of increased androgen action. The combination of obesity and elevated androgens seems especially likely to be associated with an unfavorable lipid profile.[55] However, it is not unusual in the author's experience to see slender women who have marked lipid abnormalities.

Current guidelines[8] that recommend a complete lipid profile only when total cholesterol is more than 239 mg/dl are based on considerations of economy rather than optimization of detection of abnormalities. Because the same total cholesterol in a woman can be associated with a low or high HDL level—and therefore a favorable or unfavorable TC/HDL ratio— total cholesterol by itself is uninformative. A complete profile consisting in measurement of triglycerides, total cholesterol, HDL cholesterol (HDL-C), with calculation of VLDL-C and LDL-C, is warranted so that women at risk can be identified. Without suggesting that women without androgenic changes need not have lipid determinations, we wish to emphasize that the presence of androgenic changes makes it important to obtain these measurements, especially with the accumulating evidence suggesting that low HDL-C levels play an important role in the risk of developing coronary heart disease (CHD). The clinical usefulness of apolipoprotein (apo) measurements and HDL subfractions is unclear at the present time, although there is some evidence that apo A1 correlates more closely with cardiovascular risk than HDL itself.[56,57] Further experience is necessary to determine when they are helpful in estimating risk and designing treatment for individuals.

Much controversy surrounds the use and interpretation of the glucose tolerance test (GTT). Once advocated for universal screening of potential diabetics, the GTT is now thought to be indicated only when there is reason to suspect the presence of diabetes. In general, obese women, especially those with an android habitus and those with ACN, should have a GTT.

Adolescent girls with obesity and ACN should be treated. Fasting blood glucose is the least sensitive measure for diabetes, as it is normal in some who have marked postprandial hyperglycemia. A 2- or 3-hour GTT is more sensitive; a value in excess of 200 mg/dl at two time points is considered diagnostic. Intermediate values suggest diabetes, especially if other signs are present. Measurement of insulin levels simultaneously with glucose is useful, as one of the earliest events in type II (maturity onset) diabetes is insulin resistance. The significance of insulin resistance is discussed earlier in this chapter. The diagnosis of diabetes in women is discussed in more detail in Chapter 8.

Treatment of Androgenic Disorders

Treatments available for androgenic disorders may be grouped into three categories:

1. Those directed at correcting the endocrine aberrations and changes in appearance
2. Those directed at restoring ovulation in order to permit fertility
3. Those directed at the metabolic complications of these conditions

We consider here the first and third aspects of treatment.

Hyperandrogenism

It is the generally accepted principle of medical therapeutics that an ideal treatment is one that corrects the underlying cause of the condition. Because the causes of androgen excess or increased target organ sensitivity are incompletely understood, treatment cannot be so directed. However, it is usually possible to correct the endocrine disturbance, at least to the extent of normalizing elevated androgens. This goal is accomplished by (1) identifying the androgens that are elevated, as discussed under laboratory evaluation; and (2) performing dexamethasone suppression testing or other maneuvers to determine whether the excessive androgen secretion is being driven primarily by ACTH, LH, or both. An 8-day dexamethasone suppression test using 0.375 mg orally qid is appropriate for this purpose. One or two days of dexamethasone administration are not sufficient to suppress adrenal androgen production, although glucocorticoid levels may suppress 12 hours after a single dose of dexamethasone. Use of gonadotropin releasing hormone (GNRH) analogues for suppression testing may permit determination of the ovarian or LH-dependent component of circulating androgen levels more readily than measures available in the past. When the adrenal is the predominant source of androgens (more precisely, when the androgens are dexamethasone-suppressible), small doses of dexamethasone can be used to bring them into the normal range. We have found that the dose requirement is usually 0.25 mg as a single bedtime dose; it is never more than 0.375 mg nightly.[58] The higher doses of 0.50 or 0.75 mg daily frequently recommended are hazardous and should be avoided.

When the ovary is the predominant source of androgens, dexamethasone or another glucocorticoid is not appropriate therapy. In this case an oral contraceptive or LRH analogue might be chosen. There have been few studies of the effects of oral contraceptives on the skin and metabolic abnormalities of androgenic disorders despite their widespread use for these conditions.

One study has shown a favorable effect on lipids when an oral contraceptive was taken by women with polycystic ovaries for 6 months.[59] However, the progestin employed was desogestrel, which is not currently available in the United States. Logic dictates choosing a relatively nonandrogenic agent for a patient who is experiencing increased androgen action. Levonorgestrel and norgestrel are more androgenic than the other progestins used in oral contraceptives in the United States. Oral contraceptives containing these progestins are popular because of their reputation for a low incidence of bleeding abnormalities. Except for the infrequent dysfunctionally bleeding patient who cannot be controlled on any other drug, use of these progestins probably should be avoided in women with androgenic disorders. It is the authors' impression that acne or alopecia may be worsened by these preparations; however, the possibility that alopecia is the natural evolution of the condition and unrelated to the oral contraceptive cannot be excluded.

The least androgenic pills in general use in the United States have 35 μg of ethinyl estradiol and either 1.0 mg of ethynodiol diacetate or 0.4 or 0.5 mg of norethindrone. These agents appear to be the most appropriate preparations for women with androgenic disorders. When ovarian suppression is desired, the choice of a progestin-dominant pill, e.g., ethinyl estradiol 0.035 mg with ethynodiol diacetate, seems appropriate. In other circumstances, (e.g., maintenance of regular menstruation in women with oligoamenorrhea), a low progestin drug (e.g., one containing ethinyl estradiol 0.035 mg and norethindrone 0.4 mg) may be a reasonable alternative. The progestins norgestimate and desogestrel have been reported to have little androgenic effect on lipid levels but, unfortunately, are not available at this time in the United States.

Although dexamethasone or an oral contraceptive, when appropriately prescribed, reduces androgen levels toward or into the normal range, there is no information on whether it results in an improvement in lipid or other metabolic parameters. The exception would be the study using desogestrel cited above. Accordingly, when these agents are prescribed, it should not be assumed that they will correct lipid or carbohydrate abnormalities. Their established role is to suppress elevated androgens, control menstrual abnormalities, and serve as adjuncts to androgen antagonists in the treatment of the skin abnormalities.

There has been considerable interest in the use of (GNRH) analogues in gynecology. These agents suppress gonadotropin secretion and essentially restore a prepubertal hormonal state. Androgens are effectively suppressed.[22] Initial reports suggest that they do not reverse the insulin-resistant diabetes associated with acanthosis nigricans.[24] Whether they would be more effective if initiated very early in the course of the disease is an important question that has not been addressed. Nor are there data concerning whether suppression of androgens by these agents has beneficial effects on lipids. It is clear that estrogens exert favorable effects on lipid parameters in the female population as a whole, but, the effect of exogenous estrogens on abnormal lipid levels has not been well studied.

Perhaps because it is impractical to lower androgen levels to undetectable amounts, the use of an androgen antagonist appears to be necessary for satisfactory treatment of acne, hirsutism, and androgenic alopecia. Spironolactone is most often used in the United States, and there is considerable evidence that it is effective.[52] Cimetidine has also been used, but its efficacy is uncertain. Cyproterone acetate is effective[53] but exhibits considerable progestogenic side effects; in any event, it is unlikely to become available in the United States, although it is used extensively in Canada and Europe. An antiandrogen that has been recently introduced is flutamide. Others that act by inhibiting conversion of testosterone to dihydrotestosterone by 5-α-alpha reductase will also become available in the near future. Use of these drugs in women with androgenic disorders is limited by concern that they would interfere with normal masculinization of a male fetus. Whether these antiandrogens have a beneficial effect on lipid metabolism remains unknown.

Hyperlipidemia

This book has emphasized that lipid metabolism in women differs from that in men because of the differing hormonal milieus. Although some disorders such as familial hypercholesterolemia are similar in both sexes, there may be other lipid disturbances that are distinctive to women as a result of alterations in androgen and estrogen secretion or action. The evidence relating high androgen levels to low levels of HDL and high levels of LDL was reviewed earlier in the chapter. However, androgens are clearly not the only factors in determining lipid levels in women. The effects of obesity, diet, exercise, smoking, and genetic factors are likely to interact with endocrine components. Accordingly, it is difficult in an individual patient to ascertain which of these factors are producing the pattern seen. Although it is plausible that in some women with unfavorable lipid changes hormonal manipulation, such as estrogen administration or androgen suppression, would be an effective means of therapy, this approach is hypothetical at the present time. Because therapy for lipid changes may be lifelong, the physician should not recommend a particular course of treatment without adequate knowledge of the benefits and risks. Although the effects of oral contraceptives and postmenopausal hormone replacement on serum lipid levels have been studied extensively, these studies have been done almost exclusively in normal women. Studies of the effects of hormonal therapy on women with lipid abnormalities are needed.

At the present time, therefore, treatment of lipid abnormalities in women must be carried out in accordance with the same principles used for treatment of male patients. However, physicians who treat women should be aware of these issues and await further developments.

Insulin-Resistant Diabetes

Although diabetes mellutus is discussed in detail in Chapter 8, a few remarks are pertinent here. Type II (maturity onset) diabetes, which accounts for most cases seen in adults, is due at least in its early stages to insulin resistance. Those with the PCOD/ACN/IR triad may have a more severe degree of insulin resistance. Because the pathogenesis of type II diabetes is thought to involve induction of insulin resistance by excessive insulin levels, there is concern that insulin administration may worsen the condition. There is also a tendency for insulin to produce weight gain, especially in women. Use of an oral agent (glipizide or glyburide) seems to be reasonably effective in our experience. Many diabetologists believe that the mild hyperglycemia characterizing the early stages of type II diabetes may be sufficient to produce eventual complications. Accordingly, the indication for starting treatment is the early diabetic state rather than the presence of symptoms, which may not be apparent until the diabetes has been present for many years. A useful way to monitor therapy is for the patient to do self blood glucose monitoring before breakfast and 1 hour afterwards 2 or 3 days a week. The 1 hour post-prondial value should be less than 140 mg/dl. Despite thelr insulin resistance, some of these patients are sensitive to oral agents, and minimal starting doses should be used.

Dietary counseling is essential. The meal plan should include a bedtime snack and advice not to skip meals, thereby reducing the risk of hypoglycemia.

Although oral sulfonylureas are effective to some degree in improving the metabolic abnormalities associated with insulin resistance in diabetes mellitus, they are far less effective than weight reduction. Even loss of 20 to 30 pounds may improve the GTT or, in some cases, result in apparent normalization of glucose metabolism. Weight reduction does not simply remove the necessity for taking medication, but it is effective in restoring normoglycemia. Unfortunately, however, only a few patients achieve weight loss. Some also lack sufficient motivation to take the medication on a regular basis. A reasonable approach is to counsel the patient regarding weight reduction but to institute drug therapy after 4 to 6 months if progress is not being made. Obesity and its treatment are discussed in Chapter 9.

Conclusion

This chapter has presented the concept that androgenic disorders comprise a broad spectrum of interrelated conditions in which there are a variety of endocrine findings and clinical manifestations. Because androgenic disorders may have profound effects on the well-being of affected women, physician attention to these conditions is justified. Treatment is available for the skin changes, as well as the anovulation, and is beneficial in most of the women treated. Treatment is also available for the associated hyperlipidemia and diabetes mellitus. It is the author's hope that the seriousness of these disorders will become more widely recognized and that research into pathogenesis and treatment will be stimulated.

References

1. Wild RA, Painter PC, Coulson PB, et al. Lipoprotein lipid concentrations and cardiovascular risk in women with polycystic ovary syndrome. J Clin Endocrinol Metab 1985;61:946–951.
2. Wild RA, Bartholomew MJ. The influence of body weight on lipoprotein lipids in patients with polycystic ovary syndrome. Am J Obstet Gynecol 1988; 159:423–427.
3. Wild RA, Grubb B, Conner C, et al. Hirsutism in women with coronary artery disease (CAD): implications of the cardiovascular risk of androgen excess. American Fertility Society Program Supplement, 1988:S15.
4. Plymate SR, Fariss BL, Bassett M, Matej L. Obesity and its role in polycystic ovary syndrome. J Clin Endocrinol Metab 1981;S2:1246–1248.
5. Lapidus L, Lindstedt G, Lundberg PA, et al. Concentrations of sex-hormone binding globulin and corticosteroid binding globulin in serum in relations to cardiovascular risk factors and to 12-year incidence of cardiovascular disease and overall mortality in postmenopausal women. Clin Chem 1986;32:146–152.
6. Godsland IF, Wynn V, Crook D, Miller NE. Sex, plasma lipoproteins and atherosclerosis: prevailing assumptions and outstanding questions. Am Heart J 1987;114:1467–1503.
7. Furman RH, Alaupovic P, Howard PP. Effects of androgens and estrogens on serum lipids and the composition and concentration of serum lipoproteins in normolipemic and hyperlipemic states. Prog Biochem Pharmacol 1967;2:21–5249.
8. Goodman DS, et al. Report of the national cholesterol education program expert panel on detection, evaluation, and treatment of high blood cholesterol in adults. Arch Intern Med 1988;148:36–69.
9. Barbieri RL, Ryan KJ. Hyperandrogenism, insulin resistance, and acanthosis nigricans syndrome: a common endocrinopathy with distinct pathophysiologic features. Am J Obstet Gynecol 1983;147:90–101.
10. Flier JS, Kahn CR, Roth J. Receptors, antireceptor antibodies and mechanisms of insulin resistance. N Engl J Med 1979;300:413–419.
11. Kahn CR, Flier JS, Bar RS, et al. The syndromes of insulin resistance and acanthosis nigricans. N Engl J Med 1976;295:739–745.
12. Rosenberg AM, Haworth JC, Degroot GW, et al. A case of leprechaunism with severe hyperinsulinemia. Am J Dis Child 1980;134:170–175.
13. Flier JS, Young JB, Landsberg I. Familial insulin resistance with acanthosis nigricans, acral hypertrophy and muscle cramps. N Engl J Med 1980;303:970–973.
14. Bar RS, Muggeo M, Roth J, et al. Insulin resistance, acanthosis nigricans, and

normal insulin receptors in a young women: evidence for a postreceptor defect. J Clin Endocrinol Metab 1978;47:620–625.

15. Pulini M, Raff SB, Chase R, Gordon EE. Insulin resistance and acanthosis nigricans. Ann Intern Med 1976;85:749–751.

16. Chang RJ, Nakamura RM, Judd HL, Kaplan SA. Insulin resistance in nonobese patients with polycystic ovarian disease. J Clin Endocrinol Metab 1983;57:356–359.

17. Chang J, Geffner M. Associated non-ovarian problems of polycystic ovarian disease: insulin resistance. Clin Obstet Gynecol 1985;12:675–684.

18. Jialal I, Naiker P, Reddi K, et al. Evidence for insulin resistance in non-obese patients with polycystic ovarian disease. J Clin Endocrinol Metab 1987; 64:1066–1069.

19. Modan M, Halkin H, Fuchs Z, et al. Hyperinsulinemia: a link between glucose intolerance, obesity, hypertension dyslipoproteinemia, elevated serum uric acid and internal cation imbalance. Diabete Metab 1987;13:375–380.

20. Jialal I, Naiker P, Reddi K, et al. Evidence for insulin resistance in non-obese patients with polycystic ovarian disease. J Clin Endocrinol Metab 1987; 64:1066–1069.

21. Fern M, Rose DP, Fern EB. Effect of oral contraceptives on plasma androgenic steroids and their precursors. Obstet Gynecol 1978;51:541–544.

22. Willemsen WNP, Franssen AMHW, Rolland R, Vemer HM. The effects of buserelin on the hormonal states in PCOD. Prog Clin Biol Res 1986;225:377–389.

23. Pasquali R, Fabbri R, Venturoli S, et al. Effect of weight loss and anti-androgenic therapy on sex hormone blood levels and insulin resistance in obese patients with polycystic ovaries. Am J Obstet Gynecol 1986,154:139–144.

24. Geffner ME, Kaplan SA, Bersch N, et al. Persistence of insulin resistance in polycystic ovarian disease after inhibition of ovarian steroid secretion. Fertil Steril 1986;45:327–333.

25. Pasquali R, Fabbri R, Venturoli S, et al. Effect of weight loss and anti-androgenic therapy on sex hormone blood levels and insulin resistance in obese patients with polycystic ovaries. Am J Obstet Gynecol 1986;154:139–144.

26. Hultquist GT, Olding LB. Endocrine pathology of infants of diabetic mothers. Acta Endocrinol (Copenh) [Suppl 241] 1981;97:64.

27. Stuart CA, Prince MJ, Peters EJ, Meyer WJ: Hyperinsulinemia and hyperandrogenemia: in vivo androgen response to insulin infusion. Clin Gynecol 1987;69:921–925.

28. Poretsky L, Smith D, Seibel M, et al. Specific insulin binding sites in human ovary. J Clin Endocrinol Metab 1982;59:809–812.

29. Veldhuis J, Kolp L, Toaff ME, Strauss JF, Demers LM. Mechanisms subserving the trophic actions of insulin on ovarian cells. J Clin Invest 1983;72:1046–1057.

30. Garzo VG, Dorrington JH: Aromatase activity in human granulosa cells during follicular development and the modulation by follicle-stimulating hormone and insulin. Am J Obstet Gynecol 1984;148;657–662.

31. Owen E, Homburg R, Eshel A, et al. Combined growth hormone and gonadotrophin treatment for ovulation induction. American Fertility Society Annual Meeting Program Supplement, 1988:Sl

32. Flier JS, Eastman RC, Minaker KL, et al. Acanthosis nigricans in obese

women with hyperandrogenism. Diabetes 1985;34:101–107.

33. Imperato-McGinley J, Peterson RF, Sturla F, Dawood Y, Bar RS. Primary amenorrhea associated with hirsutism, acanthosis nigricans, dermoid cyst of the ovaries and a new type of insulin resistance. Am J Med 1978;65:389–395.

34. Tatna FM, Graharn RAC, Dandona P, Sarkany I. The syndrome of acanthosis nigricans, hyperandrogenism and insulin resistance. Clin Exp Dermatol 1984;9:526–531.

35. Kahn CR, Flier JS, Bar RS, et al. The syndrome of insulin resistance and acanthosis nigricans: insulin receptor disorders in man. N Engl J Med 1976;294: 739–745.

36. Ferriman D, Gallwey JD. Clinical assessment of body hair growth in women. J Clin Endocrinol Metab 1961;21:1440–1447

37. Foster DW. Insulin resistance—a secret killer? N Engl J Med 1989;320:733–734.

38. Stout RW. Insulin and atheroma—an update. Lancet 1987;1:1077–1079.

39. Zavaroni I, Bonorae G, Pagliara M, et al. Risk factors for coronary artery disease in healthy persons with hyperinsulinemia and normal glucose tolerance. N Engl J Med 1989;320:702–706.

40. Givens JR, Andersen RNI Umstot ES, et al. Clinical findings and hormonal responses in patients with polycystic ovarian disease with normal versus elevated LH levels. Obstet Gynecol 1976;47:388–394.

41. Berger MJ, Taymor ML, and Patton WC. Gonadotrophin levels before and after luteinizing hormone-releasing hormone in the investigation of amenorrhea. Br J Obstet Gynaecol 1978;85:945–956.

42. Barbieri RL, Hornstein MD. Hyperinsulinemia and ovarian hyperandrogenism: cause and effect. Endocrinol Metab Clin North Am 1988;17:685–703.

43. Redmond GP, Gidwani G, Bergfeld W, et al. Regulation of excessive androgen secretion in women: role of ACTH responsive endocrine tissue. American Fertility Society Annual Meeting Program Supplement, 1987:83.

44. Huseman C, Johanson A, Varma M, Blizzard RM: Congenital lipodystrophy: an endocrine study in three siblings. J Pediatr 1978;93:221–226.

45. D'Ercole AJ, Underwood LE, Groelke J, Plet A. Leprechaunism: studies on the relationship among hyperinsulinism, insulin resistance and growth retardation. J Clin Endocrinol Metab 1979;48:495–502.

46. Taylor SI, Dons RF, Hernandez E, et al. Insulin resistance associated with androgen excess in women with autoantibodies to the insulin receptor. Ann Intern Med 1982;97:851–855.

47. Kellett HA, Collier A, Taylor R, et al. Hyperandrogenism, insulin resistance, acanthosis nigricans and systemic lupus erythematosus associated with insulin receptor antibodies. Metabolism 1988;37:656–659.

48. Harrison LC, Dean B, Peluso I, et al. Insulin resistance, acanthosis nigricans and polycystic ovaries associated with a circulating inhibitor of postbinding insulin action. J Clin Endocrinol Metab 1985;60:1047–1052.

49. Dunaif A, Hoffman AR, Scully RE, et al. Clinical, biochemical, and ovarian morpholosic features in women with acanthosis nigricans and masculinization. Obstet Gynecol 1985;66:545–552.

50. Marynik SP, Chakmakjian ZH, McCaffree DL, et al. Androgen excess in cystic acne. N Engl J Med 1983;308:981–986.

51. Levell MJ, Cawood ML, Burke B, Cunliffe WJ. Acne is not associated with abnormal plasma androgens. Br J Dermatol 1989;120:649–654.
52. Cumming DC, Yang JC, Rebar RW, et al. Treatment of hirsutism with spironolactone. JAMA 1982;247:1295–1298.
53. Hammerstein J, Mickies J, Leo-Rossbert I, et al. Use of cyproterone acetate (CPA) in the treatment of acne, hirsutism and virilism. J Steroid Biochem 1975;6:827–836.
54. Bergfeld WF, Redmond GP. Androgenic alopecia. Dermatol Clin 1986;5:491–500.
55. Redmond GP, Gidwani G, Gupta M, et al. Cardiovascular risk factors in androgenic disorders: correlation of higher testosterone with lower HDL and higher LDL cholesterol. American Fertility Society Annual Meeting Program Supplement, 1989:S125.
56. Maciejko JJ, Holmes DR, Kottle BA, et al. Apolipoprotein A-1 as a marker of angiographically assessed coronary-artery disease. N Engl J Med 1983; 309:385–389.
57. Burkman RT, Robinson JC, Kruszon-Moran D, et al. Lipid and lipoprotein changes associated with oral contraceptive use: a randomized clinical trial. Obstet Gynecol 1988;71:33–38.
58. Redmond GP, Gidwani GP, Gupta MK, et al. Treatment of androgenic disorders with dexamethasone: Dose-response relationship for suppression of dehydroepiandrosterone sulfate. Acad Dermatol 1990;22:91–93.
59. Rojanasakul A, Chailurkit L, Sirimongkolkasem R, Chaturachinda K. Effects of combined desogestrel-ethinylestradiol treatment on lipid profiles in women with polycystic ovarian disease. Fertil Steril 1987;48:581–585.

8
Diabetes Mellitus in Women

BYRON J. HOOGWERF

Diabetes mellitus is a risk factor for atherosclerotic vascular disease in women due to both an independent contribution of the diabetes and the associated dyslipidemia. This chapter discusses diabetes mellitus in general, with emphasis on these issues. Data are derived from studies in both men and women, but there is special emphasis on the impact in women.

There are three features of diabetes mellitus in women that should be borne in mind when reading this chapter. First, gestational diabetes is a unique form of diabetes associated with pregnancy. In addition to the inherent risk to the pregnancy, gestational diabetes is associated with an increased risk to develop type 2 diabetes mellitus in the future. Second, in young adult women diabetes is a major contributing risk factor for the development of atherosclerotic vascular disease. Young women with diabetes mellitus are at five to six times the risk for coronary heart disease as their nondiabetic counterparts. Third, with increasing interest in the association of clustering of coronary heart risk factors (obesity, hypertension, hyperlipidemia), it should be noted that such clustering occurs more frequently in women.

Classification

Although there are several types of diabetes mellitus terms of pathophysiology of the disease, the hallmark of all diabetes is hyperglycemia. On that basis all of the major clasification schemes have utilized hyperglycemia as the way to establish the diagnosis of diabetes. Over the years a number of systems and classification schemes have evolved, but currently the schemes proposed by the National Diabetes Data Group[1] and the World Health Organization[2] are the most widely accepted. The National Diabetes Data Group has proposed three ways to make the diagnosis of diabetes in nonpregnant persons. First is evidence of marked hyperglycemia, usually with glycosuria, in the face of symptoms of elevated glucose. Second is fasting plasma glucose determinations of more than 140 mg/dl on two occasions. Third is the glucose levels after a 50-g oral glucose load, with the demonstration of the 2-hour plasma glucose being more than 200 mg/dl and any one of the preceding plasma glucose values (obtained at 30-minute intervals) also over 200 mg/dl. This classification also characterizes persons who have elevated glucose levels in the absence of clear evidence of diabetes and calls this lesser degree of hyperglycemia "impaired glucose tolerance." Impaired glucose tolerance is based on a fasting plasma glucose level of less than 140 mg/dl, a 2-hour plasma glucose value between 140 and 200 mg/dl, and one of the preceding plasma glucose values over 200 mg/dl. A normal oral glucose tolerance test by the National Diabetes Data Group classification includes a fasting plasma glucose of less than 115 mg/dl, a 2-hour plasma glucose of less than 140 mg/dl, and all other values less than 200 mg/dl. All other possible combinations were characterized as nondiagnostic.

The major types of diabetes mellitus defined by pathophysiology include type I, or insulin-dependent, diabetes mellitus (IDDM, formerly called juvenile-onset diabetes mellitus); type II, or non-insulin-dependent, diabetes mellitus (NIDDM, formerly called adult-onset diabetes mellitus); gestational diabetes mellitus; and secondary forms of diabetes such as those caused by pancreatitis or pancreatectomy.

Type I diabetes is a genetic disease with an immunological basis. Although the diabetes gene has not been definitely localized, it has been established to be on the short arm of chromosome 6 in the HLA region.[3] There is progressive beta cell destruction of the islets,[4,5] which ultimately results in a loss of beta cell function, i.e., the capability to produce insulin. Type I diabetes typically comes on before age 20, although it may appear as late as the eighth decade. It seems that the development of diabetes is more precipitous in young people than in adults. Marked insulinopenia frequently results in marked hyperglycemia as well as the predisposition to develop ketosis and ketoacidosis. Type I diabetic patients require insulin for maintenance of glycemic control and, in fact, to survive. Type I diabetes occurs in approximately two to four persons per thousand in the typical United States population with a slight excess incidence in males.[6]

Type II diabetes mellitus occurs in about 6.6% of the adult population in the United States and increases in incidence with increasing age.[7] The NHANES II data showed a slightly higher prevalence of diabetes in women than men (7.4% versus 5.7% between the ages of 20 and 74 years), with most of the difference in young to middle-aged women. By the ages of 65 to 74 years, a greater percentage of men (19.2%) than women (16.5%) have diabetes mellitus. The higher prevalence in women has been confirmed in a number of other studies, although it may be modified by such factors as obesity, parity, and longevity.[6] The pathophysiological mechanism of type II diabetes mellitus is one in which there is impaired insulin action (called *insulin resistance*) and a progressive loss of beta cell function over time. The exact nature of the impaired insulin action is not known;

however, most of it appears to be a post-insulin-receptor defect.[8] Type II diabetes mellitus is also a genetic disease, as demonstrated by the monozygotic twin studies of Tattersall and Pyke,[9] as well as a strong family history of diabetes in many patients. There is a definite relation between obesity and type II diabetes. Estimates vary, but at least 40 to 80% of all type II diabetic patients are obese.[10] The National Health and Nutrition Examination Survey II demonstrated that approximately one-half of persons with type II diabetes in the United States are not aware that they have hyperglycemia.[7] This point highlights the fact that in many patients the disease may be asymptomatic.

Gestational diabetes is the type of diabetes that occurs during the course of pregnancy. The blood glucose values for diagnosis are lower than those used to make the diagnosis of other forms of diabetes.[11-13] Gestational diabetes mellitus is distinct from diabetes mellitus, which may have existed prior to the onset of pregnancy (type I or type II). Hyperglycemia appears to be the result of pregnancy-related hormones, including human placental lactogen, which cause relative insulin resistance. Therefore this mechanism is similar to that of type II diabetes. Women who have gestational diabetes are at increased risk to develop type II diabetes in the future. Although estimates vary, it appears that up to 30% of women with gestational diabetes may develop type II diabetes mellitus later.[11] Women who have gestational diabetes require serial follow-up to detect the possible early development of type II diabetes mellitus. Furthermore, special efforts should be made to encourage weight reduction, to monitor other cardiovascular risk factors (e.g., lipids, blood pressure), and to be cautious with regard to drugs that may impair glucose tolerance (e.g., glucocorticoids, thiazides).

There are a number of secondary forms of diabetes. Pancreatitis and pancreatectomy result in an insulinopenic form of diabetes. However, frequently because of loss of glucagon, insulin requirements are much lower in such patients. Other forms of secondary diabetes include those induced by glucocorticoids. For example, prednisone administration in conjunction with renal transplantation results in approximately 15% of transplant recipients having diabetes mellitus.[14] Secondary forms of diabetes are not discussed further in this chapter.

Impaired Glucose Tolerance

Impaired glucose tolerance is characterized by elevations of plasma glucose after the ingestion of oral glucose. The values are not as markedly elevated as those that characterize diabetes mellitus.[1,2] Impaired glucose tolerance is characterized by an increased risk of developing type II diabetes in the future. Furthermore, it appears to be accompanied by an increased risk for atherosclerotic vascular disease. Whether either of these risks is greater in women is not clear. Because impaired glucose tolerance may be associated with other cardiovascular risk factors, including obesity, hypertension, and hyperlipoproteinemia, treatment of these risk factors may need to take the glucose values into account. Treatment of hypertension, for example, should probably be undertaken by avoiding the use of thiazide diuretics, which have a tendency to cause glucose elevations. Lipid disorders should not be treated with nicotinic acid unless serial glucose determinations are followed. This drug has a propensity to elevate glucose (probably on the basis of causing insulin resistance). Although no standard guidelines have been established for following patients with impaired glucose tolerance, the fact that fasting plasma glucose concentrations are remarkably reproducible (i.e., have a low coefficient of variation) suggests that serial laboratory determinations of fasting plasma glucose may be a reasonable way to follow this entity. It appears that hemoglobin AlC's are too insensitive to distinguish either impaired glucose tolerance or type II diabetes from normal glucose tolerance with any degree of sensitivity and reliability.

Risk Factors

Both type I and type II diabetes mellitus have an associated genetic predisposition, as noted above. For type I diabetes there appear to be environmental triggers (e.g., viral illness), which may play a role in the development of the disease, although acute viral illness may more often unmask the diabetic condition than cause it. For type II diabetes, there is a clear increased risk associated with increasing age[7] and obesity.[8,10] Furthermore, when obesity is associated with increased atherogenicity in the lipid profiles and documented atherosclerosis, there is an associated increased risk to have diabetes.[15] Increasing body weight has also been associated with a greater risk for progression from impaired glucose tolerance to diabetes mellitus.[16] Furthermore, an increased waist/hip ratio is associated with increased risk for diabetes, and this risk increases across the range of adiposity from nonobese to markedly obese.[17,18] Women with increased waist/hip ratios are at increased risk to develop diabetes than comparably obese women with lower waist/hip ratios. The increase in intraabdominal fat is also associated with lipid profiles characterized by increased atherogenicity.[19] The relation of body habitus to cardiovascular risk is discussed in Chapter 9.

Complications

All types of diabetes mellitus are characterized by the same spectrum of complications, which has led to the conclusion that hyperglyceria in some way is the major culprit. The severity of the complications may vary with the type of diabetes mellitus. Microvascular complications in general are more severe in patients with type I diabetes, whereas macrovascular complications seem to be more evident in patients with type II diabetes. The largest reported longitudinal data set suggesting an association between the level of hyperglycemia and the risk for complications is that of Pirart, who reported 4400 patients followed over several decades.[20] He showed a definite relation between all complications of diabetes and the level of glycemic control. There are accumulating animal data that also show clear relations between the degree of hyperglycemia and the risk for microvascular complications. These data are not discussed here. Currently the Diabetes Control and Complications Trial (DCCT) is the largest prospective study designed to answer the question of whether rigorous glycemic control reduces the risk for complications in type I diabetic patients. The results from this study will not be available for several years.[21,22]

The chronic complications of diabetes can be classified into microvascular complications (which are essentially unique to diabetes mellitus), neuropathy, and macrovascular disease.[23] Microvascular complications include diabetic retinopathy and nephropathy. Diabetic retinopathy may be evident long before it results in symptoms or loss of visual acuity. Because diabetes is the leading cause of blindness in young people, and because of the clear evidence that laser therapy in appropriately selected patients helps to protect vision, routine ophthalmologic examinations are currently recommended for all patients with diabetes mellitus.[10] The hallmark of diabetic nephropathy is proteinuria. A number of studies have demonstrated the importance of blood pressure regulation in slowing down the progression of diabetic nephropathy.[24,25] Nevertheless, diabetic nephropathy is one of the leading causes of end-stage renal disease resulting in the need for dialysis or transplantation. Diabetic neuropathy may affect both the peripheral nervous system and the autonomic nervous system. The commonest feature is loss of sensation in the lower extremities. This loss of sensation has as its major adverse outcome an increased risk of callous formation or foot deformities, which in turn predispose to skin breakdown. The loss of integument increases the risk for infection. The sequence of events frequently leads to amputation of the lower extremities.

For each of the above complications, there does not appear to be any particular predisposition for them to occur in either sex. This finding is in contrast to the macrovascular complications of diabetes, where the relative risk for atherosclerotic disease as a result of diabetes mellitus is substantially greater in women.

The macrovascular complications of diabetes include atherosclerotic coronary artery disease, cerebral vascular disease, and peripheral vascular disease. The atherosclerotic lesions in patients with diabetes mellitus are much more likely to be diffuse. Furthermore, diabetes mellitus substantially increases the risk for atherosclerotic disease, especially coronary heart disease, in women. Data from the Framingham Study show that this risk is especially evident in young to middle-aged women, in whom the relative risk of coronary heart disease for a woman with diabetes is six times that of her nondiabetic counterpart.[26] It is approximately the same as her diabetic male counterpart. Therefore diabetes has been characterized as the great equalizer of coronary heart disease risk. This risk is compounded by the observation that risk factors may "cluster" in persons with diabetes mellitus, at least type II diabetes mellitus.[27] Accumulating data suggest that several coronary heart disease risk factors tend to coexist in the same person: obesity, hypertension, hyperlipoproteinemia, and hyperglycemia. Such clustering is especially evident in persons with hyperglycemia, who are much more likely to have hyperlipoproteinemia or hypertension even when the contribution of obesity is taken into account. Furthermore, such clustering of risk factors is more common in women than in men with diabetes mellitus. This observation has clear implications for the overall management of women with diabetes mellitus. There is accumulating evidence that diabetes mellitus may be associated with low HDL cholesterol concentrations.[28] Because women in general have higher HDL cholesterol levels (at least in the premenopausal state) than men, this reduction in HDL cholesterol may also contribute to the increased risk for atherosclerotic vascular disease in women. There is a frequent association of low HDL cholesterol levels in patients with both type I and type II diabetes meilitus.[29-31] Insulin treatment of type I diabetes mellitus consistently raises HDL cholesterol levels.[32] In type II diabetes mellitus, there is limited effect on HDL cholesterol with diet or sulfonylurea treatment. An HDL response seems somewhat more likely to occur if triglycerides are high and improve with therapy.[31] Insulin-treated type II diabetic patients demonstrate an increase in HDL cholesterol. The changes observed are similar in both men and women, although some investigators have concluded that weight loss in women may more effectively improve the lipid profile than a corresponding weight loss in men.[33]

Treatment

The overall treatment of diabetes mellitus is an attempt to normalize glycemic control. However, because of the associated metabolic abnormalities with diabetes, there may also be improvement in other aspects of the diabetic syndrome, including dyslipidemia.

The three major components of the management of diabetes mellitus are proper diet, exercise, and pharmacotherapy. The overall goal of dietary therapy is to achieve and maintain desirable body weight. For type I diabetic patients, who are typically not overweight, adequate calories should be given to maintain body weight. All too frequently, inappropriate caloric restriction is initiated as part of the program. For example, active women may require up to 30 to 40 kcal/kg body weight. For type II diabetic patients, who are much more likely to be obese, an important component of the diet is caloric restriction to ensure weight loss. Because obesity contributes to the insulin resistance, weight reduction, frequently results in substantial improvement in glycemic control. Furthermore, weight loss may be associated with a reduction in hyperlipidemia [both very low density lipoproteins (VLDL) and low density lipoproteins (LDL)]. The diet composition for patients with diabetes was recommended in the most recent American Diabetes Association statement[34] and agrees closely with those recommended for the Step One American Heart Association Diet[35] (see Chapter 11). The emphasis is on achieving a carbohyrate intake of more than 50% of total calories largely in the form of complex carbohydrate while reducing fat intake to 30% or less. Protein intake should be 12 to 20% of the total calories. The concept of restricting carbohydrate, especially simple sugar, is popular among patients with diabetes. This notion had its roots during the preinsulin era at a time when there was no knowledge of a distinction between type I and type II diabetes. The observation had been made that high fat diets improved survival of children who developed diabetes. This was likely the result of lower insulin needs than those associated with carbohydrate or protein ingestion. However, since that time, a number of studies have demonstrated that type II diabetes overall is better controlled with higher percentages of carbohydrates, especially complex carbohydrate.

There are still a number of controversies regarding the proper diet for patients with diabetes mellitus, especially for those with dyslipidemias. For example, studies (in men) have suggested that increasing the amount of fat, especially in a mononsaturated form, may benefit both glycemic control and lipid profiles in diabetic subjects.[36] There are also controversies about the role of simple carbohydrates in the diabetic diet. It appears that moderate amounts of sucrose can be added to mixed meals without serious deterioration of glycemic control.[37] This finding is not consistent, however, as both sucrose[38] and complex carbohydrate[39] have been associated with worsening of the lipid profile in type II diabetic subjects. Consequently, the role of sucrose and fructose[40] as nutritive sweeteners and total carbohydrate content in the diet are still the subject of investigation in diabetes mellitus. The concept that foods of similar caloric content may have a different effect on glycemic excursion has been popularized under the notion of "glycemic index."[41,42] Many of the studies investigating this concept have been done with single food entities and not in conjunction with a mixed meal. Consequently, the concept seems to offer little if any advantage over current dietary concepts.

The role of exercise in the management of diabetes has been studied more in men than in women.[43] Nevertheless, these observations are likely to be valid for both sexes. In obese (typically type II) diabetic persons, the major benefit of exercise is to facilitate weight reduction. Weight reduction is clearly associated with improvement in glycemic control. In the absence of weight reduction, regular exercise may have little if any impact on improvement in blood glucose control.[44] In type I diabetic patients, a number of effects of exercise may be noted.[43] First, in persons whose glycemic control is satisfactory, there is a general reduction in blood glucose during the time of exercise. Second, there is evidence that there may be a delayed effect of exercise with the possibility of hypoglycemia occurring many hours after engaging in exercise. Some of these effects may be a result of increased insulin absorption. (Higher skin temperature associated with exercise may facilitate such increase in insulin absorption.) Finally, there is evidence in persons who are underinsulinized and moderately hyperglycemic at the time of initiating exercise that their blood glucose levels may in fact worsen during the course of exercise. This finding is associated with some ketosis, suggesting mobilization of fat to meet the energy needs of the body.

Current drug therapy for diabetes is sulfonylureas,[45] the only oral agents currently available in the United States. Sulfonylureas stimulate insulin secretion from the pancreas and as such are useful only in persons with type II diabetes. They are generally initiated only after diet and exercise have been implemented and demonstrated to not achieve satisfactory control. Sulfonylureas also seem to improve insulin sensitivity. Insulin stimulation is an early effect, and reduction in insulin resistance seems to be a later effect. Sulfonylureas are not effective in patients with type I diabetes. Furthermore, they are contraindicated in any pregnant diabetic patient. In type II diabetic patients with hypertriglyceridemia, there is evidence that improvement of glycemic control in conjunction with sulfonylureas may result in a reduction of triglyceride levels as well. Many physicians utilize sulfonylureas in the face of mild hyperglycemia and moderate hypertriglyceridemia rather than initiate specific lipid-lowering therapy. When this treatment is not effective, other agents can be added to lower specific lipoproteins.

Sulforylureas have been categorized as "first generation" (tolbutamide, tolazamide, chlorpropamide, acetohexamide) and "second generation" (glipizide, glyburide) agents. The second generation agents have the advantages of fewer side effects, reduced effects on the action of other drugs that are protein-bound, and, in general, increased potency at the therapeutic doses when compared to first generation agents. Whereas chlorpropamide tends to be slightly more potent than either of the second generation agents, it has been associated with a worse sice effect profile as well. Hypoglycemia may occur with any sulfonylurea, but the frequency and severity of hypoglycemia are worst with chlorpropamide. Furthermore, chlorpropamide may cause hyponatremia because of impaired free water clearance. This problem is not seen with the other agents, as they tend to have a diuretic effect and do not impair free water clearance. At equivalent doses glyburide may have a slightly greater effect on lowering blood glucose than glipizide. Glyburide seems to have a slightly greater effect on lowering fasting blood glucose levels, whereas glipizide has a slight greater effect on postprandial glucose levels. The ability of these agents to lower insulin resistance seems to be mediated by enhanced secretion of insulin into the portal system and the associated effect on the liver. There are no studies that document the advantage of one agent over another in achieving this effect; however, because there is a direct correlation between fasting blood glucose levels and hepatic glucose production, glyburide may have a slightly greater effect than glipizide in this regard.

Insulin therapy is always indicated in patients with type I diabetes. Approximately one half of all patients with type II diabetes of more than 10 years' duration also require insulin for satisfactory glycemic control. In addition to regulating glucose, insulin may be associated with a reduction in triglyceride levels and in some cases with elevations of HDL cholesterol. These effects may be a result of modulating lipid-regulating enzymes, e.g., lipoprotein lipase.

Two confounding variables must be considered in the pharmacotherapy of diabetes mellitus. First, the University Group Diabetes Program (UGDP) raised the question about whether use of sulfonylureas increased the risk for coronary heart disease.[47] This statement is incorporated in all the package inserts; however, there are numerous articles criticizing study design. In essence, it seems that the most widely held belief is that attempts at rigorous glycemic control may be more important than any contribution of sulfonylurea to the risk for coronary heart disease. Second, hyperinsulinemia has been suggested since the 1970s as a possible contributor to increased risk for atherosclerotic disease.[48] Evidence in some animal models appears convincing, and there are a number of studies suggesting that elevated plasma insulin levels are associated with an increased risk for coronary heart disease in humans. Because both sulfonylureas and subcutaneous insulin administration (especially the latter) increase peripheral insulin concentration, the possibility of adverse effects from hyperinsulinism must be considered. No studies have addressed this point directly. The insulin arm of the UGPD did not demonstrate any increased risk (or benefit) from insulin administration targeted to lower blood glucose to a predetermined level when compared to to fixed insulin doses or the oral agent placebo.[49,50]

Summary

Currently, the general treatment of diabetes mellitus and its complications are essentially the same in both sexes. However, some aspects of how diabetes affects women may provide useful insights into our understanding of diabetes—especially type II diabetes—and its role in increasing the risk for atherosclerotic vascular disease. The observations that parity and gestational diabetes are both associated with an increased risk to develop type II diabetes raises some intriguing questions about the possible contributory role of temporary hormonal changes on body weight and the future risk for glucose intolerance. The marked increase in risk for coronary heart disease in women with diabetes also raises questions about the impact of the female hormonal milieu and hyperglycemia on the atherosclerotic process. Studies in women may provide useful insights into some basic mechanisms of disease.

The clinician who deals with a large number of women must be particularly attuned to the associated risk factors that predispose to the development of diabetes. Inferential evidence suggests that aggressive efforts at weight management would reduce the risk for the development of diabetes mellitus and the risks for atherosclerotic complications in women who have diabetes. Most clinicians think of atherosclerotic disease as a problem of men. The clinician who takes care of a woman with diabetes must always be cognizant of the fact that her risk for coronary heart disease is essentially the same as that for her male counterpart. Furthermore, the possibility of "silent" myocardial disease in patients with diabetes mellitus means that even symptoms that are not always "textbook" must be appropriately evaluated. Symptoms suggestive of angina or congestive heart failure must be aggressively evaluated in women with diabetes mellitus.

References

1. National Diabetes Data Group. Classification and diagnosis of diabetes mellitus and other categories of glucose intolerance. Diabetes 1979;28:1039–1057.
2. Harris MI, Haden WC, Knowler WC, Bennett PH. International criteria for the diagnosis of diabetes and impaired glucose tolerance. Diabetes Care 1985;8:562–567.
3. Rotter JI, Rimoin DL. Heterogeneity in Diabetes Mellitus Update 1978: evidence for further genetic heterogeneity with juvenile-onset, insulin dependent diabetes mellitus. Diabetes 1978;27:595–605.
4. Srikanta S, Ganda OP, Eisenbarth GS, Soeldner JS. Islet cell antibodies and beta-cell function in monozygotic triplets and twins initially discordant for type I diabetes mellitus. N Eng J Med 1983;308:322–325.
5. Srikanta S, Ganda OP, Jackson RA, et al. Type I diabetes mellitus in monozygotic twins: chronic progressive beta-cell dysfunction. Ann Intern Med 1983;99:320–326.
6. Barrett-Connor E, Wingard DL. Sex differences in diabetes mellitus. In: Gold EB, ed. The Changing Risk of Disease in Women. Lexington, MA: Collamore Press, 1984:257–286.
7. Harris MI, Hadden WE, Knowler WC, Bennett PH. Prevalence of diabetes and impaired glucose levels in U.S. population age 20–74 years. Diabetes 1988;36:1595–1607.
8. Reaven GM. The role of insulin resistance in human disease (Banting Lecture 1988). Diabetes 1988;37:1595–1607 [excellent review of the topic with 71 references].
9. Tattersall RB, Pyke D. Diabetes in identical twins. Lancet 1972;2:1120–1124.

10. Lebovitz H, ed. Physicians Guide to non-Insulin Dependent (Type II Diabetes Mellitus). Diagnosis and Treatment. 2nd Ed. Alexandria, VA: American Diabetes Association, 1988.
11. O'Sullivan JB, Mahan CM. Criteria for the oral glucose tolerance test in pregnancy. Diabetes 1964;13:278–285.
12. O'Sullivan JB. Establishing criteria for gestational diabetes. Diabetes Care 1980;3:437–439.
13. Taylor CD. Diagnosing gestational diabetes: Is the gold standard valid? Diabetes 1989;12:565–572.
14. Friedman EA, Shuh T, Beyer MM, Morris T, Britt KMH. Post-transplant diabetes in kidney transplant recipients. Am J Nephrol 1985;5:196–202.
15. Snaten RJ, Willis PK, Fajans S. Atherosclerosis in diabetes mellitus: correlations with serum lipid levels, adiposity and serum insulin levels. Arch Intern 1972;130:835–843.
16. Kadowaki T, Miyake Y, Hagura R, et al. Risk factors for worsening to diabetes subjects with impaired glucose tolerance. Diabetoloaia 1984;20:44–49.
17. Hartz A, Rupley DC, Rimm AA. The association of girth measurement with disease in 32,856 women. Am J Epidemiol 1984;119:71–80.
18. Friedman DS, Rimm AA. The relation of body fat distribution as assessed by six girth measurements to diabetes mellitus in women. AM J Public Health 1989;79:715–720.
19. Peiris AN, Sothman MS, Hoffman RG, et al. Adiposity, fat distribution and cardiovascular risk. Ann of Intern Med 1989;110:867–872.
20. Pirart J. Diabetes mellitus and its degenerative complications: a prospective study of 4400 patients observed between 1947 and 1973. Diabetes Care 1978;1:168–188, 225–263.
21. DCCT Research Group. The Diabetes Control and Complications Trial (DCCT): design and methodologic considerations for the feasibility phase. Diabetes 1985;35:530–545.
22. DCCT Research Group. Diabetes Control and Complications Trial (DCCT): results of feasibility study. Diabetes Care, 1987;10:1–19.
23. Watkins PJ, ed. Long-term complications of diabetes. Clin Endocrinol Metab, 1986;15:715–1001.
24. Parvings HH, Anderson AR, Smidt U, Svendsen PA. Early aggressive antihypertensive treatment reduces the rate of decline in kidney function in diabetic nephropathy. Lancet 1983;00:1175–1178.
25. Parving HH, Andersen AR, Smidt UM, et al. Diabetic nephropathy and arterial hypertension: the effect of antihypertensive treatment. Diabetes 1983;32(suppl 2):83–87.
26. Castelli WP, Doyle JT, Gordon T, et al. HDL cholesterol, and other lipids in coronary heart disease. Circulation. 1977;55:767–777.
27. Wingard DL, Barrett-Connor E, Crigui M, Suarez L. Clustering of heart disease risk factors in diabetic compared to non-diabetic adults. Am J Epidemiol 1983;117:19–26.
28. Howard BV, Savage P, Bennion W, Bennett PH. Lipoprotein composition in diabetes mellitus. Atherosclerosis 1978;80:153–162.
29. Schmitt JK, Poole JR, Lewis SB, et al. Hemoglobin A-1 correlates with the ratio of low to high density lipoprotein cholesterol in normal weight type II diabetes. Metabolism 1982;31:1084–1089.

30. Breyman M, Gidez LI, Eder HA. High density lipoprotein subclasses in diabetes. Am J Med 1986;81:488–491.
31. Nikkila EA. High density lipoproteins in diabetes. Diabetes 1981;30:82–87.
32. Eckel RH, Elbers J, Chung M, et al. High density lipoprotein composition in insulin-dependent diabetes mellitus. Diabetes 1981;30:132–138.
33. Kennedy L, Walshe K, Hadden DR, et al. The effect of intensive dietary therapy on serum high density lipoprotein cholesterol in patients with type II (non-insulin dependent) diabetes mellitus: a prospective study. Diabetologia 1982;23:24–27.
34. American Diabetes Association. Nutritional recommendations and principles for individuals with diabetes mellitus: 1986. Diabetes Care 1987;10:126–132.
35. Expert Panel. Report of the National Cholesterol Education Program Expert Panel on detection, evaluation, and treatment of high blood cholesterol in adults. Arch Intern Med 1988;148:36–69.
36. Garg A, Nonanome A, Grundy SM, et al. Comparison of a high carbohydrate diet with a high-monosaturated fat diet with non-insulin dependent diabetes mellitus. N Engl J Med 1988;319:829–834.
37. Bantle JP, Laine DC, Castle GW, et al. Post prandial glucose and insulin responses to meals containing different carbohydrates in normal and diabetic subjects. N Engl J Med 1983;309:7–12.
38. Hollenbeck CB, Coulston AM, Reaven GM. Effects of sucrose on carbohydrate and lipid metabolis, in NIDDM patients. Diabetes Care 1989;12(suppl 1):62–66.
39. Coulston AM, Hollenbeck CB, Swislocki ALM, Reaven GM. Persistence of the hypertriglyceridemic effect cf low fat-high carbohydrate diets in NIDDM patients. Diabetes Care 1989;12:94–101.
40. Bantle JP. Clinical aspects of sucrose and fructose metabolism. Diabetes Care 1989;12(suppl 1):56–61. [References 38 and 40 are from a symposium on sweeteners in diabetes and contain a number of references on the topic.]
41. Jenkins DJA, Wolever TMS, Taylor RH, et al. Glycemic index of foods: a physiological basis for carbohydrate exchange. Am J Clin Nutr 1981;34:362–366.
42. American Diabetes Association: Glycemic effects of carbohydrates. Diabetes Care 1984;7:607–608.
43. Richter EA, Ruderman NB, Schneider SH. Diabetes and exercise. Am J Med 1987;70:201–209.
44. Leon AS, Conrad JC, Casal DC, et al. Exercise for diabetes: effects of conditioning at constant body weight. J Cardiac Rehabil 1984;4:278–286.
45. Gerich JE. Drug therapy—oral hypoglycemic agents. N Engl J Med 1989;321:1231–1245.
46. University Group Diabetes Program. A study of the effects of hypoglycemic agents on vascular complications in patients with adult-onset diabetec. II. Mortality results. Diabetes 1970;19(suppl 12):785–830.
47. Stout RW. The role of insulin in atherosclercsis in diabetes and non-diabetics: a review. Diabetes 1981;30:(suppl 2):54–57.
48. Stout, RW. Insulin and atheroma: 20-yr perspective. Diabetes Care 1990;13:631–654.
49. University Group Diabetes Program: Effects of hypoglycemic agents of vascular complications in patients with adult-onset diabetes. VII. Mortality and

selected non-fatal events with insulin treatment. JAMA 1978;240:37–42.
50. University Group Diabetes Program. Effects of hypoglycemic agents on vascular complications in patients with adult onset diabetes. VIII. Evaluation of insulin therapy: final report. Diabetes 1982;31(suppl 15):1–77.

Selected References on Glycemic Control and Diabetic Complications

DCCT Research Group. Diabetes Control and Complications Trial (DCCT): results of feasibility study. Diabetes Care 1987;10:1–19.

Fuhrmann K, Reiher H, Semmler K, et al. Prevention of congenital malformations in infants of insulin-dependent diabetic mothers. Diabetes Care 1983;6:219–223. [This study was one of the earlier clinical studies in humans supporting the role of rigorous glycemic control in reducing the risk for congenital anomalies.]

Hanssen KF, Dahl Jorgensen K, Lauritzen T, et al. Diabetic control and microvascular complications: the near-normoglycaemic experience. Diabetologia 1986;29:677–684. [This report is a good review of the literature on microvascular complications. There is an extensive bibliography summarizing most of the major studies that have addressed this issue.]

Pirart J. Diabetes mellitus and its degenerative complications: a prospective study of 4400 patients observed between 1947 and 1973. Diabetes Care 1978;1:168–188.

9
Obesity in Women

GEOFFREY P. REDMOND

Obesity is caused by a food intake greater than is needed for maintenance and energy expenditure. The excess of energy taken in over that expended is stored in the form of adipose tissue. Obesity may be cured simply by reducing food intake below energy requirements. When this measure is taken there is gradual but progressive diminution of adipose tissue mass. This treatment has always been available, requires little or no technology, and is cost-effective. Moreover, the treatment reduces the associated risk for cardiovascular disease, several forms of cancer, hypertension, diabetes mellitus, gout, and several other diseases.

The above paragraph summarizes all that is easy to understand about obesity. Because cures of this condition are infrequent, obesity remains a major cause of misery for the patient and frustration for the physician. The persistence of the obese state despite the will of the patient and the physician remains unexplained. This chapter reviews the pathophysiology, psychology, and treatment of obesity. It reviews relevant research briefly but critically. There are many misconceptions regarding obesity in the minds of both lay and professional people. Success in working with the obese patient can be enhanced by understanding of the nature of the condition.

Definitions

It is well to begin with the definition of obesity because even here there has been some confusion. Obesity is an excessive amount of adipose tissue. Accordingly, being overweight is not always indicative of obesity, especially in the case of athletic males whose muscle mass may put them over the recommended ideal weight on the scale. Because women do not "bulk up" as much as men it is uncommon for women to exceed the normal weight ranges because of muscle rather than fat. For this reason, a variety of techniques have been introduced to determine body composition. The most accurate is underwater weighing, but this technique requires special equipment. Measurement of skin folds with calipers is simple but less accurate. These methods have importance as research techniques but are not necessary for the clinician. Simple visual inspection of the patient together with an accurate weight measurement indicates the presence of excessive adiposity. In the infrequent cases in which excessive weight is due to "fluid retention" or increased muscle mass, it is obvious during the physical examination. The use of the body mass index, discussed below, is the most useful way to assess body weight in a clinical setting.

It now remains to define what is "excessive" in terms of body fat stores. Though it may be forgotten in these days of weight consciousness, it is necessary for health that there be some stored body fat. Accordingly, the healthy body is not fatless. There are several distinct conceptions of ideal weight that are not always distinguished. Many women define ideal weight for themselves in terms of fashion. Unfortunately, the idealization of thinness continues, even as the American population becomes heavier. Many women who are normal in terms of body habitus regard themselves as overweight and feel they should be making more effort to diet or exercise. It is the author's impression that the idealization of thinness is a worldwide phenomenon even though in the past some populations may have been more tolerant of obesity.[1] Needless distress occurs when women of normal habitus regard themselves as obese. This personal definition frequently differs from the social definition of obesity, which is when an individual looks "fat" to others. Other adults are usually more lenient in the definition of obesity than the woman herself. Some women of normal adiposity regard themselves as obese when they are not so regarded by others. Adolescence, when body consciousness is at its peak, is an exception. Some teenage girls of normal habitus are teased about being "fat." A weight consistent with good health may be heavier than the apparent norms of the fashion magazines. Whether extreme thinness has any health advantages is controversial with some studies showing lower[2] and others higher[3] mortality. One proposed explanation is that increased mortality in markedly thin individuals reflects a high proportion of smokers in this group.

Although the ideal weights in the life insurance tables are widely used, they are stringent.[4] What is more pertinent is to have a formula that relates weight to health risks for the individual patient. A useful measure is the body mass index (BMI), which is the weight in kilograms divided by the height in meters squared (kg/M^2).[5,6] The normal female BMI is 18.5 to 22.5. Mortality risk begins to increase over the general population when the BMI exceeds 30. Accordingly, for health reasons a patient should strive to have her body mass index below 30. A lighter weight is desirable and probably does have health benefits, but it is less urgent. Use of this formula allows a physician to set *realistic* goals for obese patients that are not as discouraging as the ones in the life insurance tables. If an adverse health effect of obesity is present, such as hyperlipidemia, hypertension or non-insulin-dependent diabetes mellitus, normal weight may be individually defined as that at which amelioration of these conditions is attained. In some cases it requires a BMI well below 30. It is a common clinical observation that weight loss of 20 to 30 pounds in an individual who is still far above ideal weight often results in improvement of these medical complications, especially glucose intolerance and hyperlipidemia. Accordingly, the trend of weight down or up may be important separately from the total degree of obesity. This point means for example, that a 250-pound patient might achieve significant health benefits by reducing to 220 pounds, even though she continues to be obese. Hypertension may be less sensitive to weight reduction than glucose intolerance, as there is evidence that the reduction in blood pressure is proportional to the amount of weight lost.[7]

Classification

It is evident that the causes of obesity are multiple and that obesity is not a single disease. A variety of approaches have been attempted to classify obesity into categories. Early work by Hirsh's group had suggested that there were fundamental differences between obesity of childhood onset and adult onset.[8] The childhood-onset type was associated with an increased number of fat cells, whereas later onset was associated with an increased size of the individual fat cells. A distinction was proposed between hyperplastic and hypertrophic obesity, with the former more often being of childhood onset and the latter being usually of adult onset. However, subsequent research has indicated that the distinctions are not so clear. Some of the differences in fat cell size and number may have to do with how recent the weight gain has been. The hypothesis that weight gained during childhood is less easily lost is popular but unproved. However, it may be more difficult to change an abnormal eating pattern that has been present from early childhood than one that has been of more recent onset.

Another important distinction between types of obesity is between android (upper segment) and gynecoid (lower segment) obesity.[5,9-11] Gynecoid obesity is associated with an exaggeration of the normal feminine fat distribution. The upper body is relatively spared, and there is considerable widening of the hips, buttocks, and thighs (Figs. 9–1A and 9–1B). In contrast, android obesity affects mostly the upper body segment, with relative thinness of the hips, buttocks, and thighs. The pattern is evident during physical examination in a woman who has a large abdominal panniculus but small buttocks and thin thighs (Figs. 9–2A and 9–2B). Obesity distribution can be quantitated by comparing the waist to hip ratio. Many studies, including one extensive one,[10] have demonstrated convincingly that health risk is far greater with android obesity. This finding suggests that although endocrine factors may not be pathogenetic in obesity they likely play some role in determining the form of obesity and hence the

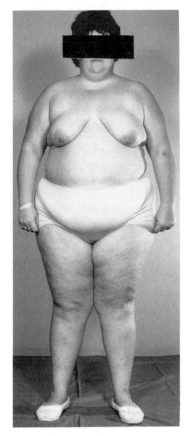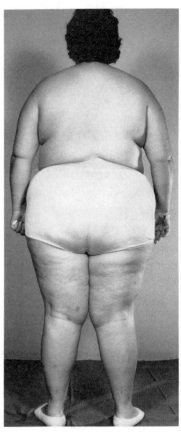

A   B

FIGURES 9.1 (A) and (B). Gynecoid obesity. In this form of obesity excessive adipose tissue is deposited so as to exaggerate the normal female habitus. There is market thickening of hips, buttocks, and upper thighs. This pattern is also referred to as lower segment obesity.

degree of health risk posed by the obesity.[9] Many women with androgen excess disorders have an android fat distribution. Whether the increased health risk is due to the fat distribution itself or is a separate effect of increased androgen secretion is unknown. A third possibility is that android fat distribution is an excessive target organ response to androgens. There is some evidence that the type of obesity is a function of age at onset. Prepubertal onset is likely to be gynecoid, whereas pubertal onset is androgynous and later onset is android.[9] If so, the pattern of fat distribution may reflect the levels of androgens at the time of onset, as they are low during childhood, moderate during early adolescence, and higher during early adulthood, especially if there is an androgenic disorder.[12] Studies of the ontogeny of fat distribution with respect to hormonal changes would be helpful.

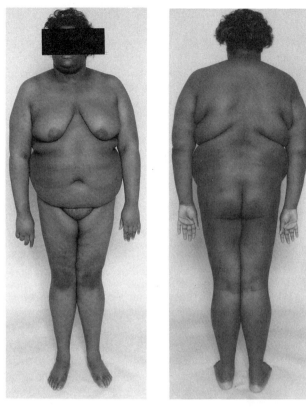

FIGURES 9.2 (A) and (B). Android obesity. Deposition of fat is increased on the upper body with relative thinning of the hips, buttocks, and thighs. This pattern is also termed upper segment obesity. Defeminization of contours is evident.

It is important for the clinician to recognize the android habitus. Women with this form of obesity should be selected for determination of cardiovascular risk factors and encouragement of weight reduction.

Etiology

Theories as to the cause of obesity are legion. The most popular are not psychological or physiological, but moral. It is generally assumed that obese people are self-indulgent or lacking in "will power." Obese patients themselves may hold this view—one that is too often shared by their physicians. Another popular theory is couched in psychological rather than moralistic terms and holds that obesity is compensation for some sort of emotional disorder. This view persists despite overwhelming evidence to the contrary.[13] Many studies indicate that psychopathology is no more prevalent in obese people than in others.[14] Hayes and Ross[15] did not find a significant effect of obesity on well-being, although exercise and good health did have a positive effect. Women's psychological well-being was not more affected by obesity than that of men, but the study employed a rather simple questionnaire administered during a telephone interview. Depression may be associated with obesity but is as likely the result of the obesity as its cause.[15] However, depression may play a role in perpetuating obesity, as some individuals eat more when depressed or anxious and others eat less.[16] The difference therefore may be less the presence of depression or stress than the individual's way of responding to it. Of course, subgroups of obese patients, such as those with bulimia, may have significant psychopathology and self-destructive behavior. Despite the considerable publicity given to eating disorders, most obese patients do not practice such bizarre behaviors. There are some women who do not have eating disorders but are worried that they do. Binging is normal in American society under some circumstances, being, for example, the expected behavior on the national holiday of Thanksgiving. Attitudes toward overeating are complex, to say the least.

Obesity results in behaviors that tend to perpetuate the obese state. Because heavy individuals feel uncomfortable with exercise and are ashamed of displaying their bodies, they may tend to stay indoors and remain inactive. Socializing outside of the home or beyond a close circle of old friends may be avoided because of a deep sense of shame about physical appearance. A rather restricted life develops in which the main source of pleasure is food. If several family members are obese, there may be mutually reenforcing behavior that perpetuates the obesity.

Although there do not seem to be clear psychological differences between obese and nonobese individuals, the same is not true for social factors. A variety of studies indicate that lower socioeconomic status is associated with a greater prevalence of obesity.[17,18] One study has found that the socioeconomic difference affects primarily weight gain during the childbearing years.[18] However, with the trend for increasing obesity, there may be some effect of socioeconomic status on childhood obesity as well. This association is particularly unfortunate, as other risk factors for early heart disease may be associated with less favorable socioeconomic status. However, socioeconomic factors account for only a limited amount of the variance between obese and nonobese populations.

Biological theories that seek to account for obesity fall into two main categories. *Metabolic theories* suggest that utilization of substrate in an obese individual is more efficient or that its efficiency increases more rapidly with weight reduction.[20-21] A common argument for this viewpoint is that obese individuals who reduce rarely maintain their lower degree of adiposity. Although there is suggestive evidence of improved metabolic efficiency in reduced obese individuals, it is far from conclusive. Not all groups have found a lower metabolic rate in obese individuals. Furthermore, it may be a misinterpretation of these studies to conclude that weight reduction is metabolically impossible. At most, the studies indicate that to reduce and then maintain the reduced state a more stringent reduction of calories is required than might otherwise be supposed to be the case.[20] It remains true that if calories are sufficiently restricted, fat stores are mobilized and adipose mass is diminished. Obesity is not seen in famine victims. Hyperphagia is an obligate factor in obesity.[22] One reason this obvious fact is sometimes questioned is that obese individuals are often embarrassed to eat publicly and therefore carry out their excessive food consumption in private.

The *set point hypothesis* is the second major biological theory of obesity.[23] This theory holds that body mass is regulated by the central nervous system. Maintenance of adiposity may be both by behavioral mechanisms. (feeding behavior and changes in activity) and metabolic adjustments. Evidence to support this theory includes that fact that adiposity is stable in most adult animals, as well as in humans, and that the level of adiposity is highly conserved.[23] When fat is surgically removed from animals, they usually restore it to its previous amount. It is not surprising that reduction of fat stores would be homeostatically resisted, as energy storage is essential for survival of any animal. The set point may be affected by environmental cues and in particular by the quantity and palatability of food available.[24] Interestingly, hypothalamic lesions in animals that alter body mass seem to do so by effects on *both* eating behavior and activity levels. Ventromedial nucleus (VMN) lesions in rats produce not only hyperphagia but decreased activity. Lateral hypothalamic lesions produce the opposite changes of hypophagia and *increased* activity. The effects of VMN lesions are strikingly similar to what is observed in human obesity, i.e., excessive food consumption and diminished physical activity. In humans, when appetite control is damaged as a result of surgery in the area of the hypothalamus, the result almost invariably is hyperphagia and obesity. It is exceedingly rare for hypophagia and emaciation to occur. Presumably evolutionary pressures strongly mitigate against survival of individuals inclined to hypophagia, resulting in a preponderance of appetite-stimulating mechanisms over inhibiting ones.

Some work has indicated a role for cholecystokinin in satiety,[25] which makes it possible to explore the attractive possibility that the increased appetite drive in obese people may be a neurochemical defect in satiety mechanisms. There is also considerable evidence for a role of insulin in the perpetuation of obesity as well as in its adverse health effects.[26–29] Insulin levels are directly correlated with adiposity. Insulin may act on the central nervous system to signal satiety. It is possible that individuals eat until they have raised their insulin to a certain level. Because obesity is associated with some degree of insulin resistance, i.e., defective tissue response to insulin, an obese individual may have to eat more so as to raise insulin levels higher in order to feel satisfied.

The set point and metabolic theories of obesity are not mutually exclusive but, rather, represent a difference of emphasis. The set point theory can explain both the strong behavioral component of obesity and its resistance to treatment directed only at behavior. It is helpful when counseling patients because it permits the patients to understand the importance of their behavior in maintaining their obese state without implying that they are weak-willed or psychologically abnormal. In this sense obesity is a handicap caused by abnormal brain function that can be overcome with effort.

Endocrine Factors

Although folk wisdom attributes massive obesity to "hormonal imbalance," there is little evidence for such a mechanism. In particular, hypothyroidism does not seem to be an important cause of obesity, and correction of the hypothyroid state does not result in long-term weight reduction.[30] There are, however, alterations of endocrine function due to the obese state itself.[31] Cortisol secretion is increased in obesity, but its metabolic clearance rate is also elevated so that serum levels are unchanged.[32,33] Despite the fact that obesity is a feature of Cushing syndrome, it is clear that increased glucocorticoid secretion is not a factor in the pathogenesis of exogenous obesity. Production of dehydroepiandrosterone sulfate (DHEA-S), testosterone, and some other androgens appears to be increased in obese women, but their metabolic clearance may be increased as well.[34] In our own experience, androgen levels are correlated with degree of obesity in women who present with androgenic disorders.[12,35] It has been proposed that the anabolic effects of androgens play a role in the pathogenesis of obesity; but if this proposal were so, males would be more obese then females. Unlike women in whom obesity may be associated with hyperandrogenism, obese men tend to have low testosterone levels.[36] Some morbidly obese men have hypogonadotropic hypogonadism due to their obesity.[37]

Growth hormone-deficient children tend to have a mild to moderate degree of obesity that may be ameliorated by growth hormone replacement. Growth hormone has some lipotropic effects. One study[38] indicated that growth hormone therapy during a hypocaloric weight reduction program accelerated the decline in adipose tissue mass. The effects, however, were not dramatic.

In conclusion, although obesity is associated with alterations of endocrine function, it is likely that the hormones studied to date are more important in the complications of obesity than in its pathogenesis. Because obesity is a disorder of regulation it is entirely plausable that other hormones, as yet undiscovered, play a role in producing or maintaining the obese state.

Obesity in Women

Because the most striking action of estrogens is to promote fat deposition in a unique configuration, some believe that female gender predisposes to obesity. Population data do not bear out this belief. However, more women than men seek to lower their weight by dieting. A feminist theory of obesity has evolved which holds that certain aspects of women's role in society predispose to obesity. These theories have been comprehensively reviewed by McBride.[39] Proposed factors include the past tendency to discourage physical exercise in girls, the role of women in preparing food and nurturing family members, and the association of importance and power with a large body. It is difficult to objectively assess the actual contribution of such factors to obesity in women. They may account, however, for how or why some women feel victimized by their obese state. Regardless of whether obesity is biologically different in the two sexes, the *experience* of being obese is clearly different for men and women.

Pregnancy appears to be associated with increasing adiposity.[18] Every physician who treats female patients is aware of the woman who has difficulty losing the weight gained with each pregnancy and so becomes progressively heavier. However, many women who have borne several children do not exhibit cumulative obesity, and therefore it is difficult to conclude that pregnancy per se is a cause of obesity. The biological factors that determine if weight is lost after pregnancy are unknown. Socioeconomic factors do play a role.[18]

Treatment

Treatment of obesity must involve induction of negative energy balance, which may be accomplished by decreasing food intake, increasing activity, or both. Exercise has positive effects on health. As a sole modality, however, it is not usually effective in causing significant weight reduction[40] simply because most individuals cannot exercise enough hours during the week to expend enough calories. However, as an adjunct to caloric restriction, exercise is helpful and may accelerate the rate of weight reduction. Furthermore, the benefits of exercise on cardiovascular health and mood are such that it should be recommended to obese individuals as part of their weight reduction program. The nature and intensity of exercise should be individualized. The morbidly obese or entirely sedentary individual may have limited exercise tolerance[41] and need the assistance of a skilled physical therapist to learn to walk even short distances. As exercise tolerance increases and weight diminishes, walking can be increased to 1 to 2 hours a day.

Highly motivated or less obese individuals may take up sports such as running, cycling, swimming, or cross-country skiing. Running and aerobics tend to be stressful to the lower extremities, especially for heavy patients. Static exercise such as using Nautilus equipment or weight lifting are not helpful in weight reduction or cardiovascular fitness to nearly the same degree as aerobic exercise. Because the time available for exercise is usually limited, it is best devoted to aerobic activity.

There are two general approaches to caloric restriction. With the conventional approach calories are restricted to a moderate or marked degree, but dietary composition is essentially normal. It results in rather slow weight reduction but allows flexibility in choice of foods. As alternatives, a variety of methods for rapid weight reduction have been promulgated. Liquid diets have had a bad reputation in the past because early forms utilized poor quality protein and so were inadequate in essential amino acids. They were also deficient in potassium and probably magnesium as well. There are suitable contemporary preparations such as Optifast (R) that appear to be nutritionally complete and to not be associated with the cardiac deaths attributed to earlier liquid protein diets.[42] In our program, we have made extensive use of a form of Protein Sparing Modified Fast,[43,44] which involves using limited portions of lean meat, fish, poultry without skin, and some vegetables. This diet is similar in composition to the better liquid diets such as Optifast in that it is high in protein and low in fat and carbohydrate. Because it uses a variety of foods it may be nutritionally more complete. It also provides some experience in food selection. It is the author's impression that this regimen is more effective than liquid diets; however, definitive data to support this belief are lacking. Unfortunately, all such programs are more successful in inducing initial weight loss than in maintaining it. Some individuals do maintain the lower weight, however, justifying the effort made by health professionals in running the program.

There has arisen a fad for pronouncing obesity incurable and recommending that treatment efforts be abandoned.[45] In the author's view this attitude is simply giving in to frustration; it is difficult to justify not attempting to treat a fatal disease because the success rate of treatment is low. There is little evidence for the idea that eating disorders are created by medically sound advice on weight control.

A common element of *all* successful weight reduction programs is frequent visits to the dietitian and physician. If the physician or other care givers are uninterested in the obese patient or project an attitude of pessimism, they are unlikely to see good results.

Surgical approaches to obesity go in and out of favor.[46] In general, they are hazardous and of questionable long-term efficacy. The use of drugs, mainly central stimulants, for suppression of appetite is no longer considered good medical practice. These agents are addicting; and although they may result in loss of few more pounds over the first several weeks, they do not seem to have long-term benefits. The antidepressant fluoxetime produces some appetite suppression and has resulted in modest weight reduction in some studies.[47] This effect is not great enough for fluoxetime to be useful by itself for the treatment of obesity. However, it is the drug of choice for depression in obese individuals. Most of the other antidepressants have a stimulatory effect on appetite and often result in worsening of obesity.

Conclusions

Seemingly the simplest of all diseases to understand, obesity is actually one of the most complex and baffling. Although evidence suggests it is a disease of the central nervous system, why some individuals eat to the point of obesity and others do not remains a mystery. Advances in understanding the pathobiology of obesity have not yet resulted in better treatments. Social and personal factors make the experience of obesity more onerous for women. Treatment of obesity consists in a variety of methods for reducing calories consumed and increasing calories expended. Attitudes of the care giver are crucial to the success of weight reduction programs. Although most obese patients are unsuccessful in losing weight, a few individuals lose large amounts and retain their healthier habitus indefinitely. Obese individuals are exposed to criticism and sarcasm to a degree rarely appreciated by those who have always been lean. Accordingly, they greatly appreciate a sympathetic and nonjudgmental attitude on the part of the physician.

References

1. Wright EJ, Whitehead TL. Perceptions of body size and obesity: a selected review of the literature. J Community Health 1987;12:117–129.
2. Lew EA. Mortality and weight: insured lives and the American Cancer Society studies. Ann Intern Med 1985;103:1024–1029.
3. Harrison GG. Height weight tables. Ann Intern Med 1985;103:989–994.
4. Andres R, Elahi D, Tobin JD, et al. Impact of age on weight goals. Ann of Intern Med 1985;103:1030–1033.
5. Hediger ML, Katz SH. Fat patterning, overweight and adrenal androgen interactions in black adolescent females. Hum Biol 1986;58:585–560.
6. Simopoulos AP. Obesity and body weight standards. Annu Rev Public Health 1986;7:481–92.
7. MacMahon S, Cutler J, Brittain E, Higgins M. Obesity and hypertension: epidemiologlcal and clinical issues. Europ Heart J 1987;8(suppl B);57–70.
8. Leibel RL, Berry EN, Hirsch J. Biochemistry and development of adipose tissue in man. In: Conn HL Jr, DeFelice EA, Kuo P, eds. Health and Obesity. New York: Raven Press, 1983.
9. Deutsch MI, Mueller WH. Androgyny in fat patterning is associated with obesity in adolescents and young adults. Ann Hum Biol 1985;12:275–286.
10. Hartz AJ, Rupley DC, Rimm AA. The association of girth measurements with disease in 32,856 women. Am J Epidemiol 1984;119:71–80.

11. Seidell JC, Deurenberg P, Hautaust JG. Obesity and fat distribution in relation to health–current insights and recommendations. World Rev Nutr Diet 1987;50:57–91.
12. Redmond GP, Bergfeld W, Gupta M, et al. Clinical and biochemical findings in 500 women with androgenic disorders. Endocrine Society Program and Abstracts, 1989:330.
13. Wadden TA, Stunkard AJ. Psychopathology and obesity. Ann NY Acad Sci 1987;499:55–65.
14. Hallstrom T, Noppa H. Obesity in women in relation to mental illness, social factors and personality traits. Psychosom Res 1981;25:75–82.
15. Hayes D, Ross CE. Body and mind: the effect of exercise, overweight, and physical health on psychological well-being. J Health Soc Behav 1986;27:387–400.
16. Baucom DH, Aiken PA. Effect of depressed mood on eating among obese and nonobese dieting and nondieting persons. J Pers Soc Psychol 1981;1:577–585.
17. Noppa H, Hallstrom T. Weight gain in adulthood in relation to socioeconomic factors, mental illness and personality traits: a prospective study of middle-aged women. J Psychosom Res 1981;24:83–91.
18. Oken B, Hartz A, Giefe E, Rimm AA. Relation between socioeconomic status and obesity changes in 9046 women. Prev Med 1977;6:447–453.
19. Sims EAH, Danforth E Jr. Expenditure and storage of energy in man. J Clin Invest 1987;79:1019–1925.
20. Leibel RL, Hirsch J. Diminished energy requirements in reduced obese patients. Metabolism 1984;33:164–170.
21. Leibel RL, Hirsch J, Berry EM, Gruen RK. Alterations in adipocyte free fatty acid re-esterification association with obesity and weight reduction in man. Am J Clin Nutr 1985;42:198–206.
22. James WPT. Nutrition: the changing scene. Lancet 1983;386–389.
23. Keesey RE. A set-point analysis of the regulation of body weight. In: Stunkard AJ, ed. Obesity. Philadelphia: Saunders, 1980;144–165.
24. Franklin KBJ, Herberg W. Ventromedial syndrome: the rat's "finickiness" results from the obesity, not from the lesions. J Comp Physiol Psychol 1974;87:410–414.
25. Smith GP, Gilebs J. The satiating effect of cholecystokinin. Curr Concepts Nutr 1988;16:35–40.
26. Foster DW. Insulin resistance-a secret killer: N Engl J Med 1989;320:733–734.
27. Ferrannini E, Buzzigoli G, Bonadonna R, et al. Insulin resistance in essential hypertension. N Engl J Med 1987;317:350–357.
28. Stout RW. Insulin and atheroma—an update. Lancet 1987;1077–1079.
29. Zavaroni I, Bonora E, Pagliara M, et al. Risk factors for coronary artery disease in healthy persons with hyperinsulinemia and normal glucose tolerance. N Engl J Med 1989;320:702–706.
30. Hoogwerf BJ, Nuttall FQ. Long-term body weight regulation in treated hyperthyroid and hypothyroid subjects. Am J Med 1984;76:963–970.
31. Henley KM, Vaitukaitis J. Hormonal changes associated with changes in body weight. Clin Obstet Gynecol 1985;28:615–631.
32. Strain GW, Zumoff B, Strain JJ, Levin J, Fukushima DK. Cortisol production in obesity. Metabolism 1980;29:980–985.
33. Streeten DHP, Stevenson CT, Dalakos TG, et al. The diagnosis of hypercorti-

solism: biochemical criteria differentiating patients from lean and obese normal subjects and from females on oral contraceptives. J Clin Endocrinol Metab 1969;29:1191–1211.

34. Parker LN. Adrenal Androgens in Clinical Medicine. Orleans: Academic Press 1989:246–262.

35. Redmond GP, Gidwani G, Gupta M, et al. Cardiovascular risk factors in androgenic disorders: correlation of higher testosterone with lower HDL and higher LDL cholesterol. American Fertility Society Annual Meeting Program Supplement, 1989:S125.

36. Strain GW, Zumoff B, Kream J, et al. Mild hypogonadotropic hypogonadism in obese men. Metabolism 1982;31:871–875.

37. Redmond GP, Thomas A. Reproductive dysfunction in males with morbid obesity. J Androl 1985;6(2 suppl):P-67.

38. Snyder DK, Clemmons DR, Underwood LE. Treatment of obese, diet-restricted subjects with growth hormone for 11 weeks: effects on anabolism, lipolysis and body composition. J Clin Endocrinol Metab 1988;67:54–61.

39. McBride AB. Obesity of women during the childbearing years: psychological and physiologic aspects. Nurs Clin North Am 1982;17:217–225.

40. Pacy PJ, Webster J, Garrow JS. Exercise and obesity. Sports Med 1986;3:89–113.

41. Garrow JS. Effect of exercise on obesity. Acta Med Scand [Suppl 711] 1986:67–73.

42. Wadden TA, Stunkard AJ, Brownell KD. Very low calorie diets: their efficacy, safety and future. Ann Intern Med 1983;99:675–684.

43. Palgi A, Read JL, Greenberg I, et al. Multidisciplinary treatment of obesity with a protein-sparing modified fast: results in 668 outpatients. Am J Public Health 1985;75:1190–1194.

44. Wadden TA, Van Itallie TB, Blackburn GL. Responsible and irresponsible use of very-low-calorie diets in the treatment of obesity. JAMA 1990;263:83–85.

45. Wooley SC, Wooley OW. Should obesity be treated at all? In: Stunkard AJ, Stellar E, eds. Eating and Its Disorders New York: Raven Press 1984:185–192.

46. Stunkard AJ, Foster GD, Grossman RF. Surgical treatment of obesity. Adv Psychosom Med 1986;15:140–166.

47. Levine S, Deo R, Mahadevan K. A comparative trial of a new antidepressant, fluoxetine. Br J Psychiatry 1987;150:653–65.

10
Lipids, Obesity, and Female Reproductive Cancer

DAVID P. ROSE

Carcinoma of the breast, endometrium, ovary, and prostate are sex hormone-related cancers. In each case there is evidence to support a causal association between these cancers, obesity, and dietary lipids. Of the three cancers occurring in women, the most important relation—because of the high and increasing incidence rate in many parts of the world—is that for breast cancer. It is also the most contentious, with regard to the role of diet, and so it is appropriate that lipid, obesity and breast cancer receive special emphasis in this review.

Support for the belief that dietary factors, specifically lipids, are involved in breast cancer etiology comes from both epidemiological studies and work with appropriate animal models. It is clear that obesity is a risk factor for postmenopausal disease, the mechanism in all probability involving excessive estrogenic stimulation of mammary tissue owing to the known effects of adiposity on estrogen production, metabolism, and biological activity. In addition to its role in causation, obesity appears to have an adverse effect on breast cancer prognosis after surgery. Here increased estrogen activity probably stimulates residual tumor tissue and so promotes clinical recurrence and disease progression.

Whether dietary fat per se influences breast cancer development or is a factor only because it is a major source of calories and the principal contributor to obesity in Western countries is currently the subject of much discussion. The author's view is that a simple caloric effect may play a part, although the evidence for this view comes largely from extreme caloric restriction in experiments with animal models, but that lipids have a more specific role. As we shall see, different levels and types of fats and fatty acids have distinct, selective effects on steroid and protein hormones, polypeptide growth factors, and prostaglandins, all of which influence breast cancer cell growth. In addition, nonendocrine mechanisms may be involved, e.g., the influence of lipids on carcinogen activation and metabolism, cell membrane function, and immune mechanisms.

These issues are not of concern only to the academic oncologist and nutritionist. The issue of diet, nutrition, and breast cancer continues to be a lively topic in newspapers and magazines and the subject of health- and science-oriented television programs. Unfortunately, the public has become somewhat confused by the expressions of diametrically opposed medical opinion, particularly with regard to general dietary recommenda- tions for cancer prevention and intervention strategies for those at high risk of developing breast cancer or of experiencing recurrence after primary treatment.

As this chapter demonstrates, the relations between obesity, lipids, and endometrial cancer are, at least from a strictly clinical viewpoint, less com- plex. That obesity is a risk factor has been established beyond reasonable doubt, and the primary mechanism appears to be the aromatization of ster- oid precursor to produce estrone. One question of interest is the role of obesity in premenopausal endometrial cancer; several investigators have described this association (which does not apply to carcinoma of the breast). Also there are few if any data dealing with dietary lipids, endo- crine function, and endometrial cancer risk in the nonobese.

In contrast to breast and endometrial cancer, we are at a primitive stage of even collecting data to explore the relation between dietary lipids and epithelial carcinoma of the ovary. However, the challenge is there because epidemiologists continue to report an association between obesity and ova- rian cancer risk, and in case-control studies they find distinctive dietary patterns in patients with these tumors whose treatment is so often unsatis- factory.

Breast Cancer

Dietary Fat and Breast Cancer Risk

Epidemiological support for an association between dietary lipid consump- tion and breast cancer risk comes from international and some intranation- al comparisons, as well as the changes in risk that occur in migrant popula- tions. Most case-control and cohort studies have either found no relation or only weak associations, but they frequently suffer from methodological problems and the confounding effects of population homogeneity.

A number of studies have shown a positive correlation between the esti- mated per capita total consumption of fat in different countries, and breast cancer incidence and mortality rates.[1-4] Obviously, some caution is needed when interpreting such comparisons because of the uneven quality of can- cer reporting and the crude estimates of consumption derived from food availability data. Nevertheless, they are instructive and provide a useful starting point for more detailed and refined investigations.

When estimates of animal and vegetable dietary fats consumed were considered separately, it became evident that there is a strong positive cor- relation with age-adjusted breast cancer mortality rate for fats from animal sources, but not for those of vegetable origin. When the data were examined according to menopausal status,[4] it was found that the correlation was stronger for postmenopausal than for premenopausal women, an observation that grows in significance later in the present discussion.

Although there is an obvious distinction in the effects of animal and vegetable fats on breast cancer risk when international comparisons are made, the real difference may be in the fatty acid composition of various dietary lipids. Polyunsaturated fatty acids, monounsaturated oils, and hydrogenated oils are encompassed by the classification "vegetable fats." Cohen et al.[5] employed a chemically induced rat mammary tumor model to compare the effects of feeding high levels of different vegetable oils on cancer development. The intakes corresponded, on a percent of total calories basis (40%), to human fat consumption in Western countries. It was found that differences in the degree of saturation of the vegetable oils consumed had a pronounced influence on their effects on tumor promotion. Whereas feeding high levels of safflower and corn oils (82% and 56% linoleic acid, respectively) significantly enhanced mammary tumor yields, this same high intake of olive oil (8% linoleic acid) was associated with a tumor incidence no different from that in animals fed low-fat diets (20% of total calories).

It is instructive to take these results from animal experiments and apply them to the international comparisons (although in truth things were done the other way round). Greece and, to a lesser extent, Spain and Portugal have high vegetable fat consumption levels and relatively low breast cancer mortality rates. These countries, however, derive 71%, 37%, and 21%, respectively, of their total vegetable fat from olive oil. Olive oil consumption is also high in Italy, but here the beneficial effect on breast cancer risk may be obscured by high animal fat consumption. This point applies particularly to northern Italy, where the breast cancer mortality rate exceeds that in the Mediterranean south.[6]

In the United States a major component of the vegetable fat consumed is in the form of polyunsaturated fatty acids, of which linoleic acid is the principal constituent. There has been a distinct trend toward an increased consumption of linoleic acid in the American diet in recent years,[7,8] and it has been associated with a decline in deaths from ischemic heart disease.[7] Unfortunately, over the same period the incidence of breast cancer has been increasing among American women, as has the incidence of prostate cancer in American men.[9,10] Obviously, a number of risk factors may be involved; for example, the postponement of first pregnancy increases breast cancer risk, but as stressed by Wynder et al.[11] the suspicion is deepening that this change in incidence rates for both cancers involves a shift in the relative dietary intakes of ω-6 fatty acids (principally linoleic acid), and ω-3 fatty acids. Kakar and Henderson[12] have pointed out that the consumption of animal fat is similar in The Netherlands and Finland but that the breast cancer incidence rate is approximately double for Dutch women. These authors emphasized the fact that the diets typical of the two countries differ in that the Dutch consume four times as much vegetable fat as the Finnish population. However, dietary patterns in The Netherlands and Finland are different in another respect; the Finnish diets contain much higher levels of fiber, which may be protective against breast cancer because of its effect on estrogen metabolism and bioactivity.[13]

Analyses of diets consumed by normal subjects in the United States, Italy, and Finland showed that Americans derive approximately 7% of their calories from linoleic acid, whereas for Finns and Italians, who are at a relatively low risk for both breast and prostate cancer, the corresponding figure is 2.4%.[14]

The animal experiments that showed the promoting effects of linoleic acid-rich safflower and corn oils on rat mammary carcinogenesis were extended to demonstrate a protective effect of marine oils, which are rich in ω-3 fatty acids.[15,16] The mechanism probably involves the prostaglandins. Linoleic acid is metabolized to form arachidonic acid, the substrate for prostaglandin synthesis; and indomethacin, an inhibitor of the first enzyme on the pathway, suppresses the stimulatory effect of corn oil on mammary tumor development in rats exposed to a chemical carcinogen.[17]

In a continuing series of studies, Rose and coworkers have shown that these differential effects of ω-6 and ω-3 fatty acids also apply to human breast cancer and prostate cancer cells grown in culture. It was found that pharmacological inhibition of prostaglandin synthesis suppresses the growth of both cell types when the drug is incorporated in the medium.[18] Connolly and Rose have now shown that linoleic acid stimulates the growth of both human breast cancer,[19] and prostate cancer cell lines (unpublished data). Once again, these results from laboratory investigations are supported by epidemiological studies. Both breast and prostate cancers are uncommon in Eskimos[20] and subpopulations of rural Japan[21] who consume large quantities of seafood.

The ethnic composition of the population in a given country may influence the observed patterns of cancer risk. An example of this point is Israel, a country that shows a higher breast cancer mortality rate than that which would correspond to estimated animal fat consumption. However, breast cancer incidence in Israel is different for the major ethnic groups, being high among women of European origin and much lower in those who originated in Asia, Africa, and Yemen.[22] These population subgroups also differ in age of completed first pregnancy, height and body weight, and age of menarche, all of which are associated with different levels of breast cancer risk. So the position of Israel may result from various interactions, including, on the one hand, the high fat–low fiber diets (which are typical of Israelis from Europe and North America and of increased breast cancer risk) and on the other hand the nondietary protective factors such as late menarche and early first pregnancy (which are operative in women of Asian or African origin).

Reference has already been made to the North-South gradient in breast cancer incidence in Italy, and how it has been related to differing dietary practices. An increase in breast cancer risk has occurred in Japan since World War II, although the incidence continues to be relatively low. This change has affected predominantly postmenopausal women, notably those in the higher socio-economic groupings resident in large cities.[23] There is a strong positive correlation between the age-adjusted breast cancer mortality rate and estimated dietary fat consumption in the 12 Japanese prefectures,[23] whereas in Japan as a whole the increasing breast cancer risk has been accompanied by an increase in animal fat consumption.[24]

The shifting patterns of cancer risk that occurred with the Japanese migration to the United States have been carefully followed and continue to provide valuable information. Waterhouse et al.[25] reported a threefold increase in breast cancer incidence among Japanese-American women compared with those resident in Japan. This increased risk affects particularly those who are beyond menopause, an age relation that is consistent with obesity and high dietary fat intake being, at least in part, the responsible factors.

Case-control and cohort studies intended to examine the relation between dietary lipids and breast cancer risk have produced inconsistent, sometimes negative, results and are frequently cited as evidence against the existence of such an association.[26] However, as discussed in depth in a review by Prentice et al.,[27] there are problems with the use of these designs in this context. First, there is little intersubject variation in dietary fat consumption for typical subgroups of the population in Western countries. This point was illustrated in the large cohort study of American nurses performed by Willett et al., which produced no evidence that dietary fat intake was related to breast cancer risk.[26] As judged from a food frequency questionnaire, the amount of calories from fat ranged from 36% to 41% across calorie-adjusted grams of fat quintiles. Second, the instruments for dietary evaluation suitable for application to large numbers of subjects are of low accuracy. Greenwald[28] has pointed out that when applied to the Willett cohort study these two problems limit its power in such a way that it was bound to be falsely negative three times out of four.

The range of dietary lipid intakes available for assessment in cohort and case-control studies performed in Western countries, where most of this work has been done, certainly represent only a small (and upper) part of the range seen in international comparisons. Cohen et al.[29] used the N-nitrosomethylurea-induced rat mammary cancer model to examine the effects of different dietary fat levels on tumorigenesis. They found that diets in which corn oil provided 33% and 46% of total energy as fat, respectively—essentially the same spread as that observed in the American nurses cohort study—had similar promoting effects, whereas feeding 21% and 10% of calories as fat resulted in the same pronounced reductions in tumor development. In this report, which was published before Willett et al.[26] reported their human cohort study, the authors predicted that reductions in dietary fat intake to a level of 20% would be effective in reducing breast cancer risk, whereas those above 30% of calories as fat would be of little or no benefit.

To achieve a greater spread in the levels of dietary fat consumed, Toniolo et al.[30] performed a carefully designed case-control study in northwestern Italy. The region incorporates both rural and urban environs and overall has a moderately high breast cancer incidence. The dietary questionnaire was especially modified for its applicability to the geographical location under investigation and provided more detailed information regarding the types of oil consumed than is usually the case. High consumption of saturated fats and animal proteins was associated with significant elevations in breast cancer risk, and these associations persisted after adjusting for caloric intake. Statistical analysis of the data indicated that a reduction in total fat intake to less than 30% of total calories and of saturated fat to less than 10% would produce a substantial reduction in breast cancer incidence in this study population, a result in keeping with the animal model experiments.

Miller et al.,[31] reporting on a case-control study performed in four locations in Canada, found that there was a weak association between dietary lipid consumption and breast cancer for both premenopausal and postmenopausal women. They noted that they had investigated a homogeneous population, and that both the cases and controls (neighbors who themselves, in fact, were at "high risk") were probably eating larger amounts of fat than was necessary for optimal breast cancer promotion. These factors, combined with the insensitivity of the dietary evaluation methods, may have resulted in a misleadingly weak association.

Another case-control study from Canada found increased breast cancer risk to be associated with high intakes of beef and pork and total consumption of animal fats and proteins,[32] but there were methodological problems that have called the conclusions into question. In northern Italy Talamini et al.[33] observed increasing risk with the more frequent consumption of milk and dairy products, the relative risk moving from 1.0 to 1.8 to 3.4 with increasing intake of these fat sources. No association of risk was observed with meat consumption in this case-control study. Another case-control study from France,[34] involving 1010 breast cancer patients and 1950 hospital controls with nonmalignant diseases, showed increased risk to be related to the frequency of cheese consumption and the level of fat in the milk consumed, but there was no association with butter consumption.

Although most of the case-control studies were performed in countries of high breast cancer risk, two others were performed in Greece[35] and Japan,[36] respectively. As we have noted, Greece has a relatively low breast cancer incidence and is unusual in terms of diet in that olive oil is a major source of dietary lipid. These factors plus the small number of subjects involved may explain why only a weak and nonsignificant association was seen between fat intake and breast cancer risk in that study. The Japanese study showed no association between dietary fat and breast cancer risk, but it was performed in Fukuoka, which even *within* Japan is located in a region of low fat consumption and low breast cancer risk.

Body Size and Breast Cancer Risk

In a previously published review, Rose[13] examined the evidence that obesity is associated with increased breast cancer risk and brought together 11 case-control studies that supported the relation.[37-47] It was concluded that obesity is truly a risk factor for breast cancer but only in postmenopausal women where it manifests particularly in those who had their last menstrual period more than 5 years before the diagnosis of breast cancer. Actual body weight appeared to be the major risk factor; indeed when the Quetelet Index (weight/height^2) was used to assess obesity, it frequently either failed to reveal the correlation seen with body weight alone,[42,43,48] or it reduced the strength of the association.[40,49] If, as is discussed shortly, obesity is a risk factor because of its influence on extraglandular estrogen production, absolute fat tissue mass should be the relevant factor and not the amount relative to height and so use of the Quetelet Index would be inappropriate.

Several investigators,[46-50] but not all,[38-39] observed that premenopausal breast cancer is associated with lower body weight. Lubin et al.[50] made a detailed analysis and found that women who developed breast cancer before menopause tended to be of relatively low body weight and to have undergone less weight gain as adults. This relation was confirmed by Hislop et al.[51]: Heavier weight during childhood and before age 20 years reduced the risk of premenopausal breast cancer, but over the age of 40 years it increased postmenopausal breast cancer risk.

Obesity, Dietary Fat, and Breast Cancer Prognosis

There have now been at least nine full reports that obesity adversely affects prognosis after the surgical treatment of breast cancer (Table 10–1).[52-60] Most of them employed an arbitrary cutoff for classifying patients according to body size,[53-55,58,59] and one defined obesity as being 20% or more above ideal body weight.[56] Eberlein et al.[57] could identify no "cutoff" value that satisfactorily predicted prognosis but did find a strong association when regression analysis was performed with body weight as a continuous variable.

As in the case of body size and risk of breast cancer, expressing body weight in relation to height, usual applying the Quetelet Index, tended to produce either a weak[60] or no association with prognosis.[61-62] An exception was the study by Boyd et al.[55] where the Quetelet Index was more strongly associated with disease-free interval than weight alone, but in the

TABLE 10–1. Body size (obesity) and breast cancer prognosis

Study (1st author)	Age range/menopausal status	Body weight (kg)	Quetelet Index[a]
Abe[52]	Pre- and postmenopausal	Percent over "standard weight"[b]	Not examined
Donagan[53]	Pre- and postmenopausal	Cutoff 59 kg	Not examined
Tartter[54]	20–80 years	Cutoff 68 kg	Not Significant
Boyd[55]	35–70 years	Cutoff 64 kg	Significant effect
Zumoff[56]	33–80 years	Deviation from IBW[c]	Not examined
Eberlein[57]	< 40 to > 60 years	No cutoff value detected	Significant effect
Greenberg[58]	24–50 years (premenopausal)	Cutoff 60.5 kg (median weight)	Not significant
Newman[59]	35–70 years	Cutoff 63 kg (mean for group)	
Hebert[60]	20–80 years	Cutoff 73 kg (75th percentile for group)	Weak effect

[a] Q.I. = weight/height^2.
[b] Standard weight (kilograms) = (height in centimeters − 100) × 0.9; obesity = > 20% overweight.
[c] Obesity is defined as 20% or more above ideal body weight (IBW).

patients studied there was, in fact, relatively little variation in height. One interesting, but at present inexplicable, difference between the influence of body size on breast cancer risk and on prognosis of the established disease relates to menopausal status. As noted earlier, the consensus is that obesity is associated only with risk of breast cancer in postmenopausal women, and indeed that the risk may be higher for those who are below their ideal body weight and still in their pre menopausal years. In contrast, as shown in Table 10–1, most investigators have found an adverse effect of obesity on prognosis in breast cancer patients without selection for menopausal status. Unfortunately, analyses after stratification for this variable were not described in any of the published reports that included both premenopausal and postmenopausal women. However, Greenberg et al.[58] restricted their study to premenopausal breast cancer and found body weight, but not the Quetelet Index, to be a significant indicator of prognosis.

Given that the adverse effect of high body weight on breast cancer prognosis is established, consideration must be given to the clinical implications of reports that weight gain frequently occurs in postmastectomy patients treated with adjuvant chemotherapy.[63–65] Although one published study found no relation between body weight gain and risk of recurrence, the maximum follow-up was only 4 years.[65] In contrast, Camoriano et al.,[66] with 646 patients and nearly 7 years of follow-up, found that premenopausal women gaining more than the median weight at one year on chemotherapy were 1.5 times more likely to have relapsed, and 1.7 times more likely to have died, than women gaining less than the median weight. Similar trends were evident for postmenopausal patients.

Whereas there is a consensus on the effect of obesity on prognosis, an influence of dietary fat is less certain. Gregorio et al.[62] used a limited food frequency questionnaire to evaluate fat intake and its effect on prognosis in 953 breast cancer patients. After controlling for age at diagnosis and initial stage of the disease, an adverse effect of dietary fat on survival was clearly evident for those who initially had distance metastases; there was a trend in the same direction for cases of regional breast cancer but no influence at all on those with local disease (no lymph node involvement). In another study by Newman et al.,[59] which used a more comprehensive assessment of intake, dietary fat had no relation to survival. However, their experimental design was different, and only those with nonmetastatic disease were included so that they could neither confirm nor refute the major observation made by Gregorio et al. Also, statistical analyses were not possible on the basis of regional lymph node involvement because this information was not available to the investigators.

A study by Verreault et al.[67] had a related, but different, objective. There was no attempt to assess the influence of dietary fat on recurrence or survival but, rather, to seek relation with established indicators of prognosis. The investigation involved 666 women who completed a food frequency questionnaire of 114 items. With appropriate adjustments for body weight and tumor size, it was found that whereas total fat consumption was not related to nodal status, higher intakes of saturated fat were associated with axillary lymph node involvement in postmenopausal patients. The converse was true for unsaturated fats, but here high intakes accompanied node-free disease in both premenopausal and postmenopausal women. This finding appears to have its parallel in the international comparisons of dietary fat consumption levels and breast cancer risk described above. Fat intake was not related to the estrogen receptor status of the tumor; although estrogen receptor-negative cancers predict a poor prognosis, it is independent of lymph node involvement.[68]

Body Size, Endocrine Function, and Breast Cancer

In postmenopausal women the circulating estrogens are produced almost exclusively by the aromatization of androstenedione. This C_{19} steroid is secreted in part by the adrenal glands, but, in addition, its production by the ovaries continues beyond menopause. The conversion of androstenedione to estrone takes place predominantly in adipose tissue; it increases with increasing body weight, and consequently plasma estrogens are elevated in obesity.[69] In addition to the aromatase that converts androstenedione to estrone, the enzyme responsible for the reduction of estrone to estradiol, 17β-hydroxysteroid dehydrogenase, is present in breast adipose tissue, where it is positively correlated with body weight.[70]

Whether the plasma estrogen concentration or local production from steroid precursor is the important factor in breast cancer development is unclear. Some investigators have reported increased levels of plasma estrone[71] and estradiol[72] in breast cancer patients, but others found them to be normal.[73,74] Plasma androstenedione levels are increased in postmenopausal breast cancer[71] and correlate with the concentrations in adipose tissue from the breast and other sites.[75] O'Neill et al.[76] assayed aromatase activity in adipose tissue from each quadrant of mastectomy specimens, and found that it was consistently highest in the breast cancer-containing quadrant. This result may be interpreted as indicating that a tumor is more likely to develop at a site of local high estrone production, but an alternative explanation is that breast cancer cells themselves may enhance aromatase activity. It has been reported that both homogenates of breast cancer tissue and transforming growth factor-α, a polypeptide secreted by some human cancers, stimulate 17β-hydroxysteroid dehydrogenase and, hence the conversion of estrone to the biologically more active estradiol.[77]

Only a portion of the circulating estradiol is available for binding to the estrogen receptor; the rest is bound to plasma sex hormone-binding globulin (SHBG) and is considered to be biologically inert. There is an inverse relation between body weight and the plasma SHBG,[78] and so another potential mechanism for the influence of obesity on breast cancer risk involves this binding protein.

Other epidemiological risk factors for breast cancer have been associated with SHBG. Bernstein et al.[79] found parous women to have higher plasma SHBG concentrations, and lower free estradiol levels than nulliparous women, an observation consistent with the well recognized protective effect of child-bearing. Also, in one British study[80] SHBG levels were higher in women with a history of late menarche, a reproductive characteristic associated with lowered breast cancer risk. However, the true relation between postmenopausal breast cancer, obesity, and the plasma SHBG level remains unclear; normal levels have been found in case-control studies despite there being elevated levels of the biologically active free estradiol fraction.[72,74]

Several groups of investigators have sought an association between estrogen receptors and body weight in breast cancer patients, with conflicting conclusions. Papatestas et al.[81] reported that 54% of their 34 patients weighing more than 68 kg had either nondetectable levels of estrogen receptor or levels below 10 fmol/mg protein, compared with only 25% of the 59 patients with lower body weights. The association was particularly strong in postmenopausal patients, but the interpretation of this result is complicated by the inclusion of 24 patients with recurrent, metastatic disease. In another study,[82] urinary estrogen excretion was determined as well as tumor estrogen receptor status, and both related to an obesity index (weight in pounds per height in inches). Here the patients had operable disease and were studied at the time of mastectomy; the relation between the tumor estrogen receptor content and obesity was found to be a direct one, the reverse of the result obtained by Papatestas et al.[81] However, the correlation was a weak one ($r = 0.17$), applying only to postmenopausal patients, and the obesity index used was that which the same investigators found not to be related to breast cancer prognosis. Total urinary estrogens for 30 postmenopausal patients were weakly correlated with the obesity index ($r = 0.32$) but not with tumor estrogen receptor status.

De Waard et al.[83] studied 163 postmenopausal patients in The Netherlands, where the association of breast cancer risk with obesity appears to be particularly strong,[42,43] and found a direct relation between an increasing Quetelet Index and frequency of estrogen receptor-positive tumors. Nomura et al.[84] observed the same relation for body weight in Japanese postmenopausal, but not premenopausal, mastectomy patients.

Lastly, Mason et al.[85] reported a lack of association between estrogen receptor status and body weight. The patients had early disease and were stratified into premenopausal and postmenopausal groups. In fact, though, these investigators did observe a significant excess of estrogen receptor-positive tumors at the higher (70–80 kg) weight range, which they ignored perhaps because they were seeking to confirm the inverse relation originally described by Papatestas et al.[81]

If it is indeed correct that obesity is associated with estrogen receptor rich tumors in postmenopausal patients, the therapeutic implications require further consideration. Taken together with the adverse influence of high body weight on recurrence rate and the previously described endocrine changes in obese women, it appears that there is a place for weight reduction in the adjuvant therapy of postmenopausal breast cancer.

Cholesterol

Dietary lipid intake is correlated with the serum cholesterol, and cholesterol provides the starting point for the biosynthesis of the steroid hormones. Smethurst et al.[86] reported that women with nonmetastatic breast cance had higher serum cholesterol levels than female patients with cancers of other sites; and in a second report from this group of investigators,[87] both the cholesterol and phospholipids were found to be elevated in breast cancer compared with other diseases. Both studies may be faulted, however, because of the small number of patients examined and the inappropriate selection of controls.

Subsequently, three cohort studies showed no association between breast cancer risk and high serum cholesterol.[49,88,89] The large cohort study performed by Törnberg et al.[49] is, however, of special interest. The Quetelet index was inversely related to breast cancer in those aged under 50 years, confirming the previously discussed association of "thinness" with increased risk in premenopausal women, and this subset also showed a negative correlation between the serum cholesterol and cancer risk. These results, the interpretation of which is unclear, merit further investigation. It may be, of course, that there is a confounding factor that is responsible for a spurious association. One possibility is that smaller body size and lower serum cholesterol were indicators of higher socioeconomic status, which itself may be associated with at least two breast cancer risk factors: lower parity and late completed first pregnancy.

Petrakis and his colleagues have taken an interesting approach to cholesterol and breast cancer risk with studies performed on breast fluid samples collected by nipple aspiration.[90,91] High levels of cholesterol occur in this material when it is obtained from older women, together with cholesterol $5\alpha,6\alpha$-epoxide and cholesterol $5\beta,6\beta$-epoxide and their corresponding triol. Cholesterol epoxides are direct-acting mutagens, and their presence in breast fluids has been associated with atypical hyperplasia and dysplasia.[90]

Regardless of whether the serum cholesterol influences breast cancer risk or prognosis,[54] another aspect of lipid biochemistry may be important in breast cancer etiology and progression. Rudling et al.[92] have assayed low density lipoprotein (LDL) receptors in breast cancer tissues and observed an inverse correlation with survival time after surgery. This finding is consistent with the known association between high LDL receptor levels and rapid cell growth, although in their study Rudling et al.[92] found the prognostic significance of tumor LDL receptor content to be independent of DNA pattern, tumor size, and axillary lymph node involvement.

Dietary Intervention Trials for Breast Cancar

We have reviewed the evidence that obesity and possibly dietary lipids per se may influence breast cancer prognosis. The original observations, however, were indirect in nature and concerned the differing survival rates from breast cancer in the United States and Japan. Wynder et al.[93] found that, regardless of disease stage, Japanese women had a better 5-year survival rate after mastectomy than did American women. These patients were not evaluated according to their menopausal status, but when this measure was included in a second, independent, study by Sakamoto et al.[94] the relatively better 10-year survival rate in favor of the Japanese patients was shown to be restricted to those beyond the menopause. This result is, of course, consistent with the previously described epidemiological data concerning obesity, dietary lipids, and breast cancer.

The epidemiological observations, which are supported by data obtained from animal models,[95,96] have stimulated interest in dietary intervention for both breast cancer prevention and adjuvant therapy. Indeed, preliminary studies of a low-fat diet have already been initiated by investigators in the United States and Canada.

The American National Cancer Institute-supported Women's Health Trial (WHT) was developed as a multicenter dietary intervention trial with the objective of determining if a low-fat diet (20% of total calories) would reduce breast cancer incidence in women aged 45 to 69 years with specific risk factors for the disease. The rationale for the study design has been discussed in detail by Prentice et al.,[27] while Greenwald[28] has described the difficulties encountered and the issues raised during the initial feasibility stage of the trial. After much discussion, the decision was made not to proceed beyond the feasibility stage and on to the full trial with reduced breast cancer incidence as the endpoint. Nevertheless, the WHT provided a stimulus for the development of reliable biochemical markers of compliance to a low-fat diet, the evaluation of potential mechanisms, endocrine and otherwise, by which dietary fat may influence breast carcinogenesis, and the identification of meaningful risk factors in order to keep the number of participants within realistic limits.

Boyd et al.[97–98] are performing an initial study to determine the effect of a low-fat diet on mammographic patterns. The risk factor for breast cancer here is the DY (dysplastic) pattern originally described by Wolfe and subsequently confirmed by other investigators.[100] The initial results from this trial showed no significant changes in the mammographic patterns after 1 year on a low-fat diet (15% of total calories).[98] However, the dietary intervention did produce a considerable improvement in patients who had premenstrual breast tenderness and swelling and reduced nodularity as judged by physical examination.[99]

Serum estrogen and prolactin levels were determined in the low-fat trial performed by Boyd et al.,[99] but no changes were observed as a result of the dietary intervention. In a study of similar experimental design, Rose et al. observed a reduction in serum estradiol and estrone,[101] and circulating bioactive lactogenic hormones[102] after 3 months on a lowfat diet (20% of total calories); radioimmunoassayable serum prolactin levels were unchanged. Gorbach and Goldin[103] reported a similar effect on estrone sulfate concentrations in serum collected from healthy premenopausal women when they were placed on a low fat/high fiber diet.

Endometrial Cancer

Nutritional Epidemiology

The association between obesity and endometrial cancer is firmly established[104–108] and extends to those cases that occur in young women.[108] The relation was particularly strong in a case-control study performed by Wynder et al.[104] Here 21% of the cases were between 9.5 to 22.7 kg overweight at age 25 to 29 years, and 9% were more than 22.7 kg overweight at that time. Only 8% and 1%, respectively, of the controls were in these same weight categories. These data translated into a threefold increase in endometrial cancer risk for those with earlier excess weights in the 9.5 to 22.7 kg range and a ninefold increase for those whose weight had exceeded the norm by more than 22.7 kg.

More recently, Henderson et al.[108] performed a case-control epidemiological study that focused on endometrial cancer occurring in women under the age of 45 years. For these young patients, there was also an association between body weight and endometrial cancer risk; a woman who weighed 86 kg or more 1 year prior to diagnosis had an almost 18-fold increase in risk compared with a woman weighing less than 59.0 kg. Amenorrhea was also found to be a risk factor for endometrial cancer in this study and interacted with obesity. Indeed, amenorrhea was found to be a risk factor only for obese women.

An inverse relation between cigarette smoking and endometrial cancer has been recognized,[109] and, as we shall see later, it may be due to an effect of the smoking on estrogen metabolism. A smoking history modifies the adverse effect of obesity on endometrial cancer risk. Lawrence et al.[110] reported that risk did not, in fact, increase with increasing body weight among smokers, whereas for nonsmokers the association was clearly evident.

Adenomatous endometrial hyperplasia, a premalignant condition considered to result from excessive estrogenic stimulation,[111] has also been associated with obesity. In a case-control study, Kreiger et al.[112] found that for postmenopausal women the mean body weight and Quetelet Index were higher in the patients, and the index was clearly a risk factor based on the odds ratio estimate of relative risk. Unexpectedly, the mean body weight and Quetelet Index were no different for premenopausal cases and controls, and excess body weight relative to height was associated with a reduced risk of endometrial hyperplasia. There is an apparent inconsistency here in that, as we have already noted, obesity appears to be a risk factor for endometrial cancer in both premenopausal and postmenopausal women. Perhaps the problem is again the confounding effect of height, which can result in misleading values for the Quetelet index when assessing obesity.

Although dietary fat consumption and endometrial cancer risk has not been studied with anything like the intensity seen for breast cancer in recent years, the data available show similar results. The incidence rates for endometrial cancer and breast cancer are of course highly correlated,[113] and international comparisons of the type already described for breast cancer show a strong positive correlation between endometrial cancer incidence and the per capita estimated fat consumption.[1] In Hawaii a comparison of dietary practices among the different ethnic groups represented on the islands showed endometrial cancer positively correlated with both unsaturated and saturated fat consumption.[114]

La Vecchia et al.[115] performed a case-control study of endometrial cancer in Italy that confirmed obesity as a strong risk factor but also demonstrated increased risk associated with high fat consumption. Statistical evaluation indicated that the association with fat was not due simply to a high caloric intake leading to obesity. Furthermore, only certain sources of fat were responsible; the relative risk of endometrial cancer was high for the greater intakes of butter, margarine, and oils (type unspecified); however, there was no relation to milk, meat, or cheese consumption; and the cases consumed milk less frequently than the controls.

Diet, Nutrition, and Hormones

There is a well recognized relation between exposure of the endometrium to unopposed estrogen activity and endometrial cancer risk.[111,116] We noted earlier the increased production of estrone from androstenedione that occurs with obesity, and that after menopause this metabolic conversion is responsible for virtually all of the circulating estrogens. Furthermore, plasma estrone and estradiol are positively correlated with body weight in postmenopausal women.[117] While these same abnormalities—increased aromatization of androstenedione[118] and elevated plasma estrogens[117]—may be present in endometrial cancer patients, they are a function of the associated obesity and are not apparent when cases and controls are matched for body weight.

Obesity is strongly associated with a reduction in plasma SHBG,[78] which provides for an increase in the biologically active non-protein-bound and albumin-bound estradiol fractions. Elevated levels of plasma free and albumin-bound estradiol have been associated with increased breast cancer risk,[72,74,119–121] but their occurrence is independent of body weight.[72,74,119,121] Davidson et al.[122] determined the free estradiol and SHBG in 25 postmenopausal endometrial cancer patients and the same number of controls matched for body weight. In contrast to breast cancer, no significant differences were observed, although there were the expected correlations with body weight. The obese women, cases and controls, had higher levels of total estradiol in their serum and proportionally greater concentrations of free estradiol than did the nonobese women. Thus obesity and altered bioavailability of estradiol are closely linked in endometrial cancer risk, whereas a more complex situation appears to hold for breast cancer.

Estrone sulfate is present in the plasma of postmenopausal women at a concentration ten times that of estrone, it is elevated in obesity and has been reported to be increased in endometrial cancer patients.[123] Although itself considered to be biologically inert, estrone sulfate is taken up by endometrial tissue and enzymatically deconjugated there to yield estrogenically active estrone.[124] The potential relation between these findings and diet and endometrial cancer risk emerged when Woods et al.[125] reported that serum estrone sulfate levels were reduced by an average

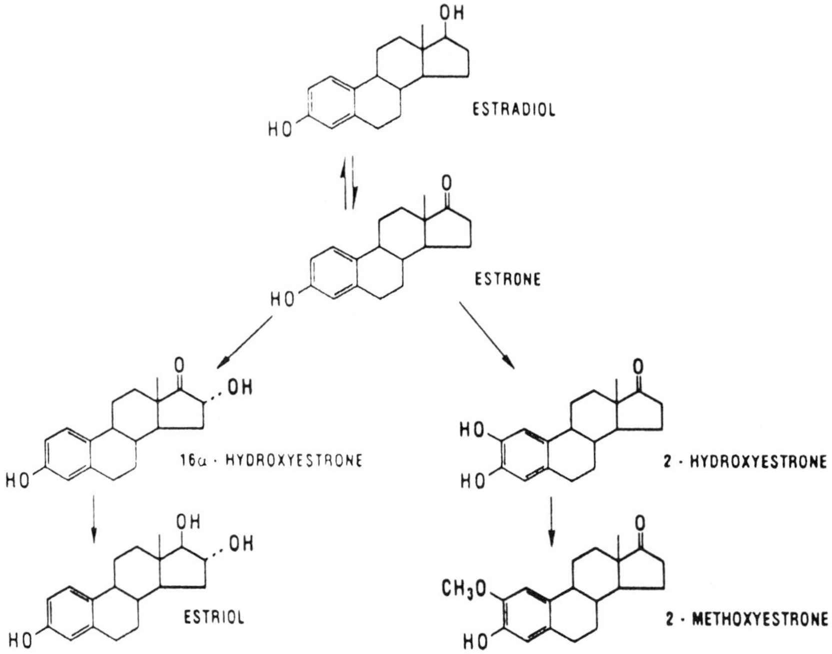

FIGURE 10–1. Metabolism of estrogens to 16α-hydroxy and catechol 2-hydroxy derivatives.

of 36% when healthy premenopausal women were transferred from a typical Western diet to one low in fat and high in fiber.

Obesity is also associated with altered hepatic metabolism of the estrogens. Estradiol is metabolized through competing pathways involving the formation of 16α-hydroxy and catechol derivatives (Fig. 10–1). Several years ago, Schneider et al.[126] used an in vivo radiometric assay to show that obese men and women have a reduced capacity for the metabolism of estradiol to the 2-hydroxylated metabolites. These compounds, principally 2-hydroxyestrone and 2-methoxyestrone, have little estrogenic activity and are rapidly cleared from the circulation. Hydroxylation at the 16α-position, however, is unaffected by obesity, and so there is a net enhancement of estrogenic activity that may contribute to the increased endometrial and breast cancer risk.

More recently, it was shown that dietary fat intake may affect estrogen metabolism in the absence of obesity. In one study,[127] healthy non-obese premenopausal women were transferred from their usual Western-type diet (providing 35–40% of calories from fat) to an isocaloric diet (25% of total calories from fat). After 2 months on the low fat diet, there was a significant decrease in the percentage of labeled estradiol excreted in urine as the 16α-hydroxylated metabolites and an increase in the excretion of 2-hydroxylated metabolites. Another study, by Hershcopf et al.,[128] evaluated the extent of 16α-hydroxylation in healthy women at increased breast cancer risk and related it to their dietary fat intakes. There were significant positive correlations between the levels of total and saturated fat consumed, expressed as percent of total calories, and formation of 16α-hydroxylated metabolites. The women in this study were not obese, and there was no correlation between the extent of 16α-hydroxylation and body weight. These two studies stress again the potential benefit of reducing dietary fat intake as an approach to the prevention of both endometrial and breast cancer. Indeed, Fishman and his colleagues[129,130] have produced evidence for the involvement of 16α-hydroxylated metabolites of estradiol in mammary carcinogenesis.

It was noted earlier that cigarette smoking appears to modify favorably the adverse effect of obesity on endometrial cancer risk. Although, of course, the health hazards associated with smoking make this effect of no practical value, it does strengthen the case for the role of abnormal estrogen metabolism in endometrial cancer risk. Thus Michnovicz et al.[131] showed that cigarette smoking produces a shift in the metabolism of estradiol to favor the formation of 2-hydroxy metabolites and away from 16α-hydroxylation. It may then reverse the excessive estrogenic activity that results from obesity-related reduced 2α-hydroxylation.

Key and Pike[132] reexamined the relation between plasma hormones and endometrial cancer risk and made a distinction between mechanisms operative in premenopausal and postmenopausal women. They considered the influence of estrogens on the endometrial cell mitotic rate and concluded that the upper limit above which plasma estrogens no longer produce a further increase in rate is set at the concentrations present during the early follicular phase of the menstrual cycle. As a result, for premenopausal women changes in the circulating estrogens with the menstrual cycle have little effect on the mitotic rate. In postmenopausal women, however, the estradiol level is set well below this upper limit, and so increases in plasma levels increase the endometrial cell mitotic rate.

This concept leads to two endocrine mechanisms by which obesity increases endometrial cancer risk. In premenopausal women, Key and Pike[132] suggested that progesterone deficiency is responsible, rather than estrogen excess, resulting in loss of the normal suppressive effect of progesterone on mitotic activity. Supporting observations include the association of obesity with amenorrhea,[133] subnormal luteal phase serum progesterone levels,[134] and irregular menstrual periods.[135] In the case of postmenopausal women, the endocrine relations already described are applicable: increased aromatization of androstenedione to yield estrone, reduced plasma SHBG levels, and increased biologically active estradiol in association with obesity.

Ovarian Cancer

As in the case of endometrial cancer, there is a strong positive correlation between the mortality rates for epithelial cancers of the ovary and breast in different countries and the same association with the level of animal fat consumption.[4] International comparisons also show positive correlations between ovarian cancer mortality rates and meat, milk, and egg consumption.[4] In Japan, where dietary habits have become closer to those of Western countries and ovarian cancer incidence is increasing among women over 50 years of age, Mori and Miyake[136] found that 19.2% of the total risk for the occurrence of this tumor in elderly women could be attributed to daily meat consumption. Decarli and La Vecchia[6] noted that the dietary patterns associated with ovarian and breast cancer risk were similar: Mortality rates for both cancers in different areas of Italy were positively correlated with the consumption of meat and dairy products.

One case-control study performed in the United States,[137] found a significant relation between ovarian cancer risk and the consumption of animal fat; the patients also consumed less vegetable fat and linoleic acid. A second study,[138] which used an abbreviated food frequency questionnaire based on 33 items, found no relation between dietary lipids and ovarian cancer, although for women in the 30- to 49-year age group there was a weak association with fiber intake and vitamin A from fruit and vegetable sources. Rose et al.,[4] in their international comparison, had also observed a strong negative correlation between ovarian cancer mortality rates and the consumption of cereals and vegetables.

Several epidemiological studies of case-control or prospective design have sought relations between body size and ovarian cancer risk;[136–142] most reported an association between obesity and risk,[137,139–142] but there are are the inevitable exceptions.[136,138] In part, the discrepancy may be related to age at diagnosis and to recent weight loss resulting from the tumor itself. Casagrande et al.[139] studied only women under 50 years of age and found a significant positive relation between excess body weight and the Quetelet Index and risk of ovarian cancer, whereas two other case-control studies that showed negative associations did so only in those over age 50.[136,137] Risch et al.[140] found obesity to be a risk factor for women aged 20 to 74 years; these authors did not stratify their data on the basis of age, but their definition of obesity was 20% or more excess body weight at age 30 or 1 year before interview for patients under age 30 at diagnosis. The case-control study performed in Boston by Cramer et al.[137] produced a trend toward higher body weight and the Quetelet's Index in ovarian cancer patients; it did not achieve statistical significance, but again the data were not reexamined in relation to age at diagnosis.

An understanding of the mechanisms by which obesity and dietary lipids may affect ovarian cancer risk must await a clearer understanding of the etiology of this tumor, which is the fourth most common cause of cancer deaths among women in Western countries.

Commentary: Recommendations for Clinical Practice

A review of the established or suspected associations between dietary lipids and sex hormone-related cancers is certainly a timely exercise. Several years ago the National Cancer Institute was sufficiently persuaded that high intakes of dietary fat constituted a significant risk factor for breast cancer to initiate a multicenter intervention trial with the objective of reducing disease incidence over a 10-year study period. The study foundered not because of difficulties in recruitment or compliance to a low-fat diet but because of reemphasized doubts by the External Advisory Group that lipids per se were responsible for enhanced risk, rather than calories and body size. Also, and perhaps more importantly, there were grave concerns about the high costs projected for completion of the trial as it evolved. These issues have been well discussed by Dr. Peter Greenwald, Director of the Division of Cancer Prevention and Control at the National Cancer Institute,[28] and by Prentice et al.[27] in their excellent review of the scientific rationale behind the trial.

Despite this false start, much was learned from the initial attempt, and several groups of investigators are now concerned with new trials in breast cancer prevention and dietary intervention as an approach to adjunctive therapy. It is recognized that there is a need to develop biochemical assays of sufficient selectivity to identify women who are truly at high risk for breast cancer, thereby reducing the numbers of participants required for statistical validity, and to define biochemical markers for the objective evaluation of compliance.

Before embarking on a new trial, more consideration must be given to the precise nature of the dietary manipulation, with regard to both the types and amount of fats consumed and the level of fiber intake. For example, is the desirable manipulation simply a reduction in total fat intake to 20% of total calories, the dietary goal in the "first generation" of low-fat trials? Or is it a decrease to only 30% of calories, together with an increase in ω-3 fatty acid-containing lipids and dietary fiber?

Clearly, these decisions cannot be made by nutritional oncologists in isolation. This point is emphasized by the beneficial effects on ischemic heart disease mortality rates that have been ascribed to an increase in vegetable oil consumption in the United States, while at the same time there is concern that linoleic acid-rich oils are associated with the increasing breast cancer incidence in American women.

While awaiting more definitive information that may be gleaned from future intervention trials, what recommendations can be made by the practicing physician on the basis of currently available data? From our critical evaluation of the literature, there appears to be a consistency concerning dietary total fat intake: A reduction to levels below 30% of total calories is likely to have a significantly beneficial effect on breast cancer incidence. This conclusion stems from a consideration of the international comparison data and the case-control and prospective studies, including the positive result obtained by Toniolo et al.[30] in northwestern Italy and the negative result obtained in Boston by Willett and coworkers.[26] It is reinforced by the results of studies of low fat diets (20–25% of total calories) on circulating hormone levels,[101–103,127] and of the animal model experiments reported by Cohen et al.[29]

With regard to the type of lipid, in contrast to the amount consumed, most of the research results emphasize saturated fats as the major cause for concern and suggest that the consumption of red meats and dairy products should be limited. Fortunately, the food industry has responded to these health concerns, and attainment of the dietary goals is being assisted by the increasing number of low fat foods available to the consumer.

The problem that quickly emerges as we think about this question is the recommendation that should be made with regard to vegetable oil consumption, specifically the intakes of ω-6 versus ω-3 fatty acids. As noted earlier, an increase in breast and prostate cancer incidence in the United States has been paralleled by increased consumption of linoleic acid, usually in the form of corn oil. Yet this shift in dietary practice has also been accompanied by a reduction in the mortality rate from cardiovascular disease. The answer may turn out to lie in recently completed and ongoing studies indicating that the *ratio* of ω-3 to ω-6 fatty acids consumed, rather than absolute amounts, may be important in influencing arachidonic acid metabolism,[143] and hence, potentially, cancer risk. Such an altered ratio, in favor of the ω-3 fatty acids, might be achieved by using both olive oil and corn oil, together with regular consumption of ω-3 fatty acid-rich fish. Blackburn and coworkers,[144] have reported on the favorable changes in serum fatty acid, lipoprotein, cholesterol, and triglyceride profiles obtained when patients with atherosclerotic disease were fed a low fat "healthy heart diet" together with fish oil supplements; and King et al.[145] described similar favorable biochemical changes when a typical American diet was modified to include two servings of fish a week.

In addition to making realistic recommendations for changes in the amount and type of dietary fats and oils, an effort should be made to increase the consumption of bran as a source of dietary fiber. This combined maneuver of reduced fat (20–25% of total calories) and increased fiber intake (25–30 g/day) may extend the benefit to include a reduction in colon cancer risk, as well as having relevance to carcinoma of the ovary in women and prostate cancer in men.

References

1. Armstrong B, Doll R. Environmental factors and cancer incidence and mortality in different countries, with special reference to dietary practices. Int J Cancer 1975;15:617–631.
2. Carroll KK. Experimental evidence of dietary factors and hormone-dependent cancers. Cancer Res 1975;35:3374–3383.
3. Hems G. The contributions of diet and childbearing to breast cancer rates. Br J Cancer 1978;37:974–982.
4. Rose DP, Boyar AP, Wynder EL. International comparisons of mortality rates for cancer of the breast, ovary, prostate and colon, and per capita food consumption. Cancer 1986;58:2363–2371.
5. Cohen, LA, Thompson, DO, Maeura Y, et al. Dietary fat and mammary cancer. 1. Promoting effects of different dietary fats on N-nitrosomethylurea-induced rat mammary tumorigenesis. JNCI 1986;77:33–42.
6. Decarli A, La Vecchia C. Environmental factors and cancer mortality in Italy: correlation exercise. Oncology 1986;43:116–126.
7. Katan MB, Beynen AC. Linoleic acid consumption and coronary heart disease in U.S.A. and U.K. Lancet 1981;1:371.
8. Handelman GJ, Epstein WL, Machlin LJ, et al. Biopsy method for human adipose with vitamin E and lipid measurements. Lipids 1988;23:598–604.
9. White E, Daling JR, Norsted TL. Rising incidence of breast cancer among young women in Washington State. JNCI 1987;79:239–243.
10. Devesa SS, Silverman DT, Young JL Jr, et al. Cancer incidence and mortality trends among whites in the United States, 1947–84. JNCI 1987;79:701–745.
11. Wynder EL, Rose DP, Cohen LA. Diet and breast cancer in causation and therapy. Cancer 1986;58:1804–1813.
12. Kakar F, Henderson M. Diet and breast cancer. Clin Nutr 1985;4:119–130.
13. Rose DP. Dietary factors and breast cancer. Cancer Surv. 1986;5:671–687.
14. Dougherty RM, Galli C, Ferro-Luzzi A, et al. Lipid and phospholipid fatty acid composition of plasma, red blood cells, and platelets and how they are affected by dietary lipids: a study of normal subjects from Italy, Finland, and the USA. Am J Clin Nutr 1987;45:443–455.
15. Jurkowski JJ, Cave WJ Jr. Dietary effects of menhaden oil on the growth and membrane lipid composition of rat mammary tumors. JNCI 1985;74:1145–1150.
16. Ip C, Ip MM, Sylvester P. Relevance of trans fatty acids and fish oil in animal tumorigenesis studies. Prog Clin Biol Res 1986;222:283–294.
17. Carter CA, Milholland RJ, Shea W, et al. Effect of the prostaglandin synthetase inhibitor indomethacin on 7,12-dimethylbenz(a)anthracene-induced mammary tumorigenesis in rats fed different levels of fat. Cancer Res 1983;43:3559–3562.
18. Reichel P, Cohen LA, Karmali R, et al. The effects of flurbiprofen on growth, prostaglandin production, and lactogenic hormone binding capacity of cultured human breast and prostate carcinoma cells. Proc Am Assoc Cancer Res 1985;26:195.
19. Rose DP, Connolly JM. Stimulation of growth of human breast cancer cell lines in culture by linoleic acid. Biochem Biophys Res Commun 1989;164:277–283.

20. Mishina T, Watanabe H, Arake H, et al. Epidemiological study of prostatic cancer by match-pair analysis. Prostate 1985;6:423–436.
21. Nielson NH, Hansen JP. Breast cancer in Greenland. Selected epidemiological, clinical and histological features. J Cancer Res Clin Oncol 1980;98:287–299.
22. Gross J, Modan B, Bertini B, et al. Relationship between steroid excretion patterns and breast cancer incidence in Israeli women of various origin. JNCI 1977;59:7–11.
23. Hirayama T. Epidemiology of breast cancer with special reference to the role of diet. Prev Med 1978;173–195.
24. Yonemoto RH. Breast cancer in Japan and the United States. Arch Surg 1980;115:1056–1062.
25. Waterhouse J, Muir CS, Corea P, et al. Cancer Incidence in Five Continents. Vol. III, Publication 15. Lyon: International Agency for Research on Cancer, 1976.
26. Willett WC, Stampfer MJ, Colditz GA, et al. Dietary fat and the risk of breast cancer. N Engl J Med 1987;316:22–28.
27. Prentice RL, Kakar F, Hursting S, et al. Aspects of the rationale for the Women's Health Trial. JNCI 1988;80:802–814.
28. Greenwald P. Issues raised by the Women's Health Trial. JNCI 1988;80:788–790.
29. Cohen, LA, Choi K, Weisburger JH, et al. Effect of varying proportions of dietary fat on the development of N-nitrosomethylurea-induced rat mammary tumors, Anticancer Res 1986;6:215–218.
30. Toniolo P, Riboli E, Protta F, et al. Calorie-providing nutrients and risk of breast cancer. JNCI 1989;81:278–286.
31. Miller AB, Kelly A, Choi W, et al. A study of diet and breast cancer. Am J Epidemiol 1978;107:499–509.
32. Lubin JH, Burns PE, Blot WJ, et al. Dietary factors and breast cancer risk. Int J Cancer 1981;28:685–689.
33. Talamini R, LaVecchia C, Decarli A, et al. Social factors, diet and breast cancer in a northern Italian population. Br J Cancer 1984;49:723–729.
34. Le MG, Moulton LH, Hill C, et al. Consumption of dairy produce and alcohol in a case-control study of breast cancer. JNCI 1986;77:633–636.
35. Katsouyanni K, Willett W, Trichopoulos D, et al. Risk of breast cancer among Greek women in relation to nutrient intake. Cancer 1988;51:181–185.
36. Hirohata T, Shigematsu T, Nomura AMY, et al. Occurrence of breast cancer in relation to diet and reproductive history: a case-control study in Fukuoka, Japan. Natl Cancer Inst Monogr 1985;69:187–190.
37. De Waard F, Baanders-van Halewijn EA, Huizinga J. The bimodal age distribution of patients with mammary carcinoma. Cancer 1964;17:141–151.
38. Valaoras VG, MacMahon B, Trichopoulos D, et al. Lactation and reproductive histories of breast cancer patients in greater Athens, 1965–67. Int J Cancer 1969;4:350–361.
39. Lin TM, Chen KP, MacMahon B. Epidemiologic characteristics of cancer of the breast in Taiwan. Cancer 1971;27:1497–1504.
40. Mirra AP, Cole P, MacMahon B. Breast cancer in an area of high parity: Sao Paulo, Brazil. Cancer Res 1971;31:77–83.

41. Ravnihar B, MacMahon B, Lindtner J. Epidemiologic features of breast cancer in Slovenia, 1965–67. Eur J Cancer 1971;7:295–306.
42. De Waard F, Baanders-van Halewijn EA. A prospective study in general practice on breast cancer risk in postmenopausal women. Int J Cancer 1974;14:153–160.
43. De Waard F, Cornelis JP, Aoki K, et al. Breast cancer incidence according to weight and height in two cities of The Netherlands and in Aichi perfecture, Japan. Cancer 1977, 40:1269–1275.
44. Staszewski J. Breast cancer and body build. Prev Med 1977;6:410–415.
45. Hirayama T. Epidemiology of breast cancer with special reference to the role of diet. Prev Med 1978;7:173–195.
46. Choi NW, Howe GR, Miller AB, et al. An epidemiologic study of breast cancer. Am J Epidemiol 1978;107:510–521.
47. Kelsey JL, Fischer DB, Holford TR, et al. Exogenous estrogens and other factors in the epidemiology of breast cancer. JNCI 1981;67:327–333.
48. Stavraky K, Emmons S. Breast cancer in premenopausal and postmenopausal women. JNCI 1974;53:647–654.
49. Tornberg SA, Holm L-E, Carstensen JM. Breast cancer risk in relation to serum cholesterol, serum beta-lipoprotein, height, weight, and blood pressure. Acta Oncol 1988;27:31–37.
50. Lubin F, Ruder AM, Wax Y, et al. Overweight and changes in weight throughout adult life in breast cancer etiology: a case-control study. Am J Epidemiol 1985;122:579–588.
51. Hislop TG, Coldman AJ, Elwood JM, et al. Childhood and recent eating patterns and risk of breast cancer. Cancer Detect Prev 1986;9:47–58.
52. Abe R, Kumagai N, Kimura M, et al. Biological characteristics of breast cancer in obesity. Tohoku J Exp Med 1976;120:351–359.
53. Donegan WL, Hartz AJ, Rimm AA. The association of body weight with recurrent cancer of the breast. Cancer 1978;41:1590–1594.
54. Tartter PI, Papetestas AE, Ioannovich J, et al. Cholesterol and obesity as prognostic factors in breast cancer. Cancer 1981;47:2222–2227.
55. Boyd NF, Campbell JE, Germanson T, et al. Body weight and prognosis in breast cancer. JNCI 1981;67:785–789.
56. Zumoff B, Gorzynski JG, Katz JL, et al. Nonobesity at the time of mastectomy is highly predictive of 10-year disease-free survival in women with breast cancer. Anticancer Res 1981;2:59–62.
57. Eberlein T, Simon R, Fisher S, et al. Height, weight and risk of breast cancer relapse. Br Cancer Res Treat 1985;5:81–86.
58. Greenberg ER, Vessey MP, McPherson K, et al. Body size and survival in premenopausal breast cancer. Br J Cancer 1985;51:691–697.
59. Newman SC, Miller AB, Howe GR. A study of the effect of weight and dietary fat on breast cancer survival time. Am J Epidemiol 1986;123:767–774.
60. Hebert JR, Augustine A, Barone J, et al. Weight, height and body mass index in the prognosis of breast cancer: early results of a prospective study. Int J Cancer 1988;42:315–318.
61. Sohrabi A, Sandoz J, Spratt JS et al. Recurrence of breast cancer: obesity, tumor size, and axillary lymph node metastases. JAMA 1980;244:264–265.
62. Gregorio DI, Emrich LJ, Graham S, et al. Dietary fat congumption and survival among women with breast cancer. JNCI 1985;75:37–41.

63. Knobf MK, Mullen JC, Xistris D, et al. Weight gain in women with breast cancer receiving adjuvant chemotherapy. Oncol Nurs Forum 1983;10:28–33.

64. Huntington MO. Weight gain in patients receiving adjuvant chemotherapy for carcinoma of the breast. Cancer 1985;56:472–474.

65. Heasman KZ, Sutherland JH, Campbell JA, et al. Weight gain during adjuvant chemotherapy for breast cancer. Breast Cancer Res Treat 1985;5:195–200.

66. Camoriano JK, Loprinzi CL, Ingle JN. Weight change in women treated with adjuvant therapy or observed following mastectomy for node-positive breast cancer. Breast Cancer Res Treat 1989;10(abstr.).

67. Verreault R, Brisson J, Deschenes L, et al. Dietary fat in relation to prognostic indicators in breast cancer. JNCI 1988;80:819–825.

68. Hawkins RA, White G, Bundred NJ, et al. Prognostic significance of oestrogen and progestogen receptor activities in breast cancer. Br J Surg 1987;74:1009–1013.

69. Vermeulen A, Verdonck L. Sex hormone concentrations in post-menopausal women. Clin Endocrinol (Oxf) 1978;9:59–66.

70. Beranek PA, Folkerd EJ, Ghilchik MW, et al. 17β-Hydroxysteroid dehydrogenase and aromatase activity in breast fat from women with benign and malignant breast tumors. Clin Endocrinol (Oxf) 1984;20:205–212.

71. Adami H-O, Johansson EDB, Vegelius J, et al. Serum concentrations of estrone, androstenedione, testosterone and sex hormone-binding globulin in postmenopausal women with breast cancer and in age-matched controls. Ups J Med Sci 1979;84:259–261.

72. Moore JW, Clark GMG, Bulbrook RD, et al. Serum concentrations of total and non-protein-bound oestradiol in patients with breast cancer and in normal controls. Int J Cancer 1982;29:17–21.

73. Thijssen JHH, Poortman J, Schwarz F. Androgens in postmenopausal breast cancer: excretion, production and interaction with estrogens. J Steroid Biochem 1975;6:729–734.

74. Reed MJ, Cheng RW, Noel CT, et al. Plasma levels of estrone, estrone sulfate, and estradiol and the percentage of unbound estradiol in postmenopausal women with and without breast disease. Cancer Res 1983;43:3940–3943.

75. Deslypere JP, Verdonck L, Vermeulen A. Fat tissue: a steroid reservoir and site of steroid metabolism. J Clin Endocrinol Metab 1985;61:564–570.

76. O'Neill JS, Elton RA, Miller WR. Aromatase activity in adipose tissue from breast quadrants: a link with tumour site. Br Med J 1988;296:741–743.

77. McNeill JM, Reed MJ, Beranek PA, et al. The effect of epidermal growth factor, transforming growth factor and breast tumour homogenates on the activity of oestradiol 17β-hydroxysteroid dehydrogenase in cultured adipose tissue. Cancer Lett 1986;31:213–219.

78. DeMoor P, Joosens JV. An inverse relation between body weight and the activity of the steroid binding β globulin in human plasma. Steroidologia 1970;1:129–136.

79. Bernstein L, Pike MC, Ross RK, et al. Estrogen and sex hormone-binding globulin levels in nulliparous and parous women. JNCI 1985;74:741–745.

80. Moore JW, Key TJA, Bulbrook RD, et al. Sex hormone binding globulin and risk factors for breast cancer in a population of normal women who had never used exogenous sex hormones. Br J Cancer 1987;56:661–666.

81. Papatestas AE, Panveliwalla D, Pertsemlidis D, et al. Association between estrogen receptors and weight in women with breast cancer. J Surg Oncol 1980;13:177–180.
82. Donegan WL, Johnstone MF, Biedrzycki L. Obesity, estrogen production and tumor estrogen receptors in women with carcinoma of the breast. Am J Clin Oncol 1983;6:19–24.
83. De Waard F, Poortman J, Collette BJA. Relationship of weight to the promotion of breast cancer after menopause. Nutr Cancer 1981;2:237–240.
84. Nomura Y, Kanda K, Shigematsu T, et al. Relation between estrogen receptors and body weight in Japanese pre- and post-menopausal breast cancer patients. Gann 1981;72:468–469.
85. Mason B, Holdaway IM, Yee L, et al. Lack of assocation between weight and oestrogen receptors in women with breast cancer. J Surg Oncol 1982;19:62–64.
86. Smethurst M, Basu TK, Williams DC. Levels of cholesterol, 11-hydroxy-corticosteroids and progesterone in plasma from postmenopausal women with breast cancer. Eur J Cancer 1975;11:751–755.
87. Basu TK, Williams DC. Plasma and body lipids in patients with carcinoma of the breast. Oncology 1975;31:172–176.
88. Williams RR, Sorlie PD, Feinleib M, et al. Cancer incidence by levels of cholesterol. JAMA 1981;245:247–252.
89. Hiatt RA, Friedman GD, Bawol RD, et al. Breast cancer and serum cholesterol. JNCI 1982;68:885–889.
90. Petrakis NL. Physiologic, biochemical and cytologic aspects of nipple aspirate fluid. Breast Cancer Res Treat 1986;8:7–19.
91. Gruenke LD, Wrensch MR, Petrakis NL, et al. Breast fluid cholesterol and cholesterol epoxides: relationship to breast cancer risk factors and other characteristics. Cancer Res 1987;47:5483–5487.
92. Rudling MJ, Stahle L, Peterson CO, et al. Content of low density lipoprotein receptors in breast cancer tissue related to survival of patients. Br Med J 1986;292:580–582.
93. Wynder EL, Kajitani T, Kuno J, et al. A comparison of survival rates between American and Japanese patients with breast cancer. Surg Gynecol Obstet 1963;117:196–200.
94. Sakamoto G, Sugano H, Hartmann WH. Comparative clinicopathological study of breast cancer among Japanese and American females. Jpn J Cancer Clin. 1979;25:161–170.
95. Cohen LA. Dietary fat and mammary cancer. In: Reddy BS, Cohen LA, eds. Diet, Nutrition and Cancer: A Critical Evaluation. Vol. 1. Boca Raton: CRC Press, 1986:77–100.
96. Katz EB, Boylan ES. Stimulatory effect of a high polyunsaturated fat diet on lung metastasis from the 13762 mammary adenocarcinoma in female retired breeder rats. JNCI 1987;79:351–358.
97. Boyd NF, Cousins M, Beaton M, et al. Methodological issues in clinical trials of dietary fat reduction in patients with breast dysplasia. Prog Clin Biol Res 1986;222:117–124.
98. Boyd NF, Cousins M, Beaton M, et al. A clinical trial of a low fat, high carbohydrate diet in patients with mammographic dysplasia: report of early

outcome. Abstract 24.3. Presented at the V International Congress of Breast Diseases, Buenos Aires, 1988.

99. Boyd NF, McGuire V, Shannon P, et al. Effect of a low-fat high carbohydrate diet on symptoms of.cyclical mastopathy. Lancet 1988;2:128–132.

100. Goodwin PJ, Boyd NF. Mammographic parenchymal pattern and breast cancer risk: a critical appraisal of the evidence. Am J Epidemiol 1988;127:1097–1108.

101. Rose DP, Boyar AP, Cohen C, et al. Effect of a low-fat diet on hormone levels in women with cystic breast disease. I. Serum steroids and gonadotropins. JNCI 1987;78:623–626.

102. Rose DP, Cohen LA, Berke B, et al. Effect of a low-fat diet on hormone levels in women with cystic breast disease. II. Serum radioimmunoassayable prolactin and growth hormone and bioactive lactogenic hormones. JNCI 1987;78:627–631.

103. Gorbach SL, Goldin BR. Diet and the excretion and enterohepatic cycling of estrogens. Prev Med 1987;16:525–531.

104. Wynder EL, Escher GC, Mantel N. An epidemiological investigation of cancer of the endometrium. Cancer 1966;19:489–520.

105. Elwood JM, Cole P, Rothman KJ, et al. Epidemiology of endometrial cancer. JNCI 1977;59:1055–1060.

106. Blitzer PH, Blitzer EC, Rimm AA. Association between teen-age obesity and cancer in 56,111 women: all cancers and endometrial cancer. Prev Med 1976;5:20–31.

107. Kelsey JL, Li Volsi VA, Holford TR, et al. A case-control study of cancer of the endometrium. Am J Epidemiol 1982;116:333–342.

108. Henderson BE, Casagrande JT, Pike MC, et al. The epidemiology of endometrial cancer in young women. Br J Cancer 1983;47:749–756.

109. Lesko SM, Rosenberg L, Kaufman DW, et al. Cigarette smoking and the risk of endometrial cancer. N Engl J Med 1985;313:593–596.

110. Lawrence C, Tessaro I, Durgerian S, et al. Smoking, body weight, and early-stage endometrial cancer. Cancer 1987;59:1665–1669.

111. Rose DP. Hormones and the etiology of endometrial cancer. In: Rose DP, ed. Endocrinology of Cancer. Vol. 1. Boca Raton: CRC Press, 1979:93–116.

112. Kreiger N, Marrett LD, Clarke EA, et al. Risk factors for adenomatous endometrial hyperplasia: a case-control study. Am J Epidemiol 1986;123:291–301.

113. Adami H-O, Krusemo UB, Bergkvist L, et al. On the age-dependent association between cancer of the breast and the endometrium: a nationwide cohort study. Br J Cancer 1987;55:77–80.

114. Kolonel LN, Hankin JH, Lee J, et al. Nutrient intakes in relation to cancer incidence in Hawaii. Br J Cancer 1981;44:332–339.

115. La Vecchia C, DeCarli A, Fasoli M, et al. Nutrition and diet in the etiology of endometrial cancer. Cancer 1986;57:1248–1253.

116. Henderson BE, Ross RK, Pike MC, et al. Endogenous hormones as a major factor in human cancer. Cancer Res 1982;42:3232–3239.

117. Judd HL, Lucas WE, Yen SSC. Serum 17β-estradiol and estrone levels in postmenopausal women with and without endometrial cancer. J Clin Endocrinol Metab 1976;43:272–278.

158   David P. Rose

118. MacDonald PC, Edman CD, Hemsell DL, et al. Effect of obesity on conversion of plasma androstenedione to estrone in postmenopausal women with and without endometrial cancer. Am J Obstet Gynecol 1978;130:448–455.
119. Moore JW, Clark GMG, Takatani O, et al. Distribution of 17β-estradiol in the sera of normal British and Japanese women. JNCI 1983;71:749–754.
120. Bernstein L, Pike MC, Ross RK, et al. Estrogen and sex hormone-binding globulin levels in nulliparous and parous women. JNCI 1985;74:741–745.
121. Jones LA, Ota DM, Jackson GA, et al. Bioavailability of estradiol as a marker for breast cancer assessment. Cancer Res 1987;47:5224–5229.
122. Davidson BJ, Gambone JC, Lagasse LD, et al. Free estradiol in postmenopausal women with and without endometrial cancer. J Clin Endocrinol Metab 1981;52:404–408.
123. Jasonni V, Bulletti C, Franceschetti F, et al. Estrone sulphate plasma levels in postmenopausal women with and without endometrial cancer. Cancer 1984;53:2698–2700.
124. Tseng L, Stolee A, Gurpide E. Quantitative studies on the uptake and metabolism of estrogens and progesterone by human endometrium. Endocrinology 1972;90:390–404.
125. Woods MN, Gorbach SL, Longcope C, et al. Low-fat, high-fiber diet reduces serum estrone sulfate in premenopausal women. Am J Clin Nutr 1989;49:1179–1183.
126. Schneider J, Bradlow HL, Strain G, et al. Effects of obesity on estradiol metabolism: decreased formation of nonuterotropic metabolites. J Clin Endocrinol Metab 1983;56:973–978.
127. Longcope C, Gorbach S, Goldin B, et al. The effect of a low fat diet on estrogen metabolism. J Clin Endocrinol Metab 1987;64:1246–1250.
128. Hershcopf RJ, Fishman J, Bradlow HL, et al. Extent of estrogen 16-alpha hydroxylation correlates with dietary saturated fat in women. Abstract 1332. Endocrinology 1988;122(suppl):353.
129. Schneider J, Kinne D, Fracchia A, et al. Abnormal oxidative metabolism of estradiol in women with breast cancer. Proc Natl Acad Sci 1982;79:3047–3051.
130. Yu SC, Fishman J. Interaction of histones with estrogens: covalent adduct formation with 16α-hydroxyestrone. Biochemistry 1985;24:8017–8021.
131. Michnovicz JJ, Hershcopf RJ, Naganuma H, et al. Increased 2-hydroxylation of estradiol as a possible mechanism for the anti-estrogenic effect of cigarette smoking. N Engl J Med 1986;315:1305–1309.
132. Key TJA, Pike MC. The dose-effect relationship between "unopposed" estrogens and endometrial mitotic rate: its central role in explaining and predicting endometrial cancer risk. Br J Cancer 1988;57:105–112.
133. Rogers J, Mitchell GW. The relation of obesity to menstrual disturbances. N Engl J Med 1952;247:53–55.
134. Sherman BM, Korenman SG. Measurement of serum LH, FSH, estradiol and progesterone in disorders of the human menstrual cycle: the inadequate luteal phase. J Clin Endocrinol Metab 1974;39:145–149.
135. Willett WC, Browne ML, Bain C, et al. Relative weight and risk of breast cancer among premenopausal women. Am J Epidemiol 1985;122:731–740.
136. Mori M, Miyake H. Dietary and other risk factors of ovarian cancer among elderly women. Jpn J Cancer Res 1988;79:997–1004.

137. Cramer DW, Welch WR, Hutchison GB, et al. Dietary animal fat in relation to ovarian cancer risk. Obstet Gynecol 1984;63:833–838.
138. Byers T, Marshall J, Graham S, et al. A case-control study of dietary and nondietary factors in ovarian cancer. JNCI 1983;71:681–686.
139. Casagrande JT, Louie EW, Pike MC, et al. "Incessant ovulation" and ovarian cancer. Lancet 1979;2:170–172.
140. Risch HA, Weiss NS, Lyon JL, et al. Events of reproductive life and the incidence of epithelial ovarian cancer. Am J Epidemiol 1983;117:128–139.
141. Tzonou A, Day NE, Trichopoulos D, et al. The epidemiology of ovarian cancer in Greece: a case-control study. Eur J Cancer Clin Oncol 1984; 20:1045–1052.
142. Garfinkel L. Overweight and cancer. Ann Intern Med 1985;103:1034–1036.
143. Boudreau M, Chanmugam P, Hwang DH. Effects of various dose levels of dietary N-3 fatty acids at a constant N-3/N-6 fatty acid ratio on arachidonic acid (AA) metabolism. Fed Proc 1989;3:A333.
144. Kowalchuk M, Plaisted C, Lopes S, et al. Evaluation of patient compliance to a low-fat healthy heart diet with fish oil supplements. Fed Proc 1989;3:A344.
145. King IB, Childs MT. The long-term effect of modifying the American diet to include moderate amounts of fish. Fed Proc 1989;3:A334.

11
Dietary Treatment of Lipids and Lipoprotein Disorders

Byron J. Hoogwerf

Several observations underlie the rationale for dietary alteration of plasma lipids and lipoproteins, especially when they are elevated. First, epidemiologically based studies and longitudinal studies of selected population cohorts have shown a relation between elevated plasma cholesterol and risk for atherosclerotic vascular disease, especially coronary heart disease. Second, clinical intervention trials using diet and drugs have shown that reduction in total cholesterol and, more particularly, a reduction in low density lipoprotein cholesterol (LDL-C) reduces the risk for coronary heart disease events. Such trials have generally used a combination of dietary and pharmacological therapy. Third, nutritional studies have shown that dietary change may significantly lower cholesterol.

Epidemiological studies have included both men and women. By contrast, the major intervention trials on which many of the current recommendations for lowering cholesterol are based have been performed with only male participants. There are a two major reasons for this fact. First, the lower incidence of coronary heart disease in women dictates that the number of women who need to be studied in an intervention trial is significantly higher than the corresponding number of men. Therefore cost and effort to perform the trial become major factors. Second, many intervention trials have been done in middle-aged men. Because this age range corresponds to the perimenopausal period and because menopause may have a significant effect on lipid and lipoprotein plasma concentrations, menopause becomes a significant confounding variable. The importance of hormonal changes in women as determinants of lipid and lipoprotein levels is now recognized and is discussed in detail elsewhere in this book. Many of the recommendations derived from intervention trials utilize information obtained in men and impute the results to women. Even in short-term nutritional studies, women are underrepresented. Most such studies involve men or groups of men and women, with only combined data being reported. Relatively few studies have evaluated women specifically, though the number has increased.

Epidemiological studies include one large study of coronary heart disease in seven countries[1] that showed a relation between a number of factors and the risk for coronary heart disease. Elevations of plasma cholesterol and the percent of caloric intake as total fat (especially as the saturated fat) were associated with increased risk for coronary heart disease. The Framingham Study, a long-term longitudinal study, has demonstrated the fact that obesity,[2,3] elevated total cholesterol,[4] increased LDL-C, and decreased high density lipoprotein cholesterol (HDL-C)[5,6] are associated with increased risk for coronary heart disease. Data from the Framingham Study have also shown that there is a relation in both men and women between total cholesterol concentrations and overall mortality. Overall deaths increase by 5% and cardiovascular deaths by 9% for each 10 mg/dl increase in cholesterol. This phenomenon holds true up to age 50 years; after age 50 the relation is less clear.[7]

In general, the relations between lipid levels and risk for coronary heart disease seem to apply to both men and women; the relative risk for any cholesterol level and at any age is lower in women. One of the largest epidemiologic studies done in women was the Walnut Creek Contraceptive Drug Study.[8] Risk factor evaluation was undertaken in more than 8900 premenopausal and 2700 postmenopausal women. Using cardiovascular mortality as an endpoint, smoking, high blood pressure, and diabetes were much more significant predictors of risk than total serum cholesterol; cholesterol was not a predictive risk factor in the postmenopausal cohort. The lack of lipoprotein subfraction determinations as predictor variables are acknowledged by the authors to be a limitation of this study.

The possibility that breast cancer in women may be linked to fat intake, especially saturated fat intake, has been controversial. Such a relation seems to exist in rodents. The issues of lipids, body weight, and female reproductive cancer are discussed more extensively by Rose in Chapter 10. His perspective is generally more supportive of the value of dietary intervention for the prevention of such malignancies. In my view, the issue is not resolved, and several negative clinical studies are mentioned here.

In extensive reviews, Hankin and Rawlings[9] and Mettlin[10] noted that both epidemiological and case-control studies showed inconsistent results but generally did not support a relation between diet composition and the risk for breast cancer. Two carefully done studies with different designs confirmed this point and deserve elaboration. Graham et al.[11] evaluated diet histories (using food frequency recall from 1 year prior to symptoms) in 2024 breast cancer cases and compared them to 1493 control patients without reproductive organ or gastrointestinal malignancy. All had been evaluated at the Roswell Park Memorial Institute. No differences in diet were detected except for somewhat decreased ingestion of vitamin A, which was associated with slightly increased risk of breast cancer in women over 55 years of age. Jones et al.[12] reported on 5485 women evaluated at the time of the National Health and Nutrition Examination Survey (NHANES I) from 1971 to 1975. Diet recall obtained at that time was compared in 99 women who developed breast cancer and women who did not have breast cancer. No significant differences were found in fat intake, total caloric intake, the amount of saturated/polyunsaturated/monounsaturated fat, or total cholesterol intake. More recent attempts to determine if diet affects the "hormonal milieu" in premenopausal women as a possible link for breast cancer have not clearly demonstrated any dietary effects.[13]

Randomized clinical trial results have also been used to demonstrate the benefits of altering lipid profiles by the associated reduction in coronary events and mortality. Although these studies were performed in men, the investigators generally attributed the results as being applicable to women. Because epidemiological data suggest similar relations between progressive worsening of lipid and lipoproteins and the risk for coronary disease in both men and women, this assumption of applicability is probably valid. Although the trials used pharmacotherapy in addition to diet, the results are likely applicable to lipid changes induced by diet only.

Three major clinical trial results are particularly important. First, data from the screenees for the Multiple Risk Factor Intervention Trial (MRFIT) showed that there was a clear relation between total plasma/serum cholesterol concentration and the risk for subsequent coronary heart disease.[14] Second, the Lipid Research Clinic's Coronary Primary Prevention Trial (CPPT) was a double-blind clinical trial in middle-aged men to test the "lipid hypothesis:" Does lowering total cholesterol and LDL-C decrease the risk for heart disease? The CPPT demonstrated that for a 9% reduction in total cholesterol—and a corresponding reduction in LDL-C—there was a 19% reduction in coronary heart disease events.[15] Furthermore, the relation between cholesterol reduction and heart disease risk reduction existed in patients who obtained substantial lipid lowering with diet alone.[16] Third, the Helsinki Heart Trial studied men with a broader range of lipid profiles and showed that decreased LDL-C and increased HDL-C as a result of a gemfibrozil treatment was associated with a reduction in coronary heart disease risk.[17] These studies, as well as a number of smaller intervention trials support the concept of dietary reduction of lipids and lipoproteins to reduce the risk of coronary heart disease.

Intervention trial data (especially MRFIT and the CPPT) are the bases for the frequently cited clinical aphorism that a 1% decrease in serum cholesterol is associated with a 2% decrease in cardiovascular disease risk. Epidemiological data support an even greater decrease: about 3% reduction in risk for each 1% reduction in serum cholesterol. These differences suggest that intervention to lower plasma cholesterol may have increased effects with increased duration of treatment.

Dietary Recommendations to Lower Cholesterol

As a result of these lines of evidence that lowering cholesterol reduces the risk for heart disease, the National Institutes of Health (NIH) issued two major reports. Dietary guidelines were outlined in a 1985 consensus con-

TABLE 11–1. Recommendations for dietary therapy of high blood cholesterol

Nutrient	Recommended intake
Total fat	< 30% of total calories
Saturated fatty acids	< 10% of total calories (step 1)
	< 7% of total calories (step 2)
Polyunsaturated fatty acids	Up to 10% of total calories
Monounsaturated fatty acids	10–15% of total calories
Carbohydrate	50–60% of total calories
Protein	10–20% of total calories
Cholesterol	< 300 mg/day (step 1)
	< 200 mg/day (step 2)
Total calories	To achieve and maintain desirable body weight

Adapted from The National Cholesterol Education Program Guidelines.[19]

ference report[18] and were reiterated in the National Cholesterol Education Program guidelines[19] for management of elevated plasma cholesterol levels, especially LDL-C. These recommendations generally conform to those proposed earlier by the American Heart Association.[20] These recommendations are summarized in Table 11–1 and are discussed in the paragraphs below.

The initial recommendation is to restrict calories in persons with obesity to achieve desirable body weight. Although it is not a consistent finding that there is a correlation of body weight and plasma cholesterol concentrations, weight loss in any individual is generally accompanied by a reduction in plasma cholesterol levels.[21,22] Such findings have not been consistent in women. Vaswani reported an initial reduction of cholesterol with weight loss, but over a 12-week period cholesterol returned to baseline.[23] Although Vaswani showed no significant change in HDL-C, others have reported an increase in HDL-C with weight loss in obese women.[24] Weight loss may alter estrogen levels in women but the impact of this change on lipoproteins has not been studied.

The second major recommendation is to reduce the total fat intake as a function of percent of calories ingested. A correlation between total fat intake and serum cholesterol levels has been shown in both epidemiological and intervention studies.[1,25–28] An initial target for total fat intake of 30% of total calories is recommended. This amount is much lower than in the average American diet in which 42% of the total calories were in the form of fat up until the early 1980s. Survey evidence suggests that dietary fat intake is now closer to 35% of calories. For example, 60% of the patients referred to The Cleveland Clinic Foundation Lipid Referral Clinic have a dietary intake of fat that is less than 30% of the total calories.[29]

TABLE 11–2. Major contributors of saturated fat and cholesterol in the U.S. diet

Saturated fat[a]	Cholesterol[b]
Hamburger meat	Eggs
Whole milk	Beef steaks, roasts
Cheeses	Hamburger meat
Beef steaks, roasts	Whole milk
Hot dogs, ham, lunch meats	Hot dogs, ham, lunch meat
Doughnuts, cookies, cake	Pork
Eggs	Doughnuts, cookies, cake
Pork	Cheeses
Butter	Liver
White bread, rolls, crackers	Chicken and turkey

Adapted from the National Health and Nutrition Examination Survey (NHANES) II, 1976–1980.
[a]These items account for 60% of the total saturated fat in the diet.
[b]These items account for 77% of the total cholesterol in the diet.

The third major component of NIH recommendations deals with the composition of fatty acid intake with special attention to saturated fat intake. It is suggested that the latter should be no more than 10% of the total calories. The rationale for this recommendation is again supported by epidemiological and intervention study data.[15,22,25,30–35] For persons whose plasma cholesterol levels do not approach acceptable levels at this quantity of saturated fat, a further lowering of saturated fat intake to 7% of total calories is advisable. It is worthwhile to note the common sources of saturated fat in the American diet (Table 11–2). The single largest source of saturated fat in the American diet is hamburger. More broadly, the commonest sources are red meats and other dairy products including milk and cheeses. Because each of these items is high in protein, appropriate changes in the diet include increasing the intake of fish and poultry and changing to lower fat forms of the dairy products (skim milk, nonfat cheeses).

Controlling dietary cholesterol intake is helpful for controlling plasma cholesterol levels.[36] Because cholesterol is a fundamental constituent of all animal cells, animal tissue is a major source of dietary cholesterol. The single largest source of dietary cholesterol in the American diet is eggs: The yolks typically contain 200 mg or more cholesterol. Concentrations of organ meats, especially liver, are also high in cholesterol, and shellfish contain moderately high concentrations. There is some suggestive evidence that cholesterol in shellfish may have an impact on overall risk different from that of other dietary sources, the reasons for which are not yet clear. Because of the high consumption of hamburger meat in the American diet, this food is also a significant source of dietary cholesterol. The current recommendations suggest limiting total daily cholesterol ingestion to a total of 300 mg daily (or no more than 100 mg/1000 kcal ingested in the diet). In women, in whom calorie requirements are lower as a result of smaller average body size, the adjustment of cholesterol intake to conform to total caloric intake is appropriate. For example, a 60-kg woman whose caloric needs are in the range of 2000 kcal/day (30–35 kcal/kg) should limit total cholesterol intake to 200 mg/day.

There is evidence that increasing dietary fiber lowers total and LDL cholesterol. It is largely an effect of soluble fiber, such as that found in lentils, beans, and such foods as oat bran.[37–39] Crude fiber has much less of an effect. It seems to require a total daily ingestion of 10 to 25 of fiber to see much of an effect on cholesterol lowering. Furthermore, the cholesterol-lowering effect of fiber seems to be less in persons who are on diets that have restricted total fat intake to levels conforming to those recommended by the American Heart Association. In fact, 11 g of soluble fiber per day lowers total cholesterol only another 3%.[39] High fiber diets exert their effects by substituting for foods containing higher quantities of fat and by binding bile salts in the gastrointestinal tract. Reduced bile salt absorption results in a loss of cholesterol in the stool and in increased conversion of cholesterol from the body pool into bile salts.[40] Such quantities of fiber predispose to significant flatulence. Such flatulence is a limiting factor in both men and women's capability to tolerate high fiber diets.

It is of interest to note that three major groups with somewhat diverse medical interests—the American Heart Association,[20] the American Diabetes Association,[41] and the National Cancer Institute—have come to recommend similar diets. The research supporting these recommendations suggests that there may be a reduction in coronary artery disease, fewer problems with hyperglycemia and its attendant secondary problems, and a reduction in risk for malignancies as a result of dietary intervention.

Magnitude of Serum Cholesterol Change with Dietary Intervention

A number of studies have been performed that help quantify the projected change in lipid levels due to a change in dietary intake. More than two decades ago Keys et al. investigated these relations in carefully controlled living arrangements in men. They showed that change in dietary saturated fat produced nearly twice the change in serum cholesterol as did a comparable change in dietary polyunsaturated fat.[42] It resulted in the following formula for change in serum cholesterol levels.

$$\Delta \text{Cholesterol (mg/dl)} = (2.7\ \Delta S) - (1.3\ \Delta P)$$

where Δ refers to the percent change in saturated fat (S) and polyunsaturated fat (P) between the two diets. Monounsaturated fats were considered to be neutral.

This group further investigated the effects of changes in dietary cholesterol intake in similar fashion[36] and showed that Δ cholesterol is equal to 1.5 times the square root of the change in dietary cholesterol (in milligrams per 1000 kcal) ingested in two diets (which they designated). The complete formula they derived was

$$\Delta\text{Cholesterol} = 1.2\ (2\Delta S - \Delta P) + 1.5\Delta Z$$

where Z is the square root of dietary cholesterol. The correlation coefficient for this formula based on 63 sets of data was 0.93. Hegsted and coworkers did a similar study[25] in institutionalized men looking at saturated fat (S), monounsaturated fat (M), polyunsaturated fat (P), and cholesterol intake (C); they derived a formula with similar degrees of change.

$$\Delta\text{Cholesterol} = 2.32\ S + 0.32\ M - 1.46\ P + 6.51\ C + 0.83$$

Neither formula was predictive of changes in other major studies of dietary intervention with the same high correlation. For example, this issue was carefully analyzed by Gordon et al., who looked at dietary changes in men participating in the Lipid Research Clinics Coronary Primary Prevention Trial. In this trial and a number of other studies summarized by these authors, there are limitations of the predictive capabilities of the formulas.[22] Nevertheless, many studies support the concept that decreasing saturated fat in the diet may have a greater impact than some other variables as predicted by both the Keys and Hegsted formulas.

Dietary Treatment to Lower Triglycerides

Dietary treatment of hypertriglyceridemia—elevations of plasma very low density lipoprotein (VLDL)—is generally the same as for elevation of total cholesterol [of which VLDL cholesterol (VLDL-C) may be a significant component] and LDL-C. In addition to weight reduction for obesity and restriction of fat intake, other dietary factors play a role in regulating triglycerides. Ethanol ingestion is associated with increased VLDL production, and restriction of ethanol may markedly decrease plasma triglyceride levels.[43,44] The impact of dietary ingestion of simple carbohydrates on elevations of triglycerides is well known,[45] especially in persons with diabetes mellitus, a disorder associated with increased risk for hypertriglyceridemia. Hypercholesterolemia may be a sign of unsuspected or uncontrolled diabetes. Control of the diabetes is essential for lowering the triglyceride level.

Studies of Lipid Lowering in Women

As noted above, most of the collective dietary recommendations are based on epidemiological data in which information from men and women are combined. This point is also true for a number of short-term intervention studies, and usually such studies do not distinguish the data from women. Some studies performed exclusively in women have supported the concept that dietary-induced lipid changes in women are likely to be comparable to those obtained in studies in men or studies combining men and women.

Kohlmeier et al.[46] compared a "normal" diet containing 43% fat, a polyunsaturated/saturated fat (P/S) ratio of 0.2, a total of 16 g of fiber, and cholesterol intake of 1 g/day with a "prudent" diet in 12 women aged 22 to 47 years. The "prudent" diet contained 31% fat, a P/S ratio of 3.2, 44 g of fiber, and a cholesterol intake of 13 mg. Lipid profiles obtained in synchrony with menstrual periods showed decreases of total cholesterol (−27.6%), LDL-C (−37.3%), and HDL-C (−16.3%) and an increase of triglycerides (+28.7%), the latter of which was not statistically significant. Such increases have been observed with increased carbohydrate intake in other studies.

Weisweiler et al.[47] evaluated the effects of three diets: (1) reference: fat 42%, P/S 0.16; (2) polyunsaturated: fat 42%, P/S 1.0; (3) polyunsaturated low fat: fat 32%, P/S 1.0 in 22 normolipidemic women (6 premenopausal). The lower saturated fat diets both showed decreases in total plasma cholesterol and LDL-C with no change in HDL-C over 6-week diet periods. Furthermore, changes in apolipoprotein B (apo B) decreased in such a way as to favor a less atherogenic composition of lipoproteins containing apo B. Jones et al.[48] randomized 31 women into one of two groups that varied in the P/S ratio (0.3 versus 1.0) and in high versus low fat content. Although not all differences were statistically significant, the low fat diets were associated with lower total plasma cholesterol concentrations. These and similar studies support the concept that diet-induced changes in plasma lipid and lipoprotein concentrations are in the expected direction in women and of approximately the expected magnitude.

Monounsaturated and ω-3 Fatty Acids in the Diet

Two areas under intense investigation include the impact of dietary monounsaturated fats and of dietary ingestion of fish oils on plasma lipid and lipoprotein concentrations and the associated risk for atherosclerotic vascular disease. Carefully performed metabolic studies suggest that equicaloric quantities of monounsaturated and polyunsaturated fats are of equal potency in lowering total cholesterol and LDL-C about the same amount when they replace saturated fats.[49] Fat composition has variable effect on triglycerides. There is a trend for HDL-C to be higher in subjects on diets with monounsaturated fats compared to those on diets with polyunsaturated fats.[50] Similar results have been found with free-living dietary studies comparing corn oil with olive oil (which contains more monounsaturated fat) in men.[51] Furthermore, when high monounsaturated fat diets (43% of total calories) were compared with low fat diets (20%) and the caloric differences were made up by carbohydrate, the monounsaturated fat diet was associated with lower plasma total cholesterol, lower LDL-C, comparable triglycerides, and higher HDL-C.[52] Most commonly used vegetable oils (corn, safflower) are high in polyunsaturated fat, and olive oil is perhaps the most commonly used source of monounsaturated fats. Some forms of safflower oils with high oleic acid levels would be considered to be high in monounsaturates. Palm oil, palm kernel oil, and coconut oils are partially hydrogenated vegetable oils and must be considered as saturated fats. Because the latter vegetable oils are more stable in storage, they are commonly used in preprepared foods as well as in the fast food industry.

Interest in a possible beneficial effect of fish oils in the diet derived from the observation that the Greenland Eskimos had a low incidence of atherosclerotic vascular disease.[53] The cold water fish, which was a major dietary constituent, contained polyunsaturated fat, but it contained the first double bond in the third position (hence the designation n-3 or ω-3) compared to the more common n-6 polyunsaturated fats, which characterize dietary polyunsaturated fats in more typical Western diets. The ingestion of this diet was associated with lower plasma levels of total cholesterol, LDL-C, VLDL-C, and triglycerides, and higher HDL-C levels. Furthermore, decreased platelet aggregation was noted. These observations have been confirmed in other clinical studies of cold water fish (commonly mackerel or salmon) or cod liver oil or other fish oil supplements. Herold and Kinsella have published an extensive review of this subject.[54] There is consistent reduction of plasma triglycerides in these studies. Of note is the observation that in subjects with markedly elevated triglycerides the reduction of plasma concentration is associated with a corresponding increase in LDL-C. No studies have demonstrated that fish oil supplement consumption reduces the risk of atherosclerotic vascular disease events. Furthermore, because of the high caloric density of fat, these supplements may become a source of additional calories.

Dietary Effects on Apoproteins

A burgeoning interest in apoproteins and their possible contribution to the risk for coronary artery disease has raised questions about whether abnormal concentrations of such apoproteins may be altered with dietary intervention. Most of the studies have focused on apo B and apo A1. Apo B is associated with LDL-C, and increased concentrations are associated with increased risk for coronary heart disease (CHD).[55,56] Apo A1 a major apoprotein of HDL, and low levels are associated with an increased risk of CHD (see Chapter 3). Other apoproteins have also been studied with various dietary perturbations. These studies have shown that dietary changes do influence plasma apoprotein levels.

An early report from Shepherd and coworkers[57] compared turnover/metabolism and plasma apo A1 concentrations in four men on saturated fat and polyunsaturated fat diets. The polyunsaturated fat diet was associated with lower triglycerides and HDL-C as well as a 21% decrease in plasma apo A1; this decrease was due largely to a decrease in synthesis. Using similar diet comparisons, Vega and coworkers showed that the higher polyunsaturated fat diet was associated with a reduction in both apo B and apo A but that the ratios of cholesterol/apo B, triglyceride/apo B, or cholesterol/apo A in HDL were not more atherogenic.[31] Dietary experiments performed by Schonfeld et al. also showed that apo A and apo B were altered by diet but that there were no significant changes in A-II, C-II, C-III, or apo E.[58] Subsequent studies have confirmed the changes for apo B in LDL and VLDL and have shown a change in apo E isoform to desialated forms with low fat diets.[59] The significance of such changes is still uncertain. Zanni et al. looked more carefully at the effects of cholesterol intake in conjunction with changes in fat composition and showed similar changes in apo B and apo A1 that corresponded with LDL and HDL.[35] Of note is the fact that their dietary manipulation resulted in changes in plasma cholesterol that closely conformed to predictions based on the Keys equation (see above).

Implementation of Dietary Recommendations

Dietary recommendations and the impact of dietary change according with these recommendations on plasma lipid and lipoprotein levels have been outlined above. Note that effective implementation frequently requires proper nutritional education from experienced nutritionists. The intense interest in "cholesterol" by the American public has been fostered not only by the medical profession but by extensive material in the lay press. It has resulted in general reduction in fat intake by the American public. In fact, 60% of people referred to a busy lipid clinic are already on diets that conform to National Cholesterol Education Program Step 1 guidelines.[29] Valuable information has been obtained from careful follow-up of the participants in the Multiple Risk Factor Intervention Trial[22,26] about the nature of dietary changes that were easiest for men to make. They included increased consumption of fish and poultry as well as changes to skim milk or low fat milk, polyunsaturated oils and margarine, fewer egg yolks, and increased low fat bread and cereals. Reducing beef, pork, and high fat cheeses and snacks was much more difficult. As an extension of these concepts, it is generally easier for people to decrease frequency of high fat foods than to decrease the quantity at a given meal. Thus it may be more effective to emphasize having eggs or red meat less frequently rather than in smaller portions. It is also easier to make small changes over longer periods of time than extensive changes all at once. A number of instructional programs have been developed that use teaching aids, dietary records, and careful assessment of dietary adherence.[60,61] Such intensive efforts do result in improved dietary compliance over a period of up to 9 months. Women have been reported to achieve better adherence to dietary recommendations than men and consequently get better cholesterol-lowering effect.[60] Because of their traditional role in food preparation, women have a major influence on their families' dietary patterns and should be included in efforts to change the diet of other family members.

Any discussion of dietary therapy for altering lipid levels would be incomplete without some brief comments about two areas: (1) eating outside the home, especially at fast food restaurants; and (2) food product marketing in a society increasingly attuned to the importance of the diet on lipid levels.

The fast food industry has been built on selling hamburgers, which is the food item heading the list for saturated fat consumption. Even well done hamburgers or other beef-based foods contain substantial calories as saturated fat. Furthermore, the most stable cooking oils are those derived from animal fats or vegetable sources that are highly saturated, such as coconut oil, palm oil, or palm kernel oil. These oils are commonly used in the frying process in the fast food industry. Restaurant dining, in general, is associated with a need to be attentive to fat intake. Even if meat entries are avoided, there are a number of sources of fat, including salad dressings, sauces and condiments, butter, and desserts. Some restaurants have begun to extend the number of low fat items beyond the typical "diet plate."

The advertising industry has tried to appeal to the consumer's desire for a lipid-altering diet but in doing so has occasionally been somewhat misleading. Many high fat foods can legitimately be advertised as having "no cholesterol." The converse may also be true, i.e., high cholesterol foods have low fat, but it has not generally been as common an advertising scheme. The proliferation of fiber-containing products, especially oat bran, has also resulted in subtle deception in advertising. Some high fiber cereals have a coconut oil content that is sufficiently high to outweigh any cholesterol-lowering effect of the fiber. In general, avoidance of saturated fat may be more important than avoidance of cholesterol when selecting preprocessed foods or those from a restaurant menu.

Many of these practices can be overcome by continued public education about all the dietary factors that contribute to changes in plasma lipid levels. Furthermore, most nutritionists who provide personal instruction emphasize the importance of reading food labels to help reduce fat and cholesterol consumption to acceptable levels.

Summary

There is evidence from both epidemiological data and intervention trial data that low blood cholesterol levels are associated with reduced risk for atherosclerotic vascular disease, especially coronary disease. Whereas most of the major intervention trials have been conducted in men, the general conclusions about a reduction in risk for coronary disease with lowering total and LDL cholesterol should be applicable to women. Efforts to lower blood cholesterol levels should always start with dietary intervention. The key features of any dietary program include weight reduction, reduction in total fat intake (especially saturated fat intake), reduction in total cholesterol intake, and an increase in fiber consumption, especially soluble fiber. Most people find it easier to reduce the frequency of food items that are high in saturated fat and cholesterol than to reduce the quantity of food with the same frequency of ingestion. The effects of dietary manipulation on plasma apoprotein levels, which may be better predictors of coronary disease risk, are currently under investigation.

References

1. Keys A. Coronary heart disease in seven countries. Circulation 1970;41(suppl 1):162–198.
2. Gordon T, Kannel WB. Diabetes, blood lipids and the role of obesity in CHD risk for women; the Framingham Study. Ann Intern Med 1977;87:393–397.
3. Hubert HB, Feinleib M, McNamara PM, Castelli WP. Obesity as an independent risk factor for cardiovascular disease: a 26 year follow-up of participants in the Framingham Heart Study. Circulation 1983;67:968–977.
4. Kannel WB, Castelli WP, Gordon T. Cholesterol in the prediction of atherosclerotic disease: new perspectives based on the Framingham Study. Ann Intern Med 1979;90:85–91.
5. Castelli WP, Abbott RD, McNamara PM. Summary estimate of cholesterol used to predict coronary heart disease. Circulation 1983;67:730–734.
6. Castelli WP, Garrison RJ, Wilson PWF, et al. Incidence of coronary heart disease and lipoprotein cholesterol levels: the Framingham Study. JAMA 1986;256:2835–2838.
7. Anderson KM, Castelli WP, Levy D. Cholesterol and mortality: 30 years of follow-up from the Framingham Study. JAMA 1987;257:2176–2180.
8. Perlman JA, Wolf PH, Ray R, Lieberknecht G. Cardiovascular risk factors, and all-cause mortality in a cohort of Northern California women. Am J Obstet Gynecol 1988;158:1568–1574.
9. Hankin JH, Rawlings V. Diet and breast cancer: a review. Am J Clin Nutr 1978;31:2005–2016.
10. Mettlin C. Diet and the epidemiology of human breast cancer. Cancer 1984;53(suppl 1):605–611.
11. Graham S, Marshall J, Mettlin C, et al. Diet in the epidemiology of breast cancer. Am J Epidemiol 1982;116:68–75.
12. Jones DY, Schatzkin A, Green SB, et al. Dietary fat and breast cancer in the National Health and Nutrition Examination Survey I epidemiologic follow-up study. JHCI 1987;79:465–471.
13. Hagerty MA, Howies BJ, Tan S, Shultz TD. Effect of low- and high-fat intakes on the hormonal milieu of premenopausal women. Am J Clin Nutr 1988; 47:653–659.

14. Stamler J, Wentworth D, Neaton JD (MRFIT Research Group). Is the relationship between serum cholesterol and risk of premature death from coronary heart disease continuous and graded? JAMA 1986;256:2823–2828.
15. Lipid Research Clinics Program. The Lipid Research Clinics Coronary Primary Prevention Trial Results. I. Reduction in incidence of coronary heart disease. JAMA 1984;251:351–364.
16. Lipid Research Clinics Program. The Lipid Research Clinics Coronary Primary Prevention Trial Results. II. The relationship of reduction in incidence of coronary heart disease to cholesterol lowering. JAMA 1984;251:365–374.
17. Frick MH, Elo O, Haapa K, et al. Helsinki Heart Study: primary prevention trial with gemfibrozil in middle-aged men with dyslipidemia. N Engl J Med 1987;317:1237–1245.
18. NIH Consensus Development Conference. Lowering blood cholesterol to prevent heart disease. JAMA 1985;253:2080–2086.
19. Expert Panel. Report of the National Cholesterol Education Program expert panel on detection, evaluation and treatment of high blood cholesterol in adults. Arch Intern Med 1988;148:1–69.
20. Nutrition Committee and the Council on Arteriosclerosis: Recommendations for treatment of hyperlipidemia in adults. Circulation 1984;69:1065A–1090A.
21. Hershcope RJ, Elahi D, Andres R, et al. Longitudinal changes in serum cholesterol in men: an epidemiologic search for an etiology. J Chronic Dis 1982;35:101–114.
22. Gordon DJ, Salz KM, Roggenhamp KJ, Franklin FA. Dietary determinants of plasma cholesterol change in the recruitment phase of the Lipid Research Clinics Coronary Primary Prevention Trial. Arteriosclerosis 1982;2:537–548.
23. Vaswani AH. Effect of weight reduction on circulating lipids: an integration of possible mechanisms. J Am Coll Nutr 1983;2:123–132.
24. Carmena R, Ascaso JF, Tebar J, Soriano J. Changes in plasma high-density lipoproteins after body weight reduction in obese women. Int J Obes 1984;8:135–140.
25. Hegsted DM, McGandy RB, Myers ML, Store FJ. Quantitative effects of dietary fat on serum cholesterol in man. Am J Clin Nutr 1965;17:281–295. [Excellent references from articles dated from 1952 to 1965 are cited in this article.]
26. Gorder DD, Dolecek TA, Coleman GC, et al. Dietary intake in the Multiple Risk Factor Intervention Trial (MRFIT): nutrient and food group changes over 6 years. J Am Diet Assoc 1986;86:744–751.
27. Daniel-Gentry J, Dolecek TA, Caggiula AW, et al. Increasing use of meatless meals: a nutrition intervention substudy in the Multiple Risk Factor Intervention Trial (MRFIT). J Am Diet Assoc 1986;86:778–781.
28. Jones DY, Judd JT, Taylor PR, et al. Influence of caloric contribution and saturation of dietary fat on plasma lipids in premenopausal women. Am J Clin Nutr 1987;45:1451–1456.
29. Cressman MD, Hoogwerf BJ, Naito HK, et al. Hypercholesterolemia: roles of the physician and registered dietitian. Cleve Clin J Med 1988;55:498–499.
30. Vessby B, Gustafsson IB, Buberg J, et al. Substituting polyunsaturated for saturated fat as a single change in a Swedish diet: effects on serum lipoprotein metabolism and glucose tolerance in patients with hyperlipoproteinemia. Eur J Clin Invest 1980;10:193–202.

31. Vega GL, Groszek E, Wolf R, Grundy SM. Influence of polyunsaturated fats on composition of plasma lipoproteins and apolipoproteins. J Lipid Res 1982;23:811–822.
32. Wolf RN, Grundy SM. Influence of exchanging carbohydrate for saturated fatty acids on plasma lipids and lipoproteins in men. J Nutr 1983;113:1521–1528.
33. Sacks FM, Ornish D, Rosner B, et al. Plasma lipoprotein levels in vegetarians: the effect of ingestion of fats from dairy products. JAMA 1985;254:1337–1341.
34. Mattson FH, Grundy SM. Comparison of effects of dietary saturated, monounsaturated and polyunsaturated fatty acids on plasma lipids and lipoproteins in men. J Lipid Res 1985;26:194–202.
35. Zanni EE, Zannis VI, Blum CB, et al. Effect of egg cholesterol and dietary fats on plasma lipids, lipoproteins and apoproteins of normal women consuming natural diets. J Lipid Res 1987;28:518–527.
36. Keys A, Anderson JT, Grande F. Serum cholesterol response to changes in the diet. II. The effect of cholesterol in the diet. Metabolism 1965;14:759–765.
37. Kelsey JL. A review of research on effects of fiber intake on man. Am J Clin Nutr 1978;31:142–159.
38. Anderson J, Story L, Sieling B, et al. Hypocholesterolemic effects of oat bran or bean intake for hypercholesterolemic men. Am J Clin Nutr 1984;40:1146–1155.
39. Van Hern BV, Liu K, Parker D, et al. Serum lipid response to the oat bran intake with a fat modified diet. J Am Diet Assoc 1986;86:759–764.
40. Kuske TT, Feldman EB. Hyperlipoproteinemia, atherosclerosis risk, and dietary management. Arch of Intern Med 1987;147:357–360.
41. American Diabetes Association. Nutritional recommendations and principles for individuals with diabetes mellitus: 1986. Diabetes Care 1987;10:126–132.
42. Keys A, Anderson JT, Grande F. Serum cholesterol response to changes in diet. I. Iodine value of dietary fat versus 25-P. Metabolism 1965;14:747–758.
43. NIH Consensus Conference. Treatment of hypertriglyceridemia. JAMA 1984;251:1196–1200.
44. Ginsberg H, Olesky J, Farquhar JW, Reaven GM. Moderate ethanol ingestion and plasma triglyceride levels. Ann Intern Med 1974;80:143–149.
45. Farquhar JW, Frank A, Gross RC, Reaven GM. Glucose, insulin, and triglyceride responses to high and low carbohydrate diets in man. J Clin Invest 1966;45:1648–1656.
46. Kohlmeier M, Stricker G, Schliert G. Influence of "normal" and "prudent" diets on biliary and serum lipids in healthy women. Am J Clin Nutr 1985;42:1201–1205.
47. Weisweiler P, Janetschek P, Schwendt P. Fat restriction alters the composition of apolipoprotein B-100 containing very low-density lipoproteins in humans. Am J Clin Nutr 1986;43:903–909.
48. Jones DY, Judd JT, Taylor PR, et al. Influence of caloric contribution and saturation of dietary fat on plasma lipids in premenopausal women. Am J Clin Nutr 1987;45:1451–1456.
49. Mattson FH, Grundy SM. Comparison of effects of dietary saturated monounsaturated and polyunsaturated fatty acids on plasma lipids and lipoproteins in man. J Lipid Res 1985;26:194–202.

50. Mensink RP, Katan MB. Effect of monounsaturated fatty acids versus complex carbohydrates on high-density lipoproteins in healthy men and women. Lancet 1987;1:122–125.

51. Sirtori CR, Tremoli E, Gatti E, et al. Controlled evaluation of fat intake in the Mediterranean diet. comparative activities of olive oil, corn oil on plasma lipids and platelets in high-risk patients. Am J Clin Nutr 1986;44:635–642.

52. Grundy SM. Comparison of monounsaturated fatty acids and carbohydrates for lowering plasma cholesterol. N Engl J Med 1986;314:745–748.

53. Dyerberg J, Bong HD. A hypothesis on the development of acute myocardial infarction in Greenlanders. Scand J Clin Lab Invest 1982;42:7–13.

54. Herold PM, Kinsella JE. Fish oil consumption and decreased risk of cardiovascular disease: comparison of findings from animal and human feeding trials. Am J Clin Nutr 1986;43:566–598.

55. Sniderman AD, Shapiro S, Marpole D, et al. Association of coronary atherosclerosis with hyperapobetalipoproteinemia (increased protein but normal cholesterol levels) in human plasma low density liproteins. Proc Natl Acad Sci USA 1980;77:604–608.

56. Sniderman AD, Wolfson C, Terg B, et al. Association of hyperapobetalipoproteinemia with endogenous hypertriglyceridemia and atherosclerosis. Ann Intern Med 1982;97:833–839.

57. Shepherd J, Packard CJ, Patch JR, et al. Effects of dietary polyunsaturated and saturated fat on the properties of high density lipoproteins and the metabolism of apolipoproteins A-1. J Clin Invest 1978;57:1582–1592.

58. Schonfeld GW, Patch W, Rudel LL, et al. Effects of dietary cholesterol and fatty acids on plasma lipoproteins. J Clin Invest 1982;69:1072–1080.

59. Weiswerter P, Janetschek P, Schwondt P. Fat restriction alters the composition of apolipoprotein B-100 containing very low-density lipoproteins in humans. Am J Clin Nutr 1986;43:903–909.

60. Majonnier MC, Hall Y, Berkson DM, et al. Experience in changing food habits of hyperlipidemic men and women. J Am Diet Assoc 1980;77:140–148.

61. DeBakey ME, Gotto AM, Scott YW, Foreyt JP. Diet, nutrition and heart disease. J Am Diet Assoc 1986;86:729–731.

12
Drugs in the Management of Lipid Disorders

DAVID W. BILHEIMER

Clinical disease can occur when certain plasma lipoprotein levels are too low or too high.[1] Frequently both abnormalities are found in the same patient, e.g., low high density lipoprotein (HDL) cholesterol and high low density lipoprotein (LDL) cholesterol in a patient at risk for atherosclerosis. The term *dyslipoproteinemia* has been used to refer to this general clinical problem, and the major clinical sequelae associated with dyslipoproteinemia include atherosclerosis, pancreatitis, and xanthoma formation.[1] Reducing the risk for these clinical sequelae is the primary goal of therapy in the dyslipoproteinemic patient. If the dyslipoproteinemia cannot be adequately controlled with appropriate life style changes, dietary therapy including calorie reduction, or control of a primary causative disorder (e.g., diabetes mellitus; hypothyroidism), drug therapy must be considered in order to achieve the desired therapeutic goals.[2,3]

The decision to use drug therapy is important for several reasons. First, drug therapy for dyslipoproteinemia is likely to be long term unless it is accompanied by other major changes such as significant weight loss or a substantial modification of eating habits. Second, drug therapy adds cost to the care of the patient, not only for the drug but for the additional laboratory tests and physician visits required for appropriate follow-up. Third, drug therapy may be associated with side effects, which can be troublesome and occasionally serious. Because lipid-lowering drugs are commonly used for years it is important to know if they are safe in long-term therapy, and this information is not always available. Fourth, the benefits of drug therapy in women, with regard to reduction of subsequent cardiovascular risk, are not established by clinical trials as they are for men. Although cardiovascular disease is the leading cause of death in women, it usually is delayed in onset about 10 years compared to men and therefore does not begin to be clinically apparent until after menopause.[4,5] This 10-year difference in age of onset of atherosclerotic disease is also observed between affected men and women in families with familial hypercholesterolemia for reasons that have yet to be defined.[6,7] These sex differences have led to the impression that women are "spared" or "protected" from the ravages of atherosclerosis for at least a decade and therefore require less aggressive therapy for their dyslipoproteinemia than do men. It is partly for this reason that women were excluded from most clinical trials of lipid-lowering drug therapy in high risk patients. Consequently, there are few data to indicate whether therapy of dyslipoproteinemia in women does lower subsequent cardiovascular risk. The decision to use drug therapy in a woman must therefore be based on the total risk factor profile of the patient, and the potential benefit of therapy must be estimated from clinical trial results involving only men.

Because coronary heart disease emerges as the leading cause of morbidity and mortality in postmenopausal women and the major cardiovascular risk factors, including hypercholesterolemia, are predictive of risk in this age group,[4,5,8] there is a growing consensus that plasma lipids should be tested as part of an evaluation of cardiovascular risk in women.[2] Women identified to be at high risk should be appropriately treated to control their cardiovascular risk factors, which includes control of hypercholesterolemia due to elevated LDL cholesterol levels.

General Approach to the Patient

A complete history and physical examination are performed along with basic laboratory tests. The history includes questions about the menstrual history (especially frequency of periods, regularity, duration, date of last normal and preceding periods, date and character of menopause), the endocrine system (especially hair distribution, goiter, dryness of skin and hair, intolerance to heat or cold, polyphagia, polydipsia, polyuria), medications taken regularly, and the cardiovascular risk factor profile (Table 12–1). The physical examination includes thyroid and pelvic examinations. Specific note is made of an arcus cornea, xanthelasmas on the eyelids, and cutaneous or tendon xanthomas on the extremities. Peripheral pulses are evaluated for intensity, and major arteries are auscultated to detect the presence of vascular bruits.

In a routine visit in a general medical practice, a nonfasting cholesterol level is the most cost-effective way to screen for hyperlipidemia. Detection of an abnormal level should be followed with additional testing as determined by the clinical setting.

However, in practices specializing in women, a simple measure of the total cholesterol level may be misleading because of the tendency for women to have higher total cholesterol levels owing to having higher HDL cholesterol levels. This situation is encountered, for example, in women receiving estrogen replacement therapy. In such cases, it is reasonable to proceed directly to a measure of the fasting cholesterol, triglyceride, and

TABLE 12-1. Major cardiovascular risk factors other than cholesterol and LDL cholesterol to consider in the evaluation and treatment of hypercholesterolemia

Male gender
Family history of premature coronary heart disease: a myocardial infarction or sudden death
    before age 55 years in a parent or sibling
Cigarette smoking: currently smokes more than ten cigarettes per day
Hypertension
Low HDL cholesterol level: below 35 mg/dl and confirmed by repeated measurement
Diabetes mellitus
History of definite cerebrovascular or occlusive peripheral vascular disease
Severe obsity ($\geq$ 30% over weight)

Adapted and modified from the Report on the National Cholesterol Education Program expert panel on detection, evaluation and treatment of high blood cholesterol in adults. Arch Intern Med 1988;148:36–69.

HDL cholesterol levels (lipoprotein measurement). It is also reasonable to proceed initially with a total lipoprotein measurement if a primary or secondary form of hyperlipidemia is suspected at the outset, if the patient has other known risk factors for cardiovascular disease, or if the patient has suspected polycystic ovarian syndrome with hyperandrogenism and a low HDL cholesterol level.[2,3,9]

It is important to detect and treat obvious lipoprotein abnormalities associated with primary forms of hyperlipoproteinemia.[3] It is also important to detect hyperlipidemia secondary to other conditions, as treatment of the primary disorder may ameliorate or correct the hyperlipidemia. In women, in whom hormonal therapy may elevate the lipoprotein levels, the potential benefits of hormone therapy must be weighed against any adverse effects on the lipoproteins, unless the changes are clearly clinically significant (e.g., triglyceride levels > 300–500 mg/dl) and require discontinuation of hormone therapy. Most patients with hyperlipidemia in routine practice have mild forms of hypercholesterolemia rather than one of the primary disorders described in Chapter 3.

Guidelines for a general approach to the patient with hypercholesterolemia have been developed by the National Cholesterol Education Program (NCEP).[2] The initial assessment of the patient over age 20 years begins with measurement of the total cholesterol level. The interpretation of the result is outlined in Table 12-2. The LDL cholesterol level is a better predictor of risk and can be calculated from the total cholesterol, HDL cholesterol, and total triglyceride levels if a fasting specimen is obtained for assay (Table 12-2). High-risk total cholesterol and LDL cholesterol levels are 240 and 160 mg/dl, respectively. These cutoff points are derived primarily from values obtained in middle-aged men. Most premenopausal women have lower LDL cholesterol levels in conjunction with a total

TABLE 12–2. Assessment of blood cholesterol levels regarding risk for CHD in adults 20 years of age and older: interpretation of total cholesterol and LDL cholesterol levels

Cholesterol level (mg/dl)		
Total	LDL[a]	Interpretation
< 200	< 130	Desirable level
200–239	130–159	Borderline high-risk level
≥ 240	≥ 160	High-risk range

Adapted and modified from the Report on the National Cholesterol Education Program expert panel on detection, evaluation and treatment of high blood cholesterol in adults. Arch Intern Med 1988;148:36–69.
[a]LDL cholesterol is calculated with the following equation:

$$\text{LDL cholesterol} = \text{total cholesterol} - \text{HDL cholesterol} - (\text{triglyceride}/5)$$

The formula loses accuracy when triglyceride levels exceed 400 mg/dl.

cholesterol of 240 mg/dl than most men due to an increased HDL cholesterol contribution to the total cholesterol level in women.

The NCEP guidelines have been criticized for placing too much emphasis on the LDL cholesterol while ignoring the predictive value of the HDL cholesterol level regarding cardiovascular risk. The beneficial effects of lowering LDL cholesterol are better established by clinical trials.[2,3] There is no clear evidence that raising the HDL cholesterol level is beneficial,[10] although the results of the Helsinki Heart Trial with gemfibrozil are suggestive.[11,12] General measures such as smoking cessation, weight loss, and aerobic exercise may raise the HDL cholesterol level. Drugs that lower the plasma cholesterol level (cholestyramine, lovastatin) also raise the HDL cholesterol level to varying degrees (see below). Two lipid-altering drugs, gemfibrozil and nicotinic acid, are especially effective in raising HDL cholesterol levels. However, because knowledge about the physiology of HDL is incomplete, a recommendation to use drug therapy to specifically raise low HDL cholesterol levels cannot be made at this time.[10]

Recommendations for the follow-up and treatment of adults classified by total cholesterol and LDL cholesterol levels are summarized in Table 12–3.[2] Note that treatment is influenced by the presence or absence of coronary heart disease or other coronary risk factors, and that minimal goals of therapy are recommended. Because the risk factors include male gender, these recommendations are more aggressive for men than for women; that is, a hypercholesterolemic man with one other risk factor is a candidate for aggressive medical intervention, whereas a hypercholesterolemic woman requires two other risk factors before more aggressive medical intervention is recommended. This difference in approach to women reflects

TABLE 12–3. NCEP recomendations for follow-up and treatment of adults classified by total cholesterol and LDL cholesterol levels: considerations based on the presence or absence of CHD and other cardiovascular risk factors

Initial finding (mg/dl)	Follow-up
Total cholesterol measurement	
< 200	Repeat total cholesterol within 5 years
200–239	
Without CHD or two other CHD risk factors[a]	Dietary information and recheck annually
With CHD or two other CHD risk factors[a]	Lipoprotein analysis; then take further action based on LDL cholesterol level (see below)
≥ 240	

Initial (mg/dl)	Suggested treatment	Minimal goal of therapy (mg/dl)
LDL cholesterol measurement[a]		
Without CHD or two other cardiovascular risk factors[b]		
≥ 160	Diet	< 160
≥ 190	Diet and drug treatment[c]	< 160
With CHD or two other cardiovascular risk factors[b]		
≥ 130	Diet	< 130
≥ 160	Diet and drug treatment[c]	< 130

Adapted and modified from the Report on the National Cholesterol Education Program expert panel on detection, evaluation and treatment of high blood cholesterol in adults. Arch Intern Med 1988;148:36–69.
[a] Risk factors include male gender, family history of premature CHD, cigarette smoking, hypertension, reduced HDL cholesterol levels, diabetes mellitus, severe obesity, definite cerebrovascular or peripheral vascular disease.
[b] LDL is calculated as described in the legend to Table 12–2.
[c] Drug treatment should not be automatically initiated but is considered if dietary therapy does not achieve desired therapeutic goals.

a lower rate of cardiovascular morbidity and mortality during middle age and later years of life.[2,4,5]

Diagnosis and treatment should not be undertaken on the basis of a single set of lipid and lipoprotein determinations. Two or three sets of measurements 2 to 8 weeks apart are recommended before diagnosing and treating the patient.[2] Spacing of measurements in this manner should minimize any minor changes in lipids and lipoproteins that occur during different phases of the menstrual cycle.[13]

The diagnostic considerations when the results of the plasma cholesterol

TABLE 12–4. Diagnostic considerations in patients with hyperlipoproteinemia

Phenotype	Lipoprotein abnormality(ies)	Typical cholesterol and triglyceride values (mg/dl)[a]	Diagnostic considerations of primary hyperlipoproteinemia	Conditions causing secondary hyperlipidemia
1	↑ Chylomicrons	Chol 300–400 Trig 3000–6000	Familial lipoprotein lipase deficiency Familial apo C-II deficiency	Systemic lupus erythematosus
2a	↑ LDL	Chol 300–400 Trig 100	Familial hypercholesterolemia Polygenic hypercholesterolemia Familial multiple lipoprotein-type hyperlipoproteinemia Familial defective apo B-100	Hypothyroidism, nephrotic syndrome, hepatoma, Cushing syndrome, dysglobulinemia, acute intermittent prophyria, contraceptive steroids, cyclosporine, anorexia nervosa, Werner syndrome, ateliotic dwarfism
2b	↑ LDL ↑ VLDL	Chol 300–400 Trig 250–500	Familial hypercholesterolemia Familial multiple lipoprotein-type hyperlipoproteinemia Familial defective apo B-100	
3	↑ Remnants of VLDL and chylomicron catabolism	Chol 300–500 Trig 300–800	Familial type 3 hyperlipoproteinemia Familial hepatic lipase deficiency	Dysglobulinemia
4	↑ VLDL	Chol 200–250 Trig 300–700	Familial hypertriglyceridemia Familial multiple lipoprotein-type hyperlipoproteinemia	Diabetes mellitus, estrogen therapy, ateliotic dwarfism, acromegaly, glucocorticoid therapy or Cushing syndrome, lipodystrophy, type I glycogen storage disease, uremia, nephrotic syndrome, acute viral hepatitis, dysglobulinemia; therapy with isotretinoin, thiazides, β-adrenergic blocking drugs, or tamoxifen; alcoholic hyperlipidemia; third trimester pregnancy
5	↑ Chylomicrons ↑ VLDL	Chol 600–800 Trig 2000–6000	Familial hypertriglyceridemia Familial multiple lipoprotein-type hyperlipoproteinemia	Poorly controlled diabetes mellitus, estrogen therapy, lipodystrophy, type I glycogen storage disease, alcoholic hyperlipidemia

Adapted and modified from Bilheimer DW. In: Kelley WN, De Vita VT Jr, DuPont HL, et al, eds. *Textbook of Internal Medicine.* Philadelphia: Lippincott, 1989:2333–2339.

[a] These values are typical ranges of results to provide perspective, but other values are possible.

and triglyceride tests document hyperlipoproteinemia are summarized in Table 12–4. This table also lists the phenotypic description of the patient based on the lipoprotein abnormalities encountered in the plasma. Lipoprotein phenotypes are declining from clinical use but are still encountered in the medical literature. In addition, many of the reports about drug efficacy describe the patients by their lipoprotein phenotypes. For these reasons, the phenotypes are provided for reference, but it should be emphasized that genetic diagnoses, when possible, are preferred for classifying patients.

Many of the severe forms of hyperlipoproteinemia require drug therapy. However, not all primary hyperlipoproteinemias respond to such treatment. A summary of the primary hyperlipoproteinemias and the suggested drug therapies for them are provided in Table 12–5.

As indicated in Table 12–3, when hyperlipidemia is confirmed in a patient and treatment is being planned, the initial step is dietary therapy, as described in Chapter 10. If dietary treatment is not adequate to lower the cholesterol level to the therapeutic goal, consideration must be given to drug treatment. The major approved drugs for hypercholesterolemia are the bile acid sequestrants (cholestyramine and colestipol), fibric acid derivatives (clofibrate and gemfibrozil), inhibitors of 3-hydroxy-3-methylglutaryl coenzyme A (HMG CoA) reductase (lovastatin), nicotinic acid, and probucol. Neomycin is occasionally used for hypercholesterolemia but does not have U.S. Food and Drug Administration (FDA) approval for this purpose. Fewer drugs are available for treating hypertriglyceridemia; they include the fibric acid derivatives and nicotinic acid. A summary of the major drugs used for hypercholesterolemia, including their doses, mechanisms of action, and common side effects, are provided in Table 12–6.

Hypolipidemic drugs are used singly or in various combinations to lower plasma lipid levels to the desired therapeutic range.[3,14] It is now clear from the results of several therapeutic trials that control of hypercholesterolemia in high risk patients does lower the subsequent risk for cardiovascular disease.[2] This long-range therapeutic benefit has been demonstrated with cholestyramine, nicotinic acid, and gemfibrozil used singly or with colestipol/nicotinic acid and colestipol/lovastatin combination therapy. The data have largely been obtained in middle-aged men, and any benefits of therapy to women must be inferred from these results. It is also not clear if any benefits of therapy apply equally to women of all ages. However, given the positive trial results in men, it is probable that women at high risk also benefit from therapy. Therefore it is increasingly important for the physician to detect hypercholesterolemia in women and to be aware of the therapeutic options available for the control of this major cardiovascular risk factor. Elevated triglyceride levels (i.e., 800–1000 mg/dl) also require medical attention because they increase the risk for pancreatitis.[2,3]

TABLE 12–5. Suggested drug therapies for the primary hyperlipoproteinemias

Primary disorder	Biochemical defect	Plasma lipoproteins elevated	Drug therapy	
			First-choice drugs	Second-line drugs
Monogenic disorders				
Familial lipoprotein lipase deficiency	Lipoprotein lipase deficiency	Chylomicrons	None	None
Familial apo C-II deficiency	Apo CII deficiency	Chylomicrons, VLDLs	None	None
Familial type 3 hyperlipoproteinemia	Abnormal apo E structure	Chylomicron and VLDL remnants	Gemfibrozil, nicotinic acid	Clofibrate, lovastatin
Familial hepatic lipase deficiency	Hepatic lipase deficiency	VLDL remnants and HDL_2	Not established	Not established
Familial hypercholesterolemia	LDL-receptor deficiency	LDLs	Colestipol, cholestyramine, lovastatin, nicotinic acid; frequently two or more drugs are combined	Probucol, neomycin

Familial defective apo B-100	Defective apo B-100 with reduced affinity for LDL receptor	LDLs	Not established but lovastatin or nicotinic acid should be tried	Unknown
Familial multiple lipoprotein type hyperlipoproteinemia	Unknown	VLDLs and LDLs; rarely chylomicrons	Nicotinic acid, gemfibrozil; frequently two drugs are combined	Lovastatin, clofibrate
Familial hypertriglyceridemia	Unknown	VLDLs; rarely chylomicrons	Nicotinic acid, gemfibrozil	Clofibrate
Multifactorial disorders Polygenic hypercholesterolemia	Unknown	LDLs	Colestipol, cholestyramine, nicotinic acid, lovastatin	Gemfibrozil, probucol
Sporadic hypertriglyceridemia	Unknown	VLDLs; occasionally chylomicrons	Similar to familial hypertriglyceridemia	

Adapted and modified from Brown MS, Goldstein JL. In: Gilman AG, Goodman LS, Rall TW, et al, eds. *Goodman and Gilman's The Pharmacological Basis of Therapeutics.* 7th Ed. New York: Macmillan, 1985:827–845.

TABLE 12–6. Summary of major drugs used for hypercholesterolemia

Drugs	Usual daily dose	Major lipoprotein decreased	Mechanism of action	Common side effects and precautions
Cholestyramine Colestipol	16–24 g 20–30 g	LDL LDL	Promotes bile acid excretion; stimulates LDL-receptor-mediated removal of LDL	Gastrointestinal symptoms, including constipation; may alter absorption of other drugs and increase triglyceride levels in patients prone to hypertriglyceridemia
Nicotinic acid	3–6 g	VLDL, LDL	Decreases VLDL synthesis	Abnormal liver function; hyperuricemia; hyperglycemia; pruritus and cutaneous flushing; heartburn
Lovastatin	20–80 mg	LDL, VLDL	Specific inhibitor of cholesterol biosynthesis; induces LDL-receptor expression	Abnormal liver function; myositis; mild gastrointestinal distress; (?) corneal opacities
Gemfibrozil	1.2 g	VLDL, LDL	Decreases VLDL synthesis; may stimulate lipoprotein lipase activity	May increase LDL cholesterol in hypertriglyceridemic patients; may promote lithogenic bile and gallstone formation; myopathy; gastrointestinal complaints
Probucol	1 g	LDL, HDL	May enhance non-LDL-receptor clearance of LDL; antioxidant properties may protect LDL from oxidation and subsequent uptake by tissue macrophages	Diarrhea and other gastrointestinal complaints; may prolong QT interval; is stored in adipose tissue and has a prolonged washout phase when discontinued

Adapted and modified from Bilheimer DW. In: Kelley WN, DeVita VT Jr, DuPont HL, et al, eds. *Textbook of Internal Medicine.* Philadelphia: Lippincott, 1989:2333–2339.

Drugs that Alter Plasma Lipoprotein Concentrations

Bile Acid Sequestrants (Cholestyramine and Colestipol)

Chemistry and Pharmacology

Bile acid sequestrants have been used to treat hypercholesterolemia for more than two decades. The drugs currently available in the United States are cholestyramine (Questran®) and colestipol (Colestid®). These two drugs have the same mechanism of action and similar therapeutic effectiveness.

Cholestyramine, which is insoluble in water, is administered orally as a suspension in a liquid selected by the patient (i.e., water, orange juice). It is not absorbed from the gastrointestinal tract.[15,16] It is eliminated in the stool and may induce constipation by reducing the intraluminal bile salt concentration. Its rate of elimination is influenced by factors that alter gastrointestinal motility (i.e., dietary fiber, Lomotil).[14]

Colestipol is a slightly yellow granular substance that, like cholestyramine, is taken orally in liquid suspension and is not absorbed from the gastrointestinal tract. Factors affecting its actions and effects in the gastrointestinal tract are similar to those for cholestyramine.[17]

Mechanism of Action

The cholesterol-lowering action of cholestyramine and colestipol relates to their properties as bile acid sequestrants. Bile acids, which facilitate digestion of dietary lipid, normally undergo an enterohepatic circulation. This process involves secretion of bile acids via the common bile duct into the intestinal lumen followed by reabsorption in the terminal ileum and return to the liver for additional cycles (Fig. 12–1A). Only a small fraction of the bile acid pool is normally excreted in the stool each day.[16] The bile acid sequestrants bind bile acids in the gut and accelerate their excretion in the stool (Fig. 12–1B), which in turn causes the hepatic bile acid pool to drop. The liver then responds by converting more cholesterol to bile acids. To meet the increased demands for cholesterol, hepatocytes express more LDL receptors to remove LDL cholesterol from the plasma, and they synthesize more cholesterol from acetate via HMG CoA (Fig. 12–1B). LDL-receptor stimulation increases the rate of removal of LDL from plasma, and the LDL cholesterol level drops.[18] Bile acid sequestrants may also alter the composition of plasma lipoproteins, but the therapeutic implications of these changes are currently unknown.[19] Bile acid sequestrants also accelerate the rate of secretion of very low density lipoprotein (VLDL) from the liver,[20] and this effect is thought to explain the increase in triglycerides that commonly occurs during treatment with these drugs.[21]

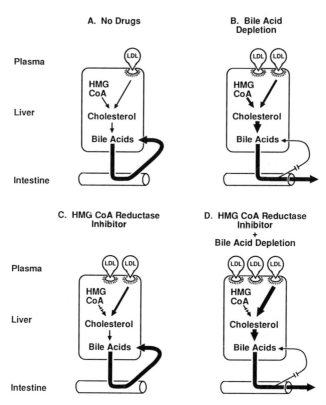

FIGURE 12–1. Hepatic LDL-receptor stimulation during therapy of hypercholesterolemia. Panel A reflects hepatic cholesterol homeostasis when no drugs are given. The other panels illustrate major changes induced by therapy with various drugs that alter cholesterol synthesis or bile acid reabsorption from the intestine. See text for details. (Reprinted from Bilheimer and East,[14] by courtesy of Marcel Dekker, Inc.)

Adverse Effects and Drug Interactions

Toxicity from cholestyramine appears to be low. Although cholestyramine has been implicated in increasing intestinal cancer in rats treated with various carcinogens,[22,23] there was no significant increase in the incidence of malignant gastrointestinal neoplasms in patients taking cholestyramine compared to placebo in the Lipid Research Clinics Coronary Primary Prevention Trial.[24]

The most common side effects are abdominal pain, belching, bloating, constipation, heartburn, and nausea.[24] In the Lipid Research Clinics Coronary Primary Prevention Trial (LRC-CPPT), the participants reporting moderate or severe side effects with cholestyramine compared to baseline before drug therapy were as follows: abdominal pain (10%), belching or bloating (17%), constipation (35%), diarrhea (5%), gas (10%), heartburn (17%), nausea (13%), and vomiting (4%). These effects were noted especially during the first year of therapy and tended to decline thereafter. Thirty-four percent of patients had at least one gastrointestinal complaint during the first year of cholestyramine treatment, but by the seventh year the percent of complaints was no greater than during the pretreatment phase of the study.[24] However, only 51% of the patients in the LRC-CPPT were able to continue with the maximum dose of cholestyramine (24 g/day) prescribed.[21] The remainder took variable amounts of the medication, ranging from none to 20 g/day.[21] Thus compliance remains a problem, but it may improve if the patient is instructed in the use of the drug, the expected side effects, and the goals of therapy.

Less common problems include aggravation of hemorrhoids and perianal rash. Rare allergic reactions occur to one or more of the components mixed with the resins.

Large doses of bile acid sequestrants may induce steatorrhea in experimental subjects,[25] but fat malabsorption has not been encountered at standard therapeutic doses.[24,26] When bile acid sequestrants have been used to treat children with familial hypercholesterolemia, there has been no evidence for sustained malabsorption or deficiency of fat-soluble vitamins.[26,27]

There are a number of drug interactions that occur as a result of altered intestinal absorption of other drugs.[14,28] These affected drugs include various antibiotics, antiinflammatory agents, cardiac glycosides, coumarin anticoagulants, diuretics, glucocorticoids, propranolol, thyroid hormones, and tolbutamide (for review, see ref. 14, 17, and 28) (Table 12–7). To reduce the magnitude of this problem, the current approach is to empirical-

TABLE 12–7. Drugs with impaired gastrointestinal absorption during bile acid sequestrant therapy

Digoxin
Digitoxin
Warfarin
Chlorothiazide
Hydrochlorothiazide
Iopanoic Acid (Telepaque)
Propranolol
Levothyroxine
Levotriiodothyronine
Glucocorticoids
Tetracycline
Potassium penicillin G

Summarized from references 14, 17, and 28.

ly separate the doses of cholestyramine by 2 to 4 hours from the administration of other medications. On occasion, hypercholesterolemic patients with complex medical problems requiring several other medications may not be able to schedule cholestyramine (or colestipol) doses adequately with the others; in such cases, another cholesterol-lowering drug should be tried if cholesterol-lowering drug therapy is clinically indicated.

Cholestyramine does not appear to affect the absorption of methyldopa, phentoin, or tolbutamide.[14,28] It also does not interfere with the therapeutic efficacy of most other lipid-lowering drugs given simultaneously.[29-33]

Although drug interactions with colestipol are often similar to those for cholestyramine, there are some differences. The rate of aspirin absorption, for example, is increased by colestipol but decreased by cholestyramine; however, neither drug significantly affects absorption of the total aspirin dose.[28] Nevertheless, unless specific data suggest otherwise, it is prudent to assume that drug interactions documented for cholestyramine are also likely to occur with colestipol[17,28] (Table 12–4). Therefore the same general recommendations and precautions given for cholestyramine also apply when using colestipol with other drugs. Colestipol may be combined with other lipid-lowering drugs to increase the lipid-lowering effect achieved using single drug therapy,[17,33,34] but colestipol may interfere with the bioavailability of gemfibrozil.[35]

Clinical Indications and Effectiveness

Cholestyramine and colestipol are indicated for the treatment of primary hypercholesterolemia, particularly that caused by heterozygous familial hypercholesterolemia or polygenic hypercholesterolemia[34,36] (Table 12–5). These drugs lower the plasma cholesterol level by up to 25% and LDL cholesterol by 30% or more.[34]

The benefits of chronic therapy with cholestyramine to control hypercholesterolemia were demonstrated by the LRC-CPPT.[21,24] In this trial 1906 middle-aged men with hypercholesterolemia were treated with a fixed dose of cholestyramine (24 g/day) and a low cholesterol, low fat diet. The control group received placebo plus diet therapy. After 7 years of follow-up, the total and LDL cholesterol levels in the cholestyramine-treated group decreased an average of 8% and 12%, respectively, compared to the placebo-treated group. The change was associated with an average 19% reduction in the incidence of CHD compared to the placebo-treated group. Subjects in this study who consistently took the maximum dose of drug prescribed (24 g/day) experienced a 19% reduction in total cholesterol, a 28% reduction in LDL cholesterol, and a 4% increase in HDL cholesterol.[21] Total plasma triglycerides increased 17% on the maximal dosage of cholestyramine. This subset of patients experienced a 39% reduction in subsequent cardiovascular risk.

Cholestyramine treatment has also reduced the rate of progression of coronary atherosclerosis in patients classified as having type II hyperlipidemia.[37,38] Although colestipol has not been as thoroughly studied, it is assumed that treatment of hypercholesterolemia with colestipol would produce results similar to those described for cholestyramine regarding cardiovascular risk.

Preparation, Dosage, and Contraindications

The unit dose of cholestyramine is 4 g, and the standard dose varies from 8 to 24 g of active drug given twice daily. Patients frequently are unable to tolerate the largest dose (24 g/day), and it is often necessary to use a maintenance dose of 16 g/day. "Low dose" therapy with 8 g/day may be nearly as effective as a dose of 16 g/day, and this approach should be considered in patients who cannot tolerate large doses of cholestyramine.[39] Low dose therapy has also been recommended for use in elderly patients with hypercholesterolemia.[40] Several formulations are available, including the standard preparation (Questran®), a low-calorie version (Questran Light®), and a flavored bar containing 4 g of active drug (Cholybar®). Patient preference and cost generally dictate the formulation selected. Powdered versions are available in unit dose packets or in bulk form where individual doses are measured by a scoop. Generally, the bulk form is less expensive than the unit dose packets. The powdered form must be mixed with liquid as a suspension before being consumed. Formulations with greater binding capacity and less bulk are under development.[41]

Colestipol (Colestid) is available in powder form at a unit dose of 5 g, and the dosage ranges from 10 to 30 g/day with a usual maintenance dose of 20 g/day given in two equal doses. Colestipol is available in 5-g packets and 500-g bottles. Each dose must be suspended in liquid before it is consumed. As with cholestyramine, the bulk form of colestipol is generally less expensive than the unit dose packets.

Cholestyramine and colestipol are contraindicated in patients with complete biliary obstruction where bile acids are unable to enter the gastrointestinal tract, but they can be used safely in most other patients with hepatic disease. These agents are also contraindicated in patients who develop hypersensitivity to any of the ingredients in the formulations. Safe use of these agents during pregnancy has not been established, and no studies on the safety of these drugs during chronic therapy in children have been published. These drugs should be avoided in patients with moderate-to-severe hypertriglyceridemia because they aggravate the hypertriglyceridemia.[42]

Fibric Acid Derivatives

Fibric acid derivatives are used throughout the world for treatment of hyperlipidemia. The group currently includes clofibrate, gemfibrozil, bezafibrate, and fenofibrate. Only clofibrate and gemfibrozil are available in the

United States. Clofibrate was the first drug in this class to be used for treating hyperlipidemia, but its use was associated with toxic effects in the World Health Organization (WHO) drug trial.[43] Consequently, it has been largely replaced by gemfibrozil in the United States. All members of the class are effective triglyceride-lowering agents, but their effects on plasma cholesterol vary. The precise mechanisms of action of this drug class are not clearly defined. A number of reviews, monographs, and symposia summarizing their mechanisms of action and use have been published.[44-61]

Clofibrate

Chemistry and Pharmacology

Clofibrate (Atromid-S®) is administered orally, and absorption from the gut is virtually complete. After absorption, clofibrate is rapidly hydrolyzed to parachlorophenoxyisobutyric acid (CPIB) by tissue and serum esterases. CPIB is the active form of the drug and is highly bound to serum proteins, especially albumin.

Approximately 60 to 95% of the drug is conjugated, primarily as glucuronide, mainly in the liver and to a limited extent in the kidney. The major route of excretion is via the kidneys, and negligible quantities appear in feces. Significant biliary secretion of the drug does occur in some species, suggesting an active enterohepatic circulation for the drug.[45] In renal failure, the half-life of CPIB is prolonged because renal clearance of the unbound drug is reduced. Clearance of the drug is also reduced in patients with cirrhosis.[45]

Mechanisms of Action

The mechanisms of action of clofibrate are not well defined. The drug produces a wide array of biochemical changes, but only a few relate clearly to changes in plasma lipid and lipoprotein levels.[44,61] Clofibrate increases tissue activity levels of both hepatic triglyceride lipase and lipoprotein lipase,[62,63] thereby enhancing the rate of catabolism of VLDL to intermediate density lipoprotein (IDL) and LDL.[64] In some patients, clofibrate reduces the production of VLDL triglyceride, but in others it has little or no effect.[65] Clofibrate may decrease the rate of formation of LDL but has little effect on the catabolism of this lipoprotein.[66]

The mechanisms of action of the fibrates are discussed in more detail in the section on gemfibrozil.

Adverse Effects and Drug Interactions

Clofibrate causes several adverse effects including an approximately twofold increase in the incidence of gallstones.[67] This effect is due to the fact that clofibrate causes human bile to become supersaturated with cholesterol, thereby promoting gallstone formation.[58] More significant was the finding in the WHO study that the patient group treated with clofibrate experienced 25% more deaths than the comparable high cholesterol placebo group.[43] No one disease accounted for this increase in deaths, and no clear explanation for the excess mortality in the drug-treated group was apparent. This adverse effect was no longer apparent in a post-trial evaluation conducted 8 years later.[68]

Clinical side effects with clofibrate are not common, and the drug is generally well tolerated. Side effects include decreased libido, breast tenderness, increased appetite, and mild gastrointestinal complaints (nausea and abdominal pain).[69] Physical findings included palpable spleen and liver enlargement. Laboratory abnormalities include lower mean bilirubin, alkaline phosphatase, hematocrit, and neutrophil counts, and higher mean levels of SGOT, creatine kinase, blood urea nitrogen, and serum potassium.[69] The reasons for the hepatic enlargement and hepatic dysfunction during clofibrate therapy are unknown. Clofibrate has been associated with the appearance of a skeletal muscle syndrome that includes myalgias, muscle stiffness, weakness, malaise, muscle tenderness, and elevated plasma levels of muscle-derived enzymes (creatine kinase and alanine aminotransferase).[70] The syndrome is reversible when the drug is withdrawn.

Clofibrate may interact with warfarin to markedly increase the anticoagulant effect. The anticoagulant dosage should be halved and the coagulation status monitored closely when clofibrate therapy is initiated. This interaction was originally thought to occur because CPIB binds to albumin at a different site than warfarin and noncompetitively inhibits its binding, thereby increasing the free warfarin concentration and its anticoagulant effect. However, with a pure displacement interaction, the increased free concentration is compensated for by increased clearance so that at steady state the free warfarin concentration and pharmacologic effect is the same as before administration of a displacing drug.[46] Therefore the enhanced effect of warfarin by clofibrate cannot be explained by a binding interaction. It is now known that clofibrate alters the metabolism of the more active s-enantiomer of warfarin, possibly increasing its concentration and anticoagulant effect.[46] However, the mechanism responsible for the interaction of warfarin with clofibrate is still not fully established. Administration of clofibrate with rifampicin, a drug that induces hepatic microsomal enzyme activity, lowers plasma CPIB levels. Plasma CPIB levels are not affected by coadministration of either cholestyramine or colestipol. Therefore clofibrate and a bile acid sequestrant can be combined to treat patients with both hypercholesterolemia and hypertriglyceridemia.[71]

Clinical Indications and Effectiveness

Indications for the use of clofibrate are becoming progressively limited. It does not appear to reduce the risk for fatal cardiovascular heart disease and has produced significant adverse side effects.[72] It is an effective triglyceride-lowering agent, but its effects on cholesterol are variable.[73] It has been used effectively in patients with type 3, type 4, or type 5 hyperlipoproteinemia.[59,73–75] These three forms of hypertriglyceridemia are the current indications for the use of clofibrate.

Clofibrate therapy may raise the HDL cholesterol in patients with hypertriglyceridemia, but this effect is variable. The drug is not recommended to treat low HDL cholesterol levels.[10,76]

Preparation, Dosage, and Contraindications

Clofibrate is dispensed as 500 mg capsules. The usual dose is 2 g/day given in two equal doses. The drug should generally be avoided in patients with renal disease; however, if it is used in such patients, the dose should be reduced as dictated by the patient's renal function. In patients with cirrhosis, the dose should be decreased by 50%.

Clofibrate is contraindicated in pregnant women because its effects on the developing fetus are not known. It is relatively contraindicated in patients with significant hepatic or renal dysfunction. It is not known to benefit patients with hyperlipidemia related to primary biliary cirrhosis.

Gemfibrozil

Chemistry and Pharmacology

Gemfibrozil (Lopid®)is a fibric acid derivative that has been available in the United States for the treatment of hyperlipidemia since 1982. The drug is administered orally and is more rapidly absorbed than clofibrate. Drug data on the pharmacokinetics of gemfibrozil in humans are limited. Peak plasma concentrations occur 1 to 2 hours after dose administration and are proportional to the dose.[50] During repeated administration, the plasma levels tend to rise but reach steady-state levels within 7 to 14 days.[50] The usual dose of gemfibrozil is 600 mg twice daily. Gemfibrozil is highly bound to serum albumin (97.0–98.6%) at therapeutic concentrations.[50]

Data on the tissue distribution of gemfibrozil in humans have not been reported, but studies in experimental animals indicate that the drug does cross the placenta.[50] Furthermore, the plasma concentration of gemfibrozil is exceeded only by its concentration in those organs involved with its metabolism and excretion (liver and kidney).[50]

Gemfibrozil is converted by the liver in humans into four major metabolites.[50] The drug and its metabolites are excreted as the glucuronide conjugates into the bile and undergo enterohepatic circulation. During chronic therapy, two-thirds of a 600-mg dose is excreted in the urine within 5 days.

Data regarding the pharmacokinetics of gemfibrozil in patients with hepatic or renal disease are limited. Clearance of gemfibrozil and its elimination half-life may be independent of renal function[77]; furthermore, the drug has been used at full dosage to treat hyperlipemia for up to 6 months in small groups of patients with uremia or nephrotic syndrome.[48] There is no evidence that peritoneal dialysis or hemodialysis affects the clearance of gemfibrozil or its principal metabolite.

Mechanisms of Action

The mechanisms of action of gemfibrozil and the other fibric acid derivatives are not completely understood. In vitro, these drugs exhibit a wide array of effects, but how these effects correlate with in vivo therapeutic changes is not clear. The effects of fibrates on plasma lipids and lipoproteins have been reviewed elsewhere.[55,59]

Gemfibrozil lowers VLDL triglyceride levels by several mechanisms. It reduces the hepatic production of VLDL triglycerides, in part by direct inhibition of hepatic triglyceride synthesis and by reduced free fatty acid substrate delivery to the liver. The latter effect is due to fibrate-induced impairment of lipolysis and release of free fatty acids from adipose tissue.[51,52,55] Gemfibrozil also stimulates lipoprotein lipase activity, which enhances the fractional catabolic rate of VLDL triglycerides.[55,78] The composition of VLDL particles, which is often abnormal in hypertriglyceridemic states, also reverts to normal during gemfibrozil therapy.[49,51,55] The magnitude of postprandial hyperchylomicronemia is also reduced by gemfibrozil therapy, but the mechanism for this effect is unknown.[79] The above changes induced by gemfibrozil also reduce the plasma concentrations of chylomicron and VLDL remnants that accumulate in patients with familial type 3 hyperlipoproteinemia.[75,80]

Gemfibrozil and the other fibrates have variable effects on plasma LDL cholesterol levels, depending on the type of patient being treated.[14] In patients with hypertriglyceridemia, gemfibrozil lowers both the production and fractional clearance rates of LDL[81]; these changes may cause an increase in the LDL cholesterol concentration during therapy.[81] Fenofibrate has similar effects on LDL metabolism in hypertriglyceridemic patients and appears to reduce the clearance of LDL through non-LDL-receptor-mediated pathways while having little effect on the fractional clearance rate via the LDL receptor pathway.[82] Fenofibrate treatment in patients with heterozygous familial hypercholesterolemia lowers the plasma LDL cholesterol level modestly by stimulating both the fractional catabolic rate and the synthetic rate for LDL apo B-100.[83] The simultaneous stimulation of LDL synthesis and catabolism have the effect of increasing the turnover of LDL in plasma without substantially lowering its steady state concentration. Fibrates may inhibit HMG CoA reductase activity and thereby stimulate LDL receptor-mediated clearance of LDL from plasma,[84] but this inhibition of the enzyme in vitro occurs only at relatively high fibrate concentrations (1–3 mM) compared to concentrations of the specific HMG CoA reductase inhibitors such as mevastatin (30 nM).[49] Thus the effects of fibrates on HMG CoA reductase activity may be nonspecific.[49]

Furthermore, the LDL lowering effects of gemfibrozil and other fibrates observed clinically are much less than those observed with HMG CoA reductase inhibitors, suggesting that inhibition of HMG CoA reductase is not a major pharmacologic action of the fibrates.[85]

Therapy with fibric acid derivatives is frequently associated with increases in HDL cholesterol levels. This change is partly related to stimulation of lipoprotein lipase and hepatic triglyceride lipase, with enhanced catabolism of VLDL and generation of HDL[55,86] (see Chapter 3). However, studies with gemfibrozil in hypertriglyceridemic patients suggest that this drug may also increase the synthetic rates for apo A-I and apo A-II, the major apoproteins in HDL.[78] A similar effect on apo A-I and apo A-II synthesis was observed during fenofibrate therapy in patients with heterozygous familial hypercholesterolemia.[83] A mechanism for this direct stimulation of HDL apoprotein synthesis has not been defined, and it may not occur in all patients. In one study of normolipidemic subjects with hypoalphalipoproteinemia, gemfibrozil therapy caused only a small increase in HDL cholesterol and no significant change in apolipoproteins A-I and A-II.[87]

Gemfibrozil treatment decreases platelet reactivity in patients during exercise,[88] and it increases plasma kallikrein inhibitory activity and kininogen levels in patients with either type 2a or 2b hyperlipidemia.[89] However, gemfibrozil does not appear to affect plasma fibrinogen levels.[88] It has been suggested that some of the beneficial effects on coronary risk observed in the Helsinki Heart Trial might be explained by gemfibrozil's effects on platelet aggregation and other hemostatic parameters, but there are no firm data available to support this hypothesis.[11]

Adverse Effects and Drug Interactions

Gemfibrozil is well tolerated by patients. The largest clinical experience with the drug has been published by the Helsinki Heart Study investigators.[12] In that study, 11.3% of subjects receiving gemfibrozil (600 mg twice daily) during the first year reported moderate to severe upper gastrointestinal complaints compared to 7% in the placebo group. During subsequent years, these rates dropped to 2.4% and 1.2%, respectively. Gemfibrozil had no effect on the frequency of constipation, diarrhea, nausea, or vomiting.[12] There was no significant increase in the incidence of cancers or in overall mortality in the gemfibrozil-treated group compared to the placebo group.[12] Thus the apparent toxic effects noted with clofibrate in the WHO study[72] were not evident with gemfibrozil.[12] Patients receiving gemfibrozil in the Helsinki Heart Study did not require significantly more gallstone surgery than patients receiving the placebo.[12] However, lithogenicity of bile is increased with gemfibrozil treatment,[90] although the degree of cholesterol saturation may not be as great as during clofibrate therapy.[91]

Myositis occasionally observed during clofibrate therapy has not been well documented in gemfibrozil-treated patients with normal renal function. However, gemfibrozil treatment was associated with episodic asymptomatic plasma creatine kinase elevations in 6 of 18 patients with chronic renal failure of various etiologies (glomerular filtration rate 27.4 ± 8.8 ml/min/1.73 M[2]).[92] Serum drug concentrations did not progressively increase during the course of this trial.[92]

Abnormal liver function occasionally occurs but rarely requires discontinuation of therapy.[93] There is no evidence for hepatic peroxisome proliferation during gemfibrozil treatment in humans.[94] Baseline and periodic liver function tests are recommended during gemfibrozil treatment.

Rarely severe anemia, leukopenia, thrombocytopenia, and bone marrow hypoplasia have been reported during gemfibrozil treatment[93]; therefore a baseline blood count is recommended prior to treatment. No toxic effects from overdosage have been reported.

Gemfibrozil potentiates the anticoagulant effects of warfarin, as already described for clofibrate.[50] It does not alter the therapeutic response to insulin or oral hypoglycemic agents.[48,50] When gemfibrozil is administered with lovastatin, there is a 5% incidence of myositis, and rhabdomyolysis may occur[95,96]; the mechanism for this adverse interaction is unknown.[95] The bioavailability of gemfibrozil may be reduced when the drug is given together with colestipol.[35] When these drugs are used together, the gemfibrozil dose should be given 1 to 2 hours before or 2 to 4 hours after the colestipol dose.

Clinical Indications and Effectiveness

Gemfibrozil is indicated for the treatment of patients with type 2b hyperlipidemia (Table 12–5), i.e., elevations of both VLDL and LDL, when standard nonpharmacologic measures (e.g., low fat/low cholesterol diet, weight loss, exercise as tolerated) and therapy with a bile acid sequestrant or nicotinic acid (or both) have not been effective.[2,10] Type 2b patients with hypertriglyceridemia, elevated LDL cholesterol levels, and low HDL cholesterol levels may show particular benefit.[11,12,97] The drug is also indicated for the treatment of patients with types 4 or 5 hyperlipidemia who are at risk for developing pancreatitis, but it is not effective in patients with lipoprotein lipase deficiency or apo C-II deficiency (Table 12–5).[1,3,98] Gemfibrozil is also effective for treating patients with type 3 hyperlipoproteinemia.[75,80]

The efficacy of gemfibrozil as a lipid-altering agent depends on the type of patient being treated. The Helsinki Heart Study results clearly illustrate this important clinical point.[11,12,97] In this trial 4081 asymptomatic men aged 40 to 55 years with non-HDL cholesterol levels greater than 200 mg/dl were randomly allocated to receive either placebo or gemfibrozil at a dose of 600 mg twice daily. Over the 5-year observation period, gemfibrozil treatment decreased the total cholesterol by 8%, the LDL cholesterol by 8 to 9%, and the triglycerides by 38%. The HDL cholesterol rose by 10%.

Cardiac endpoints (including fatal and nonfatal myocardial infarction and sudden cardiac death) were decreased by 34%, and mortality from coronary heart disease declined 26%. Significant reduction in risk occurred primarily in patients with the type 2b lipoprotein phenotype and low HDL cholesterol levels.[97] Patients with low initial HDL cholesterol levels tended to benefit more in terms of risk reduction than those with higher initial HDL cholesterol levels (e.g., > 55 mg/dl).[11,97] Therefore the current indications for gemfibrozil are in patients with the type 2b lipoprotein phenotype *and* low HDL cholesterol levels.

The value of gemfibrozil in reducing cardiovascular risk in hyperlipidemic women is not established. If risk reduction with this drug does relate in a major way to raising the HDL cholesterol level, and the benefit is least in those with HDL cholesterol levels of more than 55 mg/dl, hyperlipidemic women with HDL cholesterol levels in this range may not show the degree of risk reduction observed in men. Only a clinical trial in women can determine if gemfibrozil therapy lowers cardiovascular risk as it does in men.

Gemfibrozil may not have shown significant risk reduction in patients with type 2a hyperlipidemia (hypercholesterolemia) because its effect on LDL cholesterol in such patients is modest and generally does not achieve the treatment goals suggested by the National Cholesterol Education Program.[2] For example, in patients with primary hypercholesterolemia, gemfibrozil (1200 mg/day) lowered total cholesterol only 16%, whereas lovastatin at a dose of 80 mg/day lowered total cholesterol levels 34%.[85] Lovastatin lowered the LDL cholesterol 42% compared to 18% for gemfibrozil and raised the HDL cholesterol 8% compared to 12% for gemfibrozil. Triglyceride reduction was greater with gemfibrozil (−39%) than with lovastatin (−14%). Thus for primary hypercholesterolemia, gemfibrozil does not appear to be the drug of first choice (Table 12–5).

In patients with type 3 hyperlipidemia, gemfibrozil lowered total cholesterol and triglycerides by 40% and 70%, respectively, and raised the HDL cholesterol 45%.[80] The effects of gemfibrozil on plasma Lp(a) levels (see Chapter 3) have not been well studied, but limited data using another fibric acid derivative (bezafibrate 200 mg tid) indicate that this drug class may not be effective in reducing Lp(a) levels.[99]

Preparation, Dosages, and Contraindications

The dose of gemfibrozil is 600 mg taken orally twice daily before the morning and evening meals. The drug is supplied as 300 mg capsules and 600 mg tablets.

Gemfibrozil is contraindicated in patients with hypersensitivity to the drug and those with severe hepatic or renal dysfunction, including primary biliary cirrhosis. It should be used with caution in patients with preexisting gallbladder disease. Safe use during pregnancy has not been established, nor has safety and efficacy in children.

Other Fibric Acid Derivatives

Bezafibrate was introduced as a lipid-lowering drug during the late 1970s in Europe, but it is not yet available in the United States. The recommended dose is 200 mg taken orally two or three times daily. Bezafibrate exhibits many of the effects on lipids and lipoproteins already described for gemfibrozil, and its mechanisms of action are similar to those of gemfibrozil. Bezafibrate has not been subjected to large scale clinical trials such as the Helsinki Heart Study, so its effects on reducing long-term cardiovascular risk in hyperlipidemic patients is not established. Bezafibrate has been discussed in several reviews.[51,52,61]

Fenofibrate was introduced as a lipid-lowering agent in France in 1975 and is now available in Europe, the Middle East, and Africa; it has not been approved for use in the United States. The drug has been the subject of several reviews.[53–60] The usual dose of fenofibrate is 100 mg taken orally three times daily. It lowers plasma triglycerides, raises the HDL cholesterol level, and has a variable effect on the LDL cholesterol level.[59,60] It also has a uricosuric effect.[53] Fenofibrate therapy has been associated with a slight increase in skin rash, abnormal liver function, and increased levels of creatine kinase, creatinine, and blood urea nitrogen compared to placebo.[57] Its current indications for use are similar to those for gemfibrozil. Fenofibrate has not been evaluated for its ability to decrease long-term cardiovascular risk in hyperlipidemic patients.

Inhibitors of HMG CoA Reductase

Lovastatin

Lovastatin (Mevacor®) inhibits HMG CoA reductase, the major rate-limiting enzyme in the pathway for cholesterol biosynthesis[100,101] (Fig. 12–2). Other members of this class of HMG CoA reductase inhibitors are mevastatin, simvastatin (Zocor®), and pravastatin.[102] Lovastatin was introduced to the U.S. market for treatment of hypercholesterolemia in September 1987. This class of drugs has been the subject of several reviews.[102–106]

Chemistry and Pharmacology

Lovastatin is a potent inhibitor of HMG CoA reductase (Fig. 12–2). It is administered as a lactone prodrug that is converted to the open acid form (active drug) by esterases in tissues.

Based on data in animals, about 30% of an oral dose is absorbed, and peak plasma levels occur 2 to 4 hours after the dose is administered. Absorption of the drug from the gut is facilitated when it is taken with meals. In limited human studies, only about 5% of an oral dose reached the plasma in the form of active inhibitor. Lovastatin and its open acid form are highly bound to plasma proteins (>95%), and the drug crosses the pla-

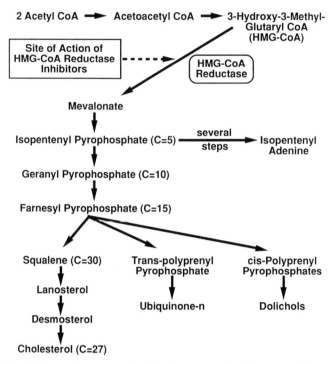

FIGURE 12–2. Pathway for synthesis of cholesterol and polyisoprenoids in mammalian tissues. The number of carbons in several of the intermediates are indicated in parentheses. Reproduced with permission from the Annual Review of Nutrition, Vol. 6, © 1986 by Annual Reviews Inc.

centa and the blood-brain barrier. Eighty percent or more of an oral dose is excreted in the stool, and only 10% is excreted in the urine.[102,105,106]

Mechanisms of Action

When intracellular cholesterol synthesis is inhibited by lovastatin, cells express more LDL receptors on their surface to obtain more LDL via the LDL receptor[107] (Fig. 12–1C). As a result of LDL receptor stimulation, especially on the liver (Fig. 12–1C), the fractional rate of catabolism of LDL (that fraction of the intravascular pool of LDL catabolized per day) increases.[107,108] Increased hepatic LDL receptor activity also enhances the clearance of IDL from the plasma, thereby leaving less for conversion to LDL (see Chapter 3). Thus the lovastatin-induced increase in hepatic LDL-receptor activity enhances LDL catabolism but also reduces the rate of LDL production from IDL. These mechanisms were defined from studies in patients with heterozygous familial hypercholesterolemia.[108] In patients with primary moderate hypercholesterolemia (? polygenic hypercholesterolemia) (see Chapter 3), lovastatin treatment may lower LDL largely by reducing LDL synthesis rather than by stimulating the fractional catabolic rate for LDL.[109] A similar effect on LDL synthesis was observed during lovastatin treatment in patients with familial type 3 hypercholesterolemia.[110] Lovastatin and other HMG CoA reductase inhibitors do not appear to lower plasma Lp(a) levels.[111,112] Although the data are less clear, lovastatin may also inhibit the synthesis and assembly of VLDL in the liver.

Data indicate that therapeutic doses of lovastatin (and perhaps other HMG CoA reductase inhibitors) apparently do not markedly impair cholesterol biosynthesis in vivo. First, lovastatin at a dose of 20 mg twice daily reduced the fecal excretion of cholesterol and bile acids in three of five patients with heterozygous familial hypercholesterolemia, but in none of these patients did the fecal output of steroids fall below the normal range, indicating that endogenous cholesterol synthesis was not markedly decreased at this drug dose.[113] Second, therapeutic doses of lovastatin in normal subjects decreased urinary mevalonate excretion levels by only 30 to 35%, suggesting that the drug did not completely block HMG CoA reductase activity.[114] Third, when a single dose of lovastatin is given to human subjects, the plasma mevalonate level drops initially but rebounds to normal within 24 hours, consistent with relatively short-lived enzyme-inhibitory effects of the drug.[114]

Adverse Effects and Drug Interactions

The most common side effects associated with lovastatin treatment involve the gastrointestinal tract; they include dyspepsia, flatus, and abdominal pain or cramps.[115–118] These symptoms are mild to moderate in severity and generally subside as therapy continues. In a long term safety study of lovastatin treatment initially involving 744 patients, only 2% of patients discontinued therapy due to drug-attributable adverse events: persistently elevated hepatic transaminases in 1.2%, rash in 0.3%, persistent gastrointestinal symptoms in 0.3%, insomnia in 0.1%, and myopathy in 0.1%.[115] Increased hepatic transaminases are usually asymptomatic and revert to normal when drug therapy is discontinued.

There was some initial concern that this class of drugs might induce cataract formation. However, in dogs the minimal toxic dose of lovastatin for cataract formation is 60 mg/kg/day and the no-effect dose is 30 mg/kg/day.[119] The therapeutic dose of lovastatin in humans is well below this range at about 1 mg/kg/day or less (70 kg human; 80 mg/day total drug dose). In clinical trials involving more than 200 patients treated with lovastatin at doses of 20 to 80 mg/day, there has been no evidence for increased cataract formation as a result of drug therapy.[116,118,120]

Because cholesterol serves as a precursor for steroid hormone production in several endocrine tissues, a number of studies have evaluated adrenal or testicular function (or both) during therapy with lovastatin and other HMG CoA reductase inhibitors. At therapeutic doses this class of drugs (lovastatin in particular) has not been shown to adversely affect either adrenal function[116,118,121–123] or gonadal function.[116,118,124] There are no published studies regarding endocrine effects in women, but menstrual irregularities have not been reported during treatment with current members of this drug class.

Several adverse drug interactions have been reported in patients receiving lovastatin. Myopathy associated with myalgias, muscle tenderness, weakness, and elevated creatine kinase (CK) levels, sometimes progressing to frank rhabdomyolysis complicated with renal failure, has occurred in patients taking lovastatin with erythromycin, niacin, gemfibrozil, or immunosuppressive therapy including cyclosporine.[95,96,125-130] The mechanism of this lovastatin-induced myopathy is not known, nor has the mechanism for any of the adverse drug interactions been explained. In a few patients who developed myopathy during simultaneous treatment with lovastatin and cyclosporine, the blood levels of lovastatin and its metabolites were significantly elevated, suggesting that cyclosporine alters the hepatic metabolism of lovastatin.[95,115] One patient taking lovastatin together with an angiotensin-converting enzyme inhibitor developed hyperkalemia along with elevated CK levels.[130] The incidence of myopathy is low when lovastatin is used alone or is unaccompanied by any of the above-mentioned drugs.[115] In one patient who developed elevated CK levels during therapy with lovastatin, rechallenge with the drug at a later date did not cause the CK level to rise again.[131]

Patients receiving coumarin anticoagulants may develop prolongation of the prothrombin time when given lovastatin therapy.[132] The basis for this change is unknown. Patients receiving coumarin anticoagulants who are about to start lovastatin therapy should have baseline prothrombin times documented and then carefully followed while lovastatin therapy is initiated. The same precaution applies if lovastatin therapy is abruptly discontinued in a patient receiving one of these anticoagulants.

Lovastatin produces skeletal malformations in rat fetuses at large doses (800 mg/kg/day) but not at doses of 80 mg/kg/day.[132] No comparable data are available for the human fetus.

Clinical Indications and Effectiveness

Lovastatin is indicated for patients with hypercholesterolemia due to an elevated LDL cholesterol level (lipoprotein phenotypes 2a and 2b)[116,117,133-135] and is particularly helpful for treating heterozygous familial hypercholesterolemia.[118,133,135] However, it has little or no effect in the rare patient with homozygous familial hypercholesterolemia, presumably because such patients cannot form adequate LDL receptors in vivo.[136] Lovastatin is effective in treating patients with familial type 3 hyperlipoproteinemia[110,137] and has also been used to treat secondary hyperlipidemia in patients with diabetes mellitus[138,139] or the nephrotic syndrome.[140] Lovastatin, when combined with colestipol, has been shown to halt progression and induce regression of coronary atherosclerosis in middle-aged men with hyperlipidemia.[141] Its ability to produce these changes in atherosclerosis when used alone are currently under study.

Lovastatin effectively reduces the total and LDL cholesterol levels.[116,118] Depending on the dose employed and the disorder in the patient, the cholesterol level may be lowered by 25 to 45%. Substantial lowering of total and LDL cholesterol levels may occur at doses of 20 mg/day, but additional lipid lowering occurs when the dose is increased to 40 or 80 mg/day.[116,117] In comparison studies with other drugs, lovastatin at a dose of 20 mg twice daily lowered total and LDL cholesterol by 27% and 32%, respectively, whereas cholestyramine (12 g twice daily) lowered these lipids by 17% and 27%, respectively.[117] When the dose of lovastatin was increased to 40 mg twice daily, the total and LDL cholesterol levels were decreased by 34% and 42%, respectively.[117] The results of comparative studies between lovastatin and gemfibrozil were described above.[85] Lovastatin (20 mg twice daily) is also more effective than neomycin (1 g twice daily) for therapy of hypercholesterolemic patients.[142]

In a comparison of lovastatin (40–80 mg/day) with probucol (1 g/day) in patients with heterozygous familial hypercholesterolemia or nonfamilial hypercholesterolemia, the LDL cholesterol was reduced 40% by lovastatin but only 10 to 17% by probucol.[143] HDL cholesterol rose 10 to 18% during lovastatin treatment but fell 27 to 33% during treatment with probucol.[143] These changes were not mediated by altered activities of hepatic lipase or lipoprotein lipase. In other studies, lovastatin also increased the HDL cholesterol by 3 to 12%, depending on the dose used and the patient group being studied.[116,117]

Preparations, Dosage, and Contraindications

Lovastatin is available in 20 mg and 40 mg tablets. The suggested starting dose is 20 mg taken with the evening meal. The dose may be adjusted upward as necessary to a maximum dose of 40 mg twice daily taken with meals. In patients taking immunosuppresive drugs (e.g., cyclosporine) the maximum dose of lovastatin should be 20 mg/day.[115] It is recommended that liver function be monitored every 4 to 6 weeks during the first 15 months of lovastatin therapy and periodically (every 3–4 months) thereafter. An eye examination with slit lamp is suggested before starting therapy with lovastatin and annually during treatment with the drug.[132] However, this recommendation for the slit lamp examination may be eliminated in the near future if ongoing safety studies continue to show no adverse effect of the drug on the human lens.

Lovastatin is contraindicated in patients allergic to the medication, and it should be avoided in patients with active liver disease. It should not be used during pregnancy because of potential hazards to the fetus.[132] When the drug is administered to women of child-bearing age, adequate birth control measures should be advised. Women who become pregnant while taking lovastatin should have the medication discontinued and be advised of the potential toxic effects to the fetus,[132] although none has been reported to date. No data are available in humans, but lovastatin appears in the breast milk of rats; therefore the drug should not be prescribed for nursing mothers. The safe use of lovastatin in children has not been established. Although lovastatin has been used without apparent incident to treat a small number of patients with the nephrotic syndrome,[140] its use in a rat model of the nephrotic syndrome induced by puromycin aminoglycoside was associated with extensive hepatocellular necrosis and death in one-half of the animals.[144] These data do not show a causal link between lovastatin and the hepatic abnormalities, but caution is suggested when using lovastatin in patients with the nephrotic syndrome and reduced plasma protein levels.[144]

Other HMG CoA Reductase Inhibitors

Simvastatin (Zocor®) was developed after lovastatin and is not yet available in the United States, although it has been released in several European countries. Early clinical experience with the drug indicates that its mechanism of action, clinical efficacy, and pattern and frequency of side effects are similar to those for lovastatin.[145-149] The dose of simvastatin is 20 or 40 mg per day given in two equal doses or as a single evening dose.

Pravastatin is not yet available in the United States but has been released in Japan. Based on published reports, including one study in non-insulin dependent diabetics, this drug is similar in efficacy to the other HMG CoA reductase inhibitors.[150-152] It is not clear if the pattern of side effects differs from those of the other HMG CoA reductase inhibitors because it is given as the open acid form rather than the lactone. This difference may alter its tissue distribution compared with that of the drugs given as lactones. The usual dose is 10 mg given twice daily.

Nicotinic Acid

Chemistry and Pharmacology

Nicotinic acid is effective in reducing both cholesterol and triglyceride levels in plasma. It is a member of the water-soluble B-complex vitamin group and is sometimes called niacin, a less specific name also applied to nicotinamide. Nicotinamide is active as a vitamin but is ineffective as a lipid-lowering agent. Extensive reviews of the literature on nicotinic acid have been published.[153-155]

Nicotinic acid is readily absorbed when given by the oral route.[156] After administration of an oral dose of 3 g of nicotinic acid, 88% of the dose appears in the urine, indicating that absorption of the drug from the gastrointestinal tract is nearly complete.[156] Blood levels of total nicotinic acid vary with the size of the oral dose. Nicotinic acid is not protein-bound, but the whole blood/serum total nicotinic acid ratio can be as much as 100:1 because intracellular nicotinic acid metabolites in the cellular elements of the blood have limited capacity to diffuse into serum.[154,156] Nicotinic acid is fairly rapidly metabolized to a variety of structurally related metabolites that are readily excreted in the urine.[153,154,156,157]

Mechanism of Action

The mechanism of action of nicotinic acid is not established, and it has multiple effects when given in pharmacological doses.[153,154] The drug lowers plasma free fatty acid (FFA) levels by inhibiting the mobilization of FFA from adipose tissue.[158] The reduced FFA substrate delivery to the liver decreases hepatic triglyceride production and in one study nicotinic acid therapy (3 g/day) reduced VLDL triglyceride synthesis by 21% in a mixed group of patients.[159] The drug exerts no consistent effect on either cholesterol synthesis or bile acid production as evaluated by sterol balance techniques,[159,160] and there is no indication that it stimulates LDL-receptor activity in vivo.[161]

Nicotinic acid raises the plasma HDL cholesterol level fairly consistently. When therapy is started the VLDL triglyceride level falls within 3 days, whereas the increase in HDL is delayed until 7 days or more.[162] Nicotinic acid does not stimulate lipoprotein lipase activity,[163,164] so the delayed increase in HDL cholesterol may not be linked to a fall in VLDL triglyceride or to accelerated catabolism of VLDL from plasma.[165] Nicotinic acid has differing effects on HDL subfractions and on the metabolism of apo A-I and apo A-II, the major apolipoproteins in HDL.[165-167] The drug decreases the fractional catabolic rate of apo A-I and thereby increases its plasma concentration; in contrast, it reduces the synthesis and plasma level of apo A-II.[165,166] The drug appears to increase the concentration of the HDL_2 subfraction while decreasing the HDL_3 subfraction,[155,166] but these changes vary and depend in part on the type of hyperlipidemia present in any given patient.[165]

Adverse Effects and Drug Interactions

Nicotinic acid in pharmacological doses can produce significant toxicity and side effects. The most common complaints include flushing, itching, and rash.[69] The flushing occurs 30 to 60 minutes after the medication is taken and is related to the rise in plasma nicotinic acid levels.[168] The flush appears to be prostaglandin-mediated and can be inhibited by pretreatment with indomethacin or aspirin.[169,170] Flushing diminishes with continued treatment beyond 3 to 4 weeks.[170] Additional cutaneous complaints include dry skin, hyperpigmentation, and acanthosis nigricans.[69,171,172] Other side effects with nicotinic acid therapy include abdominal pain, heartburn, indigestion, loss of appetite and activation of peptic ulcer.[69,171,172]

Liver function abnormalities occur with elevated liver enzymes (AST), alkaline phosphatase, and bilirubin levels.[69,171,172] In a few cases jaundice occurred and was associated with structural changes suggesting viral hepatitis[171,172] or cholestatic hepatitis.[173,174]

Hyperuricemia, sometimes with acute gouty athritis, may occur during nicotinic acid therapy.[69,175] Hyperglycemia and elevated plasma insulin levels are more common during therapy with nicotinic acid.[69,176] Diabetic patients receiving nicotinic acid therapy may need to have their insulin dosage adjusted, and patients receiving oral hypoglycemic agents may require a shift to insulin therapy for better diabetic control. Nicotinic acid therapy does not appear to cause diabetes mellitus but apparently unmasks latent diabetes.[15] In that regard, hyperinsulinemia and hyperglycemia are common in the untreated obese patient with hyperlipoproteinemia, especially hypertriglyceridemia. Although there are few studies on this topic, it is possible that existing baseline hyperinsulinemia in a hyperlipidemic patient may be made worse by nicotinic acid therapy. Whether these metabolic changes will ultimately prove harmful is currently not known.[177,178]

Nicotinic acid therapy may produce a cystoid macular edema presenting with progressive loss of visual acuity and other visual symptoms, which is reversible if nicotinic acid therapy is promptly stopped.[175,179]

The Coronary Drug Project data demonstrated elevated CK levels in patients receiving nicotinic acid therapy.[69] Possible nicotinic acid-associated myopathy with nocturnal cramps, muscle aches, myalgias, and muscle tenderness was described in three patients.[180] They exhibited elevated alanine transaminase (ALT) and CK levels that decreased when the drug was discontinued.[180]

Nicotinic acid therapy was associated with a greater frequency of ventricular premature beats and atrial fibrillation in the Coronary Drug Project, which involved patients with preexisting coronary heart disease.[69] Note that nicotinic acid was used effectively and appeared to be safe in combination with colestipol to aggressively control hypercholesterolemia in two studies in men with coronary heart disease.[141,175]

Few drug interactions have been reported with nicotinic acid. There may be a slightly increased incidence of drug-induced myopathy when nicotinic acid is used in combination with lovastatin.[127] When combined nicotinic acid-colestipol therapy was used to treat hyperlipidemia for a period of 1 year, serum thyroxine levels were decreased and triiodothyronine ratios were increased, apparently because serum thyroxine-binding globulin levels were decreased.[175,181] The reason for these changes is unknown, *but* the patients did not become clinically hypothyroid.

Clinical Indications and Effectiveness

Nicotinic acid is indicated for treating significant hyperlipidemia unresponsive to appropriate diet therapy and weight loss. It lowers plasma VLDL and LDL levels and raises the HDL concentration. It is not effective for hypertriglyceridemia caused by a deficiency of lipoprotein lipase or apo C-II (see Chapter 3) (Table 12–5).

Nicotinic acid is effective in the treatment of hypercholesterolemia.[171,172,182–184] Because the nicotinic acid dose is titrated in individual patients, response to therapy in any given patient depends on several factors, including the dose of the drug used and the type of hyperlipidemia being treated. In one study, a 3 g daily dose of nicotinic acid for 1 month reduced plasma cholesterol and triglycerides by 8 to 25%, and 26 to 38%, respectively, in patients with type 2a hyperlipidemia; reductions of 20% and 40%, respectively, were seen with type 2b hyperlipidemia; reductions of 50% and 62%, respectively, occurred in four patients with type 3 hyperlipidemia; reductions of 7 to 10% and 29 to 39%, respectively, occurred in those with "moderate" type 4 hyperlipidemia; reductions of 16 to 26% and 55 to 60%, respectively, occurred in those with "severe" type 4 hyperlipidemia; and reductions of 65% and 90%, respectively, occurred in those with type 5 hyperlipidemia.[184] In this study, the response in women was somewhat better than that in men. Note that the absolute response in patients with type 2a hyperlipidemia was relatively poor at the 3-g dose. These results collectively indicate that the onset of action of nicotinic acid is relatively prompt and can be pronounced after 1 month of therapy.

In terms of lipoproteins, nicotinic acid therapy for 6 months at a dose of 3 g/day lowered the LDL cholesterol 21% in type 2a patients, 20% in type 2b patients, and 15% in type 4 patients.[185] In this same study, HDL cholesterol levels during nicotinic acid therapy increased 31% in type 2a patients, 42% in type 2b patients, and 32% in type 4 patients.[185] Nicotinic acid therapy decreases plasma levels of apolipoproteins B-100, C-I, C-II, C-III, and E,[185,186] and it lowers serum Lp(a) levels when used in combination with neomycin.[187]

In the Coronary Drug Project, nicotinic acid therapy at a daily dose of 3 g for 5 years in middle-aged men significantly reduced long-term cardiovascular risk.[69] At the end of the 5-year trial, the nicotinic acid-treated group experienced a significantly lower incidence of nonfatal myocardial infarction (8.9% versus 12.2% in placebo controls), but total mortality and cardiovascular mortality were not improved.[69] However, at 15 years of follow-up the nicotinic acid-treated group experienced an 11% reduction in all-cause mortality and a 12% reduction in deaths related to coronary heart disease compared to the placebo-treated group.[188] Because nicotinic acid had been discontinued after 5 years, the precise reason for this reduction in mortality at 15 years cannot be established, but it is possible that the lipid reduction induced by nicotinic acid therapy accounted for this long-term benefit.[188] In a relatively small controlled trial in survivors of a myocardial infarction, combined therapy with nicotinic acid (up to 3 g/day) and clofibrate (2 g/day) in addition to diet therapy was associated with a significant decline in both fatal and nonfatal coronary events.[189,190] This combination drug therapy is no longer recommended because of the toxic effects associated with clofibrate therapy in the WHO Trial discussed previously.[72]

Nicotinic acid is not effective when used alone to treat patients with homozygous familial hypercholesterolemia.[191] However, it does lower lipids somewhat when combined with a bile acid sequestrant.[15,129]

Preparations, Dosages, and Contraindications

Nicotinic acid is available in 50, 100, 200, 250 and 500 mg tablets from various suppliers. Prescriptions should specify nicotinic acid rather than niacin to avoid confusion with nicotinamide, which is ineffective in lowering lipids.

The therapeutic dose of nicotinic acid varies but generally ranges from 1 to 2 g three times daily. To minimize side effects, therapy is started with low doses that are gradually increased. For example, one may start treatment with 100 mg three times daily for the first week, increase to 200 mg three times daily the second week, and so on until a dose of 500 mg three times daily is reached. At this point the dose is maintained for 1 month, during which time the patient is observed for both therapeutic and adverse effects. If the therapeutic response is inadequate but the patient tolerates the dose, the dose can be increased in stepwise fashion to the range of 3 to 6 g/day. The final dose required must be individualized to account for patient tolerance and the disease being treated. Nicotinic acid is taken with meals to reduce gastrointestinal side effects, and simultaneous consumption of hot beverages should be avoided to minimize the intensity of the flush. If flushing is severe, one aspirin tablet (325 mg) may reduce its intensity if taken 30 minutes before the nicotinic acid dose. This requirement for aspirin therapy should decline after the first month of nicotinic acid therapy.

Nicotinic acid is contraindicated in patients allergic to the drug, in those with abnormal liver function, or in patients with active peptic ulcer. It should be used cautiously in patients with hyperuricemia and gout and in those with diabetes mellitus. When used in combination with antihypertensive drugs, especially β-blockers, it may induce severe hypotension with syncope. Hyperlipidemic patients prone to cardiac arrhythmias should be considered for therapy other than nicotinic acid.

The use of nicotinic acid in patients with renal disease has not been adequately studied.

Sustained-release preparations of nicotinic acid, which may cause less flushing, show greater hepatic toxicity and gastrointestinal side effects as larger doses are used.[192] Thus unmodified nicotinic acid is preferred to treat hyperlipidemia.[192]

Probucol

Chemistry and Pharmacology

Probucol (Lorelco®) is used to treat hypercholesterolemia and has no significant effect on plasma triglyceride concentrations. The drug is an antioxidant structurally similar to another widely used antioxidant, butylated hydroxytoluene.[193]

Published data on the pharmacokinetics of probucol are limited largely to data on file with the manufacturer.[194–196] Intestinal absorption of probucol following an oral dose is both limited and variable. In normal humans receiving 1000 mg of probucol daily for 21 days, a single oral dose of radioactive probucol produced peak plasma levels 8 to 24 hours after administration, and absorption ranged from 0.7 to 14.0% of the radioactive dose administered.[194] When the drug was administered at a dose of 500 mg twice daily for up to 1 year, plasma levels increased gradually to steady-state levels within 3 to 4 months.[194] After 1 year of treatment, the blood levels of probucol ranged from 7.3 to 29.8 μg/ml (mean 19.0 μg/ml).[194]

Probucol is largely bound to plasma lipoproteins.[196] In one study 75% of the probucol was contained in LDL and the remainder was in VLDL and HDL,[197] but the amount of probucol bound did not correlate with the degree of cholesterol reduction. The drug is highly concentrated in adipose tissue and the adrenal gland.[194]

Probucol is slowly eliminated from the body largely via the feces. When probucol was discontinued after up to 1 year of treatment, plasma levels decreased by 60% in 6 weeks and by 80% in 6 months.[194] Metabolites of probucol in man have not been identified.

The mechanisms of action of probucol are not well defined.[196] The drug has no consistent effect on neutral steroid production, bile acid production, gallbladder bile composition, intestinal cholesterol absorption, lipoprotein lipase activity, or hepatic lipase activity.[198]

The effects of probucol on lipoprotein metabolism in humans have been reviewed elsewhere.[196,199] The drug increases the fractional catabolic rate but has no effect on the production rate of LDL. The enhanced rate of catabolism of LDL is not due to LDL-receptor stimulation because probucol also increases the rate of LDL catabolism in receptor-deficient Watanabe heritable hyperlipidemic (WHHL) rabbits.[200] The nature of the LDL clearance pathway(s) stimulated by probucol in this animal model is not known. Probucol appears to lower HDL by decreasing the rate of production of apolipoproteins A-I and A-II.[196,199]

Probucol is a potent antioxidant that associates with LDL and the other lipoproteins in plasma and protects these particles from oxidation.[196,201] Experimental studies indicate that probucol halts the progression of atherosclerosis in WHHL rabbits[202,203] and primates fed an atherosclerotic diet.[204] It is not known whether this effect is due to the antioxidant properties or to some other effect of probucol on tissue lipid accumulation.

Probucol treatment causes regression of tendon and cutanous xanthomas in patients with heterozygous or homozygous familial hypercholesterolemia.[205] This resolution of xanthomas may result from both reduced uptake and enhanced removal of cholesterol from macrophages within these lesions,[206] but the cellular mechanisms responsible for this mobilization of cholesterol are not well understood.

Adverse Effects and Drug Interactions

Probucol is generally well tolerated by patients. The most frequent side effects are diarrhea and flatulence.[195,196] In one large study, 8% of patients discontinued the drug because of side effects.[195] There are no reports of adverse reactions during probucol treatment in patients with hepatic or renal disease. Probucol has been used without incident in 12 patients with hyperlipidemia related to the nephrotic syndrome.[207]

In several animal models (rhesus monkey, beagle dog), probucol in conjunction with a high fat diet produced prolongation of the QT interval and death.[196] The drug also produces prolongation of the QT interval in humans but the effect is slight and no adverse effects, arrhythmias, or sudden deaths have been reported during probucol treatment.[196] Nevertheless, periodic electrocardiograms are recommended during treatment with the drug and care must be taken when prescribing probucol in combination with other drugs that also prolong the QT interval, such as tricyclic antidepressants, class I and III antiarrhythmics, and phenothiazines.[208] It should also be used with caution in conjunction with drugs that produce bradycardia (β-blockers) or atrioventricular block (digitalis preparations).

No acute toxicity from overdosage has been reported in humans. Its safe use during pregnancy or in children has not been established. Furthermore, the effects of probucol accumulation in adipose tissue during long-term therapy are unknown.

Adverse interactions of probucol with other drugs appear to be infrequent. When probucol and clofibrate are administered together for treatment of hyperlipemia, HDL cholesterol levels are markedly reduced.[209–211] Although the clinical significance of this change is unclear, this drug combination for treatment of hyperlipidemia is not recommended because of the increased cardiovascular risk associated with low HDL cholesterol levels.[212]

Clinical Indications and Effectiveness

Probucol is indicated for the treatment of hypercholesterolemia caused by an increase in the LDL cholesterol concentration (type 2a and 2b phenotypes), but it is ineffective for treating hypertriglyceridemia[196] (Table 12–5). Because probucol only modestly lowers the LDL cholesterol compared to other drugs and also lowers HDL cholesterol levels, it is not currently considered a first-line drug for treatment of hypercholesterolemia (Table 12–5). It should be considered for use when dietary therapy alone has not produced the desired therapeutic effect and when patients are unable to tolerate other drugs such as the bile acid sequestrants, nicotinic acid, or an HMG CoA reductase inhibitor.[2] It is helpful in patients with homozygous familial hypercholesterolemia, where it lowers the plasma cholesterol modestly and promotes the resolution of both cutaneous and tendon xanthomas.[205]

The therapeutic response to probucol varies and depends in part on the type of patient being treated. In patients with type 2a or 2b hypercholesterolemia, probucol lowers the total cholesterol about 5 to 15%, but in a few subjects reductions of more than 20% occur.[196] Reductions in LDL cholesterol vary from 14% to 20%.[196] Total and LDL cholesterol reductions may be slightly greater in patients with type 2b hyperlipidemia than in those with type 2a hyperlipidemia.[196] Some variability in drug response may relate to the apo E genotype of the individual patients (see Chapter 3). In one study, probucol produced the greatest cholesterol reduction in patients with the E4 allele.[213] HDL cholesterol levels decline 20 to 40% during therapy with probucol.[196]

In a study of patients with diabetes and hyperlipidemia, 16 weeks of therapy with probucol at a dose of 500 mg/day lowered the total plasma cholesterol by 14% and the HDL cholesterol by 16%.[196] In nine cardiac transplant patients with hyperlipidemia (type 2a or 2b), probucol produced a mean 13% reduction in total cholesterol, a 15% reduction in LDL cholesterol, and a 16% reduction in HDL cholesterol.[214] The long-term benefit of this therapy is unknown, but probucol was well tolerated when administered with prednisone and azathioprine; the patients in this study did not receive cyclosporine.[214] In 12 patients with nephrotic syndrome and hyperlipidemia (primarily phenotypes 2a or 2b), 12 weeks of probucol therapy lowered the total plasma cholesterol a mean of 30%, the LDL cholesterol a mean of 25%, the HDL cholesterol a mean of 25%, and total triglycerides a mean of 28%[196]; the long-term benefits of these changes in nephrotic patients are unknown.

Probucol is less effective than either colestipol or lovastatin in lowering the LDL cholesterol level.[196] In hypercholesterolemic patients, colestipol (10 g bid) lowered the plasma LDL cholesterol a mean of 23%, whereas probucol (500 mg bid) lowered the LDL fraction only 12%.[196] HMG CoA reductase inhibitors typically reduce the LDL cholesterol about 25 to 38%, whereas probucol lowers this fraction only 8 to 17%.[196]

Probucol was not effective in lowering cardiovascular morbidity and mortality in one 5-year multifactorial clinical trial.[210] A second trial is currently in progress.[215] More studies are required to determine if probucol is effective in humans as an antioxidant to prevent atheroma formation, and if it has a therapeutic role in the mobilization of cholesterol from tissue sites (atheromas and xanthomas).

Preparations, Dosage and Contraindications

Probucol is available in either 250 or 500 mg tablets. The standard dose is 500 mg orally twice daily with meals. A low fat, low cholesterol diet should be administered concurrently. The maximum cholesterol-lowering effect of the drug may not be apparent for several months.[196] Probucol may be used with bile acid sequestrants to enhance the cholesterol-lowering effects of either drug administered alone.[196] However, probucol has little additional effect when added to lovastatin plus colestipol in patients with heterozygous familial hypercholesterolemia.[216]

Probucol is contraindicated in patients hypersensitive to the drug. It is also not indicated in a patient with a ventricular arrhythmia or a preexisting conduction abnormality with prolongation of the QT interval.

Combination Drug Therapy for Hyperlipidemia

Two or more lipid-lowering drugs may be given together to control hyperlipidemia unresponsive to a single agent.[2,14] Combined drug therapy is most often employed in patients with severe heterozygous familial hypercholesterolemia or familial combined hyperlipidemia; or it is used to control severe hypertriglyceridemia not caused by lipoprotein lipase deficiency or apo C-II deficiency[1] (see Chapter 3). Combined drug treatment may also allow the physician to effectively treat a patient with submaximal doses of individual medications, thereby reducing the frequency and severity of adverse side effects. For example, if a hypercholesterolemic patient is intolerant of maximal doses of a bile acid sequestrant, the patient may respond to smaller doses of the sequestrant if it is combined with nicotinic acid or lovastatin. Often the second medication can also be employed at submaximal doses. Combined drug therapy for hyperlipidemia is described in several reviews[14,33,34,217-220] and is summarized in Table 12-8.

Triple drug therapy is sometimes required in patients with severe hypercholesterolemia. The combination of lovastatin, colestipol, and nicotinic acid lowers LDL cholesterol levels up to 62%,[34,218] but the risk for myositis may increase.

Aggressive combination drug therapy with either colestipol and nicotinic acid or colestipol and lovastatin in middle-aged men reduces the rate of progression and promotes regression of coronary atherosclerosis over a period of 2.0 to 2.5 years.[141,175] The colestipol/nicotinic acid combination produced similar changes in coronary bypass grafts.[175] Combination therapy for 5 years with clofibrate and nicotinic acid in survivors of myocardial infarction below 70 years of age lowered plasma cholesterol 13% and triglycerides 19% compared to controls.[190] The drug-treated group, which consisted of 21% women, experienced a 26% reduction in total mortality ($p < 0.05$) and a 36% reduction in ischemic heart disease mortality ($p < 0.01$).[190] These results collectively support the hypothesis that aggressive control of hyperlipidemia can arrest the progression of atherosclerosis and in some cases induce regression of lesions as well.

Several drug combinations do not appear to work well in selected patient groups. The combination of cholestyramine and neomycin in patients with type 2 hyperlipidemia is not more effective than cholestyramine alone, and this combination is not recommended because neomycin lowers the HDL cholesterol without further decreasing the LDL cholesterol.[30] Lovastatin

TABLE 12–8. Considerations for combined drug therapy in patients with lipoprotein disorders

Drug combination	Comment[a]
Bile acid sequestrant plus	
Nicotinic acid	Greater reduction of LDL-C and elevation of HDL-C. Reduces hypertriglyceridemia caused by resins. Has been shown to promote regression and halt progression of coronary atherosclerosis. Useful for combined hyperlipidemia.
Lovastatin	Greater reduction of LDL-C (Fig. 12–1D) and reduces hypertriglyceridemia caused by resins. Patient acceptance is better than with nicotinic acid. May allow dose of resin to be decreased.
Probucol	Greater reduction of LDL-C, but effect is relatively modest. HDL-C also drops. Does not affect triglycerides.
Gemfibrozil	Greater reduction of LDL-C than when gemfibrozil is used alone. HDL-C level usually increases. Reduces hypertriglyceridemia caused by resins.
Lovastatin plus	
Gemfibrozil	Greater reduction of LDL-C and raises HDL-C. Hypertriglyceridemia is better controlled. Especially useful for combined hyperlipidemia. Major drawback is 5% risk of myopathy with potentially severe side effects; therefore patient education and close monitoring are required when using this therapy. Combination is not better than lovastatin alone for heterozygous familial hypercholesterolemia.
Nicotinic acid	Useful for severe hypercholesterolemia if patient is intolerant of bile acid sequestrants. Greater LDL-C reduction and HDL-C elevation. Risk of myositis appears to be enhanced, but incidence is not well established.
Nicotinic acid plus neomycin	Lowers LDL-C and VLDL-C levels. Raises HDL-C levels that are lowered when neomycin is used alone. Lowers Lp(a) levels, but benefits of this therapy regarding cardiovascular risk are not established.

Adapted and modified from Bilheimer DW, East C. In: Williams RL, Brater DC, Mordenti J, eds. *Rational Therapeutics. A Clinical Pharmacologic Guide for the Health Professional.* New York: by courtesy of Marcel Dekker Inc., 1990:689–755.
[a]See text for additional details and references.

and neomycin are no better than lovastatin alone in patients with type 2 hyperlipoproteinemia.[142] Gemfibrozil and lovastatin are no better than lovastatin alone in reducing LDL cholesterol in patients with heterozygous familial hypercholesterolemia.[219] Because this drug combination increases the risk for myositis[95] and does not have a clear therapeutic advantage, it is not recommended for treatment of patients with familial hypercholesterolemia.[219]

Other Drugs with Lipid-Altering Potential

Neomycin

Neomycin, a nonabsorbable broad spectrum aminoglycoside antibiotic, lowers the plasma total cholesterol an average of 22% by reducing the LDL and HDL fractions.[221–224] The drug has no effect on plasma triglyceride levels. A neomycin dose of 1.5 g/day increases the fecal excretion of neutral sterols (cholesterol) but not of bile acids.[225,226] The drug also decreases cholesterol absorption from the gut.[226] During therapy, the production rate of LDL is decreased, but there is no consistent change in the fractional catabolic rate.[226] Neomycin may cause mild increases in hepatic transaminases, increased stool frequency, and nausea.[224] Stool flora are altered, but the clinical significance of this change is unknown.[223] Small amounts of the drug are absorbed and might theoretically produce ototoxicity or renal toxicity, but these complications were not observed at neomycin doses of 1.5 to 2.0 g/day.[224] The drug now has limited use in type 2 hyperlipoproteinemia,[224] especially in rare patients intolerant of any of the first-choice medications (Table 12–5). The drug is not approved by the FDA for treating hypercholesterolemia.

Dextrothyroxine

Dextrothyroxine (Choloxin®) has been used to treat hypercholesterolemia but its indications are restricted because of adverse side effects.[15,227] It lowers LDL cholesterol levels and HDL cholesterol levels, but its effect on VLDL cholesterol and plasma triglycerides are variable.[228–230] The drug appears to enhance LDL catabolism via hepatic LDL-receptor stimulation. The starting dose of dextrothyroxine is 1 mg/day, and it is gradually increased to 4 to 8 mg/day in increments of 1 mg/month. The drug potentiates the effects of coumadin anticoagulants. In the Coronary Drug Project, this drug, given at a dose of 6 mg/day, was associated with a greater frequency of angina pectoris, congestive heart failure, arrhythmias, decreased glucose tolerance, and abnormal liver function in the placebo group.[231] The rate of mortality was also greater than that of the placebo group and for these reasons the trial with dextrothyroxine was discontinued.[231] It was a trial of secondary prevention, so the subjects enrolled already had coronary heart disease (CHD). Therefore dextrothyroxine is contraindicated in patients with CHD.

Estrogens

Estrogen therapy in postmenopausal women with type 2 hyperlipoproteinemia lowers the total cholesterol by 11% and the LDL cholesterol by 23% while raising the HDL cholesterol by 12%.[232] Estrogen therapy is also effective in reducing the plasma lipids in women with type 3 hyperlipoproteinemia.[233,234] These effects appear to be due to stimulation of hepatic LDL receptor activity.[235,236] Despite these effects on plasma lipids, estrogen therapy for hyperlipidemia is usually not recommended for several reasons. First, results from the Coronary Drug Project in men indicated that conjugated estrogens at doses of 2.5 and 5.0 mg/day were associated with adverse effects necessitating early cessation of the use of these drugs in the trial.[237,238] There was no apparent benefit regarding CHD; and the incidence of thromboembolism, pulmonary embolism, nonfatal myocardial infarctions, and thrombophlebitis increased over that in the placebo-treated group.[237,238] Comparable data in postmenopausal women are not available.

Second, patients, male or female, who are predisposed to hypertriglyceridemia may develop massive hypertriglyceridemia during treatment with estrogens. This effect is related to increased hepatic VLDL production and may cause pancreatitis.[1] Thus estrogens are not employed as lipid-altering drugs per se. However, there are indications that estrogens in postmenopausal women do reduce cardiovascular risk. The data were obtained in women receiving unopposed estrogen therapy, and it is not known if a similar benefit would occur if the estrogens were cycled with progestational agents, as is now recommended.[239,240] Risks associated with estrogen therapy (breast or uterine cancer) must be weighed against potential benefit regarding cardiovascular risk in individual patients.

β-Sitosterol

β-Sitosterol is a plant-derived sterol that is structurally related to cholesterol.[24] β-Sitosterol is poorly absorbed from the intestine and inhibits cholesterol absorption from the gut.[241,242] The drug may lower the total cholesterol 6 to 12%,[242,243] but it also lowers the HDL cholesterol.[243] It is administered in a liquid suspension at a dose of 3 to 6 g/day. It may cause mild constipation but is otherwise well tolerated.[241,242] β-Sitosterol has little clinical use in hypercholesterolemic patients and is contraindicated in patients with β-Sitosterolemia, a rare genetic disorder characterized by increased intestinal absorption of dietary sterols and the accumulation of sitosterol and other plant sterols in blood and tissues.[1]

References

1. Bilheimer DW. Disorders of lipid metabolism. In: Kelly WN, ed. Textbook of Internal Medicine. Philadelphia: Lippincott, 1989:2258–2269.
2. Expert Panel. Report of the National Cholesterol Education Program Expert

Panel on detection, evaluation and treatment of high blood cholesterol in adults. Arch Intern Med 1988;148:36–69.

3. Bilheimer DW. Evaluation of abnormal lipid profiles. In: Kelly WN, ed. Textbook of Internal Medicine, Philadelphia: Lippincott, 1989:2333–2339.

4. Lerner DJ, Kannel WB. Patterns of coronary heart disease morbidity and mortality in the sexes: a 26-year follow-up of the Framingham population. Am Heart J 1986;111:383–390.

5. Castelli WP. Cardiovascular disease in women. Am J Obstet Gynecol 1988;158:1553–1560.

6. Slack J. Risks of ischaemic heart-disease in familial hyperlipoproteinemic states. Lancet 1969;2:1380–1382.

7. Stone NJ, Levy RI, Frederickson DS, et al. Coronary artery disease in 116 kindred with familial type II hyperlipoproteinemia. Circulation 1974;49:476–488.

8. Wong ND, Cupples A, Ostfeld AM, et al. Risk factors for long-term coronary prognosis after myocardial infarction: the Framingham Study. Am J Epidemiol 1989;130:469–480.

9. Wild RA, Painter PC, Coulson PB, et al. Lipoprotein lipid concentrations and cardiovascular risk in women with polycystic ovary syndrome. J Clin Endocrinol Metab 1985;61:946–951.

10. Grundy Sm, Goodman DS, Rifkind BM, et al. The place of HDL in cholesterol management: a perspective from the national cholesterol education program. Arch Intern Med 1989;149:505–510.

11. Manninen V, Elo O, Frick H, et al. Lipid alterations and decline in the incidence of coronary heart disease in the Helsinki heart study. JAMA 1988;260:641–651.

12. Frick MH, Elo O, Haapa K, et al. Helsinki heart study: primary prevention trial with gemfibrozil in middle-aged men with dyslipidemia. N Engl J Med 1987;317:1237–1245.

13. Knopp RH. Cardiovascular effects of endogenous and exogenous sex hormones over a woman's lifetime. Am J Obstet Gynecol 1988;158:1630–1643.

14. Bilheimer DW, East C. Lipid-lowering agents. In: Williams RL, Brater DC, Mordenti J, eds. Rational Therapeutics. A Clinical Pharmacological Guide for the Health Professional. New York: Marcel Dekker, 1990:689–755.

15. Levy RI, Fredrickson DS, Shulman R, et al. Dietary and drug treatment of primary hyperlipoproteinemia. Ann Intern Med 1972;77:267–294.

16. Grundy SM. Treatment of hypercholesterolemia by interference with bile acid metabolism. Arch Intern Med 1972;130:638–648.

17. Heel RC, Brogden RN, Pakes GE, et al. Colestipol: a review of its pharmacological properties and therapeutic efficacy in patients with hypercholesterolemia. Drugs 1980;19:161–180.

18. Brown MS, Goldstein JL. A receptor-mediated pathway for cholesterol homeostasis. Science. 1986;232:34–47.

19. Grundy SM. Bile acid resins: mechanisms of action. In: Fears R, ed. Pharmacological Control of Hyperlipidaemia. Barcelona: JR Prous Science Publishers, 1986:3–19.

20. Angelin B, Einarsson K, Hellstrom K, et al. Effects of cholestyramine and chenodeoxycholic acid on the metabolism of endogenous triglyceride in hyperlipoproteinemia. J Lipid Res 1978;19:1017–1024.

21. Lipid Research Clinics Program. The Lipid Research Clinics Primary Prevention Trial Results. II. The relationship of reduction in incidence of coronary heart disease to cholesterol lowering. JAMA 1984;251:365–374.
22. Asano T, Pollard M, Madsen DC. Effects of cholestyramine on 1,2-dimethylhydrazine-induced enteric carcinoma in germfree rats. Proc Soc Exp Biol Med 1975;150:780–785.
23. Nigro ND, Bhadrachari N, Chromchai C. A rat model for studying colonic cancer: effect of cholestyramine on induced tumors. Dis Colon Rectum 1973;16:438–443.
24. Lipid Research Clinics Program. The Lipid Research Clinics Coronary Primary Prevention Trial results. I. Reduction in incidence of coronary heart disease. JAMA 1984;251:351–364.
25. Hashim SA, Bergen SS Jr, Van Itallie TB. Experimental steatorrhea induced in man by bile acid sequestrant. Proc Soc Exp Biol Med 1961;106:173–175.
26. Kwiterovich PO Jr. Bile acid sequestrant resin therapy in children. In: Fears R, ed. Pharmacological Control of Hyperlipidemia. Barcelona: JR Prous Science Publishers, 1986:55–66.
27. West RJ, Lloyd JK. The effect of cholestyramine on intestinal absorption. Gut 1975;16:93–98.
28. Hunninghake DB. Resin therapy: adverse effects and their management. In: Fears R, ed. Pharmacological Control of Hyperlipidemia. Barcelona: JR Prous Science Publishers, 1986:67–89.
29. Boyden TW, Totman L. Synergistic effects of probucol and cholestyramine to lower serum cholesterol. J Clin Pharmacol 1981;21:48–51.
30. Hoeg JM, Maher MB, Bailey KR, et al. Effects of combination cholestyramine-neomycin treatment on plasma lipoprotein concentrations in type II hyperlipoproteinemia. Am J Cardiol 1985;55:1282–1286.
31. Angelin B, Ericksson M, Einarsson K. Combined treatment with cholestyramine and nicotinic acid in heterozygous familial hypercholesterolaemia: effects on biliary lipid composition. Eur J Clin Invest 1986;16:391–396.
32. Series JJ, Caslake MJ, Kilday C, et al. Effect of combined therapy with bezafibrate and cholestyramine on low-density lipoprotein metabolism in type IIa hypercholesterolemia. Metabolism 1989;38:153–158.
33. Witztum JL. Intensive drug therapy of hypercholesterolemia. Am Heart J 1987;113:603–609.
34. Illingworth DR, Bacon S. Treatment of heterozygous familial hypercholesterolemia with lipid-lowering drugs. Arteriosclerosis 1989;9(suppl I):I121–I134.
35. Forland SC, Feng Y, Cutler RE. Apparent reduced absorption of gemfibrozil when given with colestipol. J Clin Pharmacol 1990;30:29–32.
36. Levy RI, Fredrickson DS, Stone NJ, et al. Cholestyramine in type II hyperlipoproteinemia: a double-blind trial. Ann Intern Med 1973;79:51–58.
37. Brensike JF, Levy RI, Kelsey SF, et al. Effects of therapy with cholestyramine on progression of coronary arteriosclerosis: results of the NHLBI type II coronary intervention study. Circulation 1984;69:313–324.
38. Levy RI, Brensike JF, Epstein SE, et al. The influence of changes in lipid values induced by cholestyramine and diet on progression of coronary artery disease: results of the NHLBI type II coronary intervention study. Circulation 1984;69:325–337.
39. Angelin B, Einarsson K. Cholestyramine in type IIa hyperlipoproteinemia: is

low-dose treatment feasible? Atherosclerosis 1981;38:33–38.

40. Witztum JL. Current approaches to drug therapy for the hypercholesterolemic patient. Circulation 1989;80:1101–1114.

41. Sirtori M, Franceshini G, Gianfranceshi G, et al. Microporous cholestyramine in suspension form. Lancet 1982;2:383.

42. Crouse JR III. Hypertriglyceridemia: a contraindication to the use of bile acid binding resins. Am J Med 1987;83:243–248.

43. Report of the Committee of Principal Investigators. W.H.O. Cooperative Trial on primary prevention of ischaemic heart disease using clofibrate to lower serum cholesterol: mortality follow-up. Lancet 1980;2:379–385.

44. Havel RJ, Kane JP. Drugs and lipid metabolism. Annu Rev Pharmacol 1973;13:287–308.

45. Gugler R. Clinical pharmacokinetics of hypolipidaemic drugs. Clin Pharmacokinet 1978;3:425–439.

46. Cayen MN. Disposition, metabolism and pharmacokinetics of antihyperlipidemic agents in laboratory animals and man. Pharmacol Ther 1985;29:157–204.

47. Witiak DT, Newman HAI, Feller DR. Clofibrate and Related Analogues. New York: Marcel Dekker, 1977.

48. Marks J, ed. Dyslipoproteinemia—aspects of gemfibrozil therapy. In: Research and Clinical Forums. Vol. 4. Kent, England: [Publisher], 1982.

49. Newton RS, Krause BR. Mechanisms of action of gemfibrozil: comparison of studies in the rat to clinical efficacy. In: Fears R, ed. Pharmacological Control of Hyperlipidaemia, Barcelona: JR Prous Science Publishers, 1986:171–186.

50. Todd PA, Ward A. Gemfibrozil: a review of its pharmacodynamic and pharmacokinetic properties, and therapeutic use in dyslipidaemia. Drugs 1988;36:314–339.

51. Eisenberg S, Gavish D, Kleinman Y. Bezafibrate. In: Fears R, ed. Pharmacological Control of Hyperlipidaemia, Barcelona: JR Prous Science Publishers, 1986:145–169.

52. Monk JP, Todd PA. Bezafibrate: a review of its pharmacodynamic and pharmacokinetic properties, and therapeutic use in hyperlipidaemia. Drugs 1987;33:539–576.

53. Blane GF, Bogaievsky Y, Bonnefous F. Fenofibrate: influence on circulating lipids and side-effects in medium and long-term clinical use. In: Fears R, ed. Pharmacological Control of Hyperlipidaemia. Barcelona: JR Prous Science Publishers, 1986:187–216.

54. Kloer HU. Structure and biochemical effects of fenofibrate. Am J Med 1987;83(5B):3–8.

55. Grundy SM, Vega GL. Fibric acids: effects on lipids and lipoprotein metabolism. Am J Med 1987;83(5B):9–20.

56. Chapman JM. Pharmacology of fenofibrate. Am J Med 1987;83(5B):21–25.

57. Blane GF. Comparative toxicity and safety profile of fenofibrate and other fibric acid derivatives. Am J Med 1987;83(5B):26–36.

58. Palmer RH. Effects of fibric acid derivatives on biliary lipid composition. Am J Med 1987;83(5B):37–43.

59. Hunninghake DB, Peters JR. Effect of fibric acid derivatives on blood lipid and lipoprotein levels. Am J Med 1987;83(5B):44–49.

60. Knopp RH, Brown WV, Dujovne CA, et al. Effects of fenofibrate on plasma

lipoproteins in hypercholesterolemia and combined hyperlipidemia. Am J Med 1987;83(5B):50–59.

61. Sirtori CR, Franceschini G. Effects of fibrates on serum lipids and atherosclerosis. Pharmacol Ther 1988;37:167–191.

62. Greten H, Laible V, Zipperle G, et al. Comparison of assay methods for selective measurement of plasma lipase: the effect of clofibrate on hepatic and lipoprotein lipase in normals and patients with hypertriglyceridemia. Atherosclerosis 1977;26:563–572.

63. Nikkila EA, Huttunen JK, Ehnholm C. Effect of clofibrate on postheparin plasma triglyceride lipase activities in patients with hypertriglyceridemia. Metabolism 1977;26:179–186.

64. Kissebah AH, Adams PW, Harrington P, et al. The mechanism of action of clofibrate and tetranicotinoylfructose (Bradilan) on the kinetics of plasma free fatty acid and triglyceride transport in type IV and type V hypertriglyceridaemia. Eur J Clin Invest 1974;4:163–174.

65. Kesaniemi YA, Beltz WF, Grundy SM. Comparison of clofibrate and caloric restriction on kinetics of very low density lipoprotein triglycerides. Arteriosclerosis 1985;5:153–161.

66. Walton KW, Scott PJ, Verrier Jones J, et al. Studies on low-density lipoprotein turnover in relation to Atromid therapy. J Atheroscler Res 1963;3:396–414.

67. Coronary Drug Project Research Group. Gallbladder disease as a side effect of drugs influencing lipid metabolism. Experience in the Coronary Drug Project. N Engl J Med 1977;296:1185–1190.

68. Report of the Committee of Principal Investigators. W.H.O. Cooperative Trial on primary prevention of ischaemic heart disease with clofibrate to lower serum cholesterol: final mortality follow-up. Lancet 1984;2:600–604.

69. Coronary Drug Project Research Group. Clofibrate and niacin in coronary heart disease. JAMA 1975;231:360–381.

70. Rimon D, Ludatscher R, Cohen L. Clofibrate-induced muscular syndrome: case report with ultrastructural findings and review of the literature. Isr J Med Sci 1984;20:1082–1086.

71. Hunninghake DB. Drug interactions involving hypolipidemic drugs. In: Petrie JC, ed. Cardiovascular and Respiratory Disease Therapy. New York: Elsevier/North Holland Biomedical Press, 1980:79–105.

72. Report from the Committee of Principal Investigators. A co-operative trial in the primary prevention of ischaemic heart disease using clofibrate Br Heart J 1978;40:1069–1118.

73. Hunninghake DB, Tucker DR, Azarnoff DL. Long-term effects of clofibrate (Atromid-S) on serum lipids in man. Circulation 1969;39:675–683.

74. Stuyt PMJ, Demacker PNM, Van't Laar A. Long-term treatment of type III hyperlipoproteinemia with clofibrate. Atherosclerosis 1981;40:329–336.

75. Hoogwerf BJ, Bantle JP, Kuba K, et al. Treatment of type III hyperlipoproteinemia with four different treatment regimens. Atherosclerosis 1984;51:251–259.

76. Nestel PJ, Hunt D7E Wahlqvist ML. Clofibrate raises plasma apoprotein A-1 and HDL-cholesterol concentrations. Atherosclerosis 1980;37:625–629.

77. Evans JR, Forland SC, Cutler RE. The effect of renal function on the pharmacokinetics of gemfibrozil. J Clin Pharmacol 1987;27:994–1000.

78. Saku K, Gartside PS, Hynd BA, et al. Mechanism of action of gemfibrozil on lipoprotein metabolism. J Clin Invest 1985;75:1702–1712.
79. Weintraub MS, Eisenberg S, Breslow JL. Different patterns of postprandial lipoprotein metabolism in normal, type IIa, type III, and type IV hyperlipoproteinemic individuals: effects of treatment with cholestyramine and gemfibrozil. J Clin Invest 1987;79:1110–1119.
80. Houlston R, Quiney J, Watts GF, et al. Gemfibrozil in the treatment of resistant familial hypercholesterolemia and type III hyperlipoproteinaemia. J R Soc Med 1988;81:274–276.
81. Vega GL, Grundy SM. Gemfibrozil therapy in primary hypertriglyceridemia associated with coronary heart disease. JAMA 1985;253:2398–2403.
82. Shepherd J, Caslake MJ, Lorimer AR, et al. Fenofibrate reduces low density lipoprotein catabolism in hypertriglyceridemic subjects. Arteriosclerosis 1985;5:162–168.
83. Malmendier CL, Delcroix C. Effects of fenofibrate on high and low density lipoprotein metabolism in heterozygous familial hypercholesterolemia. Atherosclerosis 1985;55:161–169.
84. Kleinman Y, Eisenberg S, Oschry Y, et al. Defective metabolism of hypertriglyceridemic low density lipoprotein in cultered human skin fibroblasts: normalization with bezafibrate therapy. J Clin Invest 1985;75:1796–1803.
85. Tikkanen MJ, Helve E, Jaattela A, et al. Comparison between lovastatin and gemfibrozil in the treatment of primary hypercholesterolemia: the Finnish multicenter study. Am J Cardiol 1988;62:35J–43J.
86. Eisenberg S. Lipoprotein abnormalities in hypertriglyceridemia: significance in atherosclerosis. Am Heart J 1987;113:555–561.
87. Vega GL, Grundy SM. Comparison of lovastatin and gemfibrozil in normolipidemic patients with hypoalphalipoproteinemia. JAMA 1989;262:3148–3153.
88. Laustiola K, Lassila R, Koskinen P, et al. Gemfibrozil decreases platelet reactivity in patients with hypercholesterolemia during physical stress. Clin Pharmacol Ther 1988;43:302–307.
89. Torstila I, Kaukola S, Manninen V, et al. Plasma prekallikrein, kallikrein inhibitors, kininogen and lipids during gemfibrozil treatment in type II dyslipidaemia. Acta Med Scand [Suppl] 1982;668:123–129.
90. Leiss O, von Bergmann K, Gnasso A, et al. Effect of gemfibrozil on biliary lipid metabolism in normolipidemic subjects. Metabolism 1985;34:74–82.
91. Hall MJ, Nelson LM, Russel RI, et al. Gemfibrozil—the effect on biliary cholesterol saturation of a new lipid-lowering agent and its comparison with clofibrate. Atherosclerosis 1981;39:511–516.
92. Pasternack A, Vantinnen T, Solakivi T, et al. Normalization of lipoprotein lipase and hepatic lipase by gemfibrozil results in correction of lipoprotein abnormalities in chronic renal failure. Clin Nephrol 1987;27:163–168.
93. Lopid (Gemfibrozil) package insert. Parke-Davis, January 1989.
94. De La Iglesia FA, Lewis JE, Buchanan RA, et al. Light and electron microscopy of liver in hyperlipoproteinemic patients under long-term gemfibrozil treatment. Atherosclerosis 1982;43:19–37.
95. Tobert JA. Letter to the editor. N Engl J Med 1988;318:48.
96. Marais GE, Larson KK. Rhabdomyolysis and acute renal failure induced by combination lovastatin and gemfibrozil therapy. Ann Intern Med 1990; 112:228–230.

97. Manninen V, Huttunen JK, Heinonen OP, et al. Relation between baseline lipid and lipoprotein values and the incidence of coronary heart disease in the Helsinki Heart Study. Am J Cardiol 1989;63:42H–47H.

98. Leaf DA, Connor WE, Illingworth DR, et al. The hypolipidemic effects of gemfibrozil in type V hyperlipidemia. JAMA 1989;262:3154–3160.

99. Kostner G, Klein G, Krempler F. Can serum Lp(a) concentrations be lowered by drugs and/or diet? In: Carlson LA, Olsson AG, eds. Treatment of Hyperlipoproteinemia. New York: Raven Press, 1984:151–156.

100. Brown MS, Goldstein JL. Multivalent feedback regulation of HMG CoA reductase, a control mechanism coordinating isoprenoid synthesis and cell growth. J Lipid Res 1980;21:505–517.

101. Rudney H, Sexton RC. Regulation of cholesterol biosynthesis. Annu Rev Nutr 1986;6:245–272.

102. Grundy SM. HMG-CoA reductase inhibitors for treatment of hypercholesterolemia. N Engl J Med 1988;319:24–33.

103. Mabuchi H, Takeda R. Inhibitors of 3-hydroxy-3-methylglutaryl coenzyme A reductase: compactin and its analogues. In: Fears R, ed. Pharmacological Control of Hyperlipidemia. Barcelona: JR Prous Science Publishers, 1986: 251–261.

104. Illingworth DR. Specific inhibitors of cholesterol biosynthesis as hypocholesterolemic agents in humans: mevinolin and compactin. In: Fears R, ed. Pharmacological Control of Hyperlipidemia. Barcelona: Prous JR Science Publishers, 1986:231–249.

105. Hoeg JM, Brewer HB Jr. 3-Hydroxy-3-methylglutaryl-coenzyme A reductase inhibitors in the treatment of hypercholesterolemia. JAMA 1987;258:3532–3536.

106. Henwood JM, Heel RC. Lovastatin: a preliminary review of its pharmacodynamic properties and therapeutic use in hyperlipidemia. Drugs 1988;36:429–454.

107. Kovanen PT, Bilheimer DW, Goldstein JL, et al. Regulatory role for hepatic low density lipoprotein receptors in vivo in the dog. Proc Natl Acad Sci USA 1981;78:1194–1198.

108. Bilheimer DW, Grundy SM, Brown MS, et al. Mevinolin and colestipol stimulate receptor-mediated clearance of low density lipoprotein from plasma in familial hypercholesterolemia heterozygotes. Proc Natl Acad Sci USA 1983;80:4124–4128.

109. Grundy SM, Vega GL. Influences of mevinolin on metabolism of low density lipoproteins in primary moderate hypercholesterolemia. J Lipid Res 1985; 26:1464–1475.

110. Vega GL, East C, Grundy SM. Lovastatin therapy in familial dysbetalipoproteinemia: effects on kinetics of apolipoprotein B. Atherosclerosis 1988; 70:131–143.

111. Thiery J, Armstrong VW, Schleef J, et al. Serum lipoprotein Lp(a) concentrations are not influenced by HMG CoA reductase inhibitor. Klin Wochenschr 1988;66:462–463.

112. Jurgens G, Ashy A, Zenker G. Raised serum lipoprotein during treatment with lovastatin. Lancet 1989;1:911–912.

113. Grundy SM, Bilheimer DW. Inhibition of 3-hydroxy-3-methylglutaryl-CoA reductase by mevinolin in familial hypercholesterolemia heterozygotes: effects on cholesterol balance. Proc Natl Acad Sci USA 1984;81:2538–2542.

114. Parker TS, McNamara DJ, Brown CD, et al. Plasma mevalonate as a measure of cholesterol synthesis in man. J Clin Invest 1984;74:795–804.
115. Tobert JA. Efficacy and long-term adverse effect pattern of lovastatin. Am J Cardiol 1988;62:28J–34J.
116. Lovastatin Study Group II. Therapeutic response to lovastatin (mevinolin) in nonfamilial hypercholesterolemia. JAMA 1986;256:2829–2834.
117. Lovastatin Study Group III. A multicenter comparison of lovastatin and cholestyramine therapy for severe primary hypercholesterolemia. JAMA 1988;260:359–366.
118. Havel RJ, Hunninghake DB, Illingworth DR, et al. Lovastatin (mevinolin) in the treatment of heterozygous familial hypercholesterolemia: a multicenter study. Ann Intern Med 1987;107:609–615.
119. MacDonald JS, Gerson RJ, Kornbrust DJ, et al. Preclinical evaluation of lovastatin. Am J Cardiol 1988;62:16J–27J.
120. Hunninghake DB, Miller VT, Stein I, et al. Lovastatin: follow-up ophthalmologic data. JAMA 1988;259:354–355.
121. Laue L, Hoeg JM, Barnes K, et al. The effect of mevinolin on steroidogenesis in patients with defects in the low density lipoprotein receptor pathway. J Clin Endocrinol Metab 1987;64:531–535.
122. Fojo SS, Hoeg JM, Lackner KJ, et al. Adrenocortical function in type II hyperlipoproteinemic patients treated with lovastatin (mevinolin). Horm Metab Res 1987;19:648–652.
123. Thompson GR, Ford J, Jenkinson M, et al. Efficacy of mevinolin as adjuvant therapy for refractory familial hypercholesterolemia. Q J Med 1986;60:803–811.
124. Farnsworth WH, Hoeg JM, Maher M, et al. Testicular function in type II hyperlipoproteinemic patients treated with lovastatin (Mevacor) or neomycin. J Clin Endocrinol Metab 1987;65:546–550.
125. Norman DJ, Illingworth DR, Munson J, et al. Myolysis and acute renal failure in a heart-transplant recipient receiving lovastatin. N Engl J Med 1988;318:46–47.
126. East C, Alivazatos PA, Grundy SM, et al. Rhabdomyolysis in patients receiving lovastatin after cardiac transplantation. N Engl J Med 1988;318:47–48.
127. Reaven P, Witztum JL. Lovastatin, nicotinic acid, and rhabdomyolysis. Ann Intern Med 1988;109:597–598.
128. Ayanian JZ, Fuchs CS, Stone RM. Lovastatin and rhabdomyolysis. Ann Intern Med 1988;109:682.
129. Corpier CL, Jones PH, Suki WN, et al. Rhabdomyolysis and renal injury with lovastatin use. JAMA 1988;260:239–241.
130. Edelman S, Witzum JL. Hyperkalemia during treatment with HMG-CoA reductase inhibitor. N Engl J Med 1989;320:1219–1220.
131. Israeli A, Raveh D, Arnon R, et al. Lovastatin and elevated creatine kinase: results of rechallange. Lancet 1989;1:725.
132. Mevacor (lovastatin) package insert, Merck Sharp & Dohme, West Point, PA (December 1988).
133. Illingworth DR. Long term administration of lovastatin in the treatment of hypercholesterolemia. Eur Heart J 1987;8(suppl E):103–111.
134. East C, Bilhelmer DW, Grundy SM. Combination drug therapy for familial combined hyperlipidemia. Ann Intern Med 1988;109:25–32.

135. Hoeg JM, Maher MB, Zech LA, et al. Effectiveness of mevinolin on plasma lipoprotein concentrations in type II hyperlipoproteinemia. Am J Cardiol 1986;57:933–939.
136. Uauy R, Vega GL, Grundy SM, et al. Lovastatin therapy in receptor-negative homozygous familial hypercholesterolemia: lack of effect on low-density lipoprotein concentrations or turnover. J Pediatr 1988;113:387–392.
137. East CA, Grundy SM, Bilheimer DW. Preliminary report: treatment of type 3 hyperlipoproteinemia with mevinolin. Metabolism 1986;35:97–98.
138. Garg A, Grundy SM. Lovastatin for lowering cholesterol levels in non-insulin-dependent diabetes mellitus. N Engl J Med 1988;318:81–86.
139. Garg A, Grundy SM. Gemfibrozil alone and in combination with lovastatin for treatment of hypertriglyceridemia in NIDDM. Diabetes 1989;38:364–372.
140. Vega GL, Grundy SM. Lovastatin therapy in nephrotic hyperlipidemia: effects on lipoprotein metabolism. Kidney Int 1988;33:1160–1168.
141. Brown BG, Lin JT, Schaefer SM, et al. Niacin or lovastatin, combined with colestipol, regress coronary atherosclerosis and prevent clinical events in men with elevated apolipoprotein B. Circulation 1989;80(suppl II):II–266.
142. Hoeg JM, Maher MB, Bailey KR, et al. The effects of mevinolin and neomycin alone and in combination on plasma lipid and lipoprotein concentrations in type II hyperlipoproteinemia. Atherosclerosis 1986;60:209–214.
143. Helve E, Tikkanen MJ. Comparison of lovastatin and probucol in treatment of familial and non-familial hypercholesterolemia: different effects on lipoprotein profiles. Atherosclerosis 1988;72:189–197.
144. Joven J, Masana L, Vilella E, et al. Lipid-lowering drugs in treatment of hyperlipidaemia associated with nephrotic syndrome. Lancet 1989;1:1029.
145. Schulzeck P, Bojanovski M, Jochim A, et al. Comparison between simvastatin and bezafibrate in effect on plasma lipoproteins and apolipoproteins in primary hypercholesterolemia. Lancet 1988;1:611–612.
146. Mol MJTM, Erkelens DW, Gevers Leuven JA, et al. Simvastatin (MK-733): a potent cholesterol synthesis inhibitor in heterozygous familial hypercholesterolemia. Atherosclerosis 1988;69:131–137.
147. Molgaard J, von Schenk H, Olsson AG. Effects of simvastatin on plasma lipid, lipoprotein and apolipoprotein concentrations in hypercholesterolemia. Eur Heart J 1988;9:541–551.
148. Leclerq V, Harvengt C. Simvastatin (MK 733) in heterozygous familial hypercholesterolemia: a two-year trial. Int J Clin Pharmacol Ther and Toxicol 1989;27:76–81.
149. Pietro DA, Alexander S, Mantell G, et al. Effects of simvastatin and probucol in hypercholesterolemia (simvastatin multicenter study group II). Am J Cardiol 1989;63:682–686.
150. Mabuchi H, Kamon N, Fujita H, et al. Effects of CS-514 on serum lipoprotein lipid and apolipoprotein levels in patients with familial hypercholesterolemia. Metabolism 1987;36:475–479.
151. Saku K, Sasaki J, Arakawa K. Long-term effect of CS-514 (HMG-CoA reductase inhibitor) on serum lipids, lipoproteins, and apolipoproteins in patients with hypercholesterolemia. Curr Ther Res 1987;42:491–500.
152. Yoshino G, Kazumi T, Iwai M, et al. Long-term treatment of hypercholesterolemic non-insulin dependent diabetics (NIDDM) with pravastatin (CS-514). Atherosclerosis 1989;75:67–72.

153. Gey KF, Carlson LA, eds. Metabolic Effects of Nicotinic Acid and Its Derivatives. Bern: H. Huber Publishers, 1971.
154. Hotz W. Nicotinic acid and its derivatives: a short survey. Adv Lipid Res 1983;20:195–217.
155. Olsson AG, Walldius G, Wahlberg G. Pharmacological control of hyperlipidaemia: nicotinic acid and its analogues—mechanisms of action, effects and clinical usage. In: Fears R, ed. Pharmacological Control of Hyperlipidaemia. Barcelona: JR Prous Science Publishers, 1986:217–230.
156. Fumagalli R. Pharmacokinetics of nicotinic acid and some of its derivatives. In: Gey KF, Carlson LA, eds. Metabolic Effects of Nicotinic Acid and Its Derivatives. Bern: H. Huber Publishers, 1971:33–49.
157. Mrochek JE, Jolley RL, Young DS, et al. Metabolic response of humans to ingestion of nicotinic acid and nicotinamide. Clin Chem 1976;22:1821–1827.
158. Carlson LA. Consequences of inhibition of normal and excessive lipid mobilization: studies with nicotinic acid. Prog Biochem Pharmacol 1967;3:151–166.
159. Grundy SM, Mok HYI, Zech L, et al. Influence of nicotinic acid on metabolism of cholesterol and triglycerides in man. J Lipid Res 1981;22:24–36.
160. Miettinen TA. Effect of nicotinic acid on the fecal excretion of neutral sterols and bile acids. In: Gey KF, Carlson LA, eds. Metabolic Effects of Nicotinic acid and Its Derivatives. Bern: H. Huber Publishers, 1971:677–686.
161. Langer T, Levy RI. The effect of nicotinic acid on the turnover of low density lipoproteins in type II hyperlipoproteinemia. In: Gey KF, Carlson LA, eds. Metabolic Effects of Nicotinic Acid and Its Derivatives. Bern: H. Huber Publishers, 1971:641–647.
162. Carlson LA, Olsson AG, Ballantyne D. On the rise in low density and high density lipoproteins in response to treatment of hypertriglyceridemia in type IV and type V hyperlipoproteinemias. Atherosclerosis 1977;26:603–609.
163. Boberg J, Carlson LA, Froberg S, et al. Effects of chronic treatment with nicotinic acid on intravenous fat tolerance and post-heparin lipase activity in man. In: Gey KF, Carlson LA, eds. Metabolic Effects of Nicotinic Acid and Its Derivatives. Bern: H. Huber Publishers, 1971:465–470.
164. Nikkila EA. Effect of nicotinic acid on adipose tissue lipoprotein lipase and removal rate of plasma triglycerides. In: Gey KF, Carlson LA, eds. Metabolic Effects of Nicotinic Acid and Its Derivatives. Bern: H. Huber Publishers, 1971:487–496.
165. Packard CJ, Stewart JM, Third JLHC, et al. Effects of nicotinic acid therapy on high-density lipoprotein metabolism in type II and type IV hyperlipoproteinaemia. Biochim Biophys Acta 1980;618:53–62.
166. Shephard J, Packard CJ, Patsch JR, et al. Effects of nicotinic acid therapy on plasma high density lipoprotein subfraction distribution and composition and on apolipoprotein A metabolism. J Clin Invest 1979;63:858–867.
167. Atmeh RF, Shepherd J, Packard CJ. Subpopulations of apolipoprotein A-1 in human high-density lipoproteins: their metabolic properties and response to drug therapy. Biochim Biophys Acta 1983;751:175–188.
168. Svedmyr N, Harthon L, Lundholm L. Dose-response relationship between concentration of free nicotinic acid concentration of plasma and some metabolic and circulatory effects after administration of nicotinic acid and pentaerythritoltetranicotinate in man. In: Gey KF, Carlson LA, eds. Metabolic

Effects of Nicotinic Acid and Its Derivatives. Bern: H. Huber Publishers, 1971:1085–1098.

169. Phillips WS, Lightman SL. Is cutaneous flushing prostaglandin mediated? Lancet 1981;1:754–756.

170. Olsson AG, Carlson LA, Anggard E, et al. Prostacyclin production augmented in the short term by nicotinic acid. Lancet 1983;2:565–566.

171. Parsons WB Jr. Studies of nicotinic acid use in hypercholesterolemia. Arch Intern Med 1961;107:653–667.

172. Berge KG, Achor RWP, Christensen NA, et al. Hypercholesterolemia and nicotinic acid: a long term study. Am J Med 1961;31:24–36.

173. Sugarman AA, Clark CG. Jaundice following the administration of niacin. JAMA 1974;228:202.

174. Einstein N, Baker A, Galper J, et al. Jaundice due to nicotinic acid therapy. Dig Dis 1975;20:282–286.

175. Blankenhorn DH, Nessim SA, Johnson RL, et al. Beneficial effects of combined colestipol-niacin therapy on coronary atherosclerosis and coronary venous bypass grafts. JAMA 1987;257:3233–3240.

176. Miettinen TA, Taskinen M-R, Pelkonen R, et al. Glucose tolerance and plasma insulin in man during acute and chronic administration of nicotinic acid. Acta Med Scand 1969;186:247–253.

177. Zavaroni I, Bonora E, Pagliara M, et al. Risk factors for coronary artery disease in healthy persons with hyperinsulinemia and normal glucose tolerance. N Engl J Med 1989;320:702–706.

178. Kaplan NM. The deadly quartet: upper-body obesity, glucose intolerance, hypertriglyceridemia, and hypertension. Arch Intern Med 1989;149:1514–1520.

179. Millay RH, Klein ML, Illingworth DR. Niacin maculopathy. Ophthalmology 1988;95:930–936.

180. Litin SC, Anderson CF. Nicotinic acid-associated myopathy: a report of three cases. Am J Med 1989;86:481–483.

181. Cashin-Hemphill L, Spencer CA, Nicoloff JT, et al. Alterations in serum thyroid hormonal indices with colestipol-niacin therapy. Ann Intern Med 1987;107:324–329.

182. Parsons WB Jr, Flinn JH. Reduction of serum cholesterol levels and beta-lipoprotein cholesterol levels by nicotinic acid. Arch Intern Med 1959; 103:783–790.

183. Parsons WB Jr. Treatment of hypercholesterolemia by nicotinic acid. Arch Intern Med 1961;107:639–652.

184. Carlson LA, Oro L. Effect of treatment with nicotinic acid for one month on serum lipids in patients with different types of hyperlipidemia. Atherosclerosis 1973;18:1–9.

185. Yovos JG, Patel ST, Falko JM, et al. Effects of nicotinic acid therapy on plasma lipoproteins and very low density lipoprotein apoprotein C subspecies in hyperlipoproteinemia. J Clin Endocrinol Metab 1982;54:1210–1215.

186. Wahlberg G, Holmquist L, Walldius G, et al. Effects of nicotinic acid on concentrations of serum apolipoproteins B, C-I, C-II, C-III and E in hyperlipidemic patients. Acta Med Scand.1988;224:319–327.

187. Gurakar A, Hoeg JM, Kostner G, et al. Levels of lipoprotein Lp(a) decline with neomycin and niacin treatment. Atherosclerosis 1985;57:293–301.

188. Canner PL, Berge KG, Wenger NK, et al. Fifteen year mortality in coronary drug project patients: long-term benefit with niacin. J Am Coll Cardiol 1986;8:1245–1255.
189. Rosenhamer G, Carlson LA. Effect of combined clofibrate-nicotinic acid treatment in ischemic heart disease. Atherosclerosis 1980;37:129–138.
190. Carlson LA, Rosenhamer G. Reduction of mortality in the Stockholm ischaemic heart disease secondary prevention study by combined treatment with clofibrate and nicotinic acid. Acta Med Scand 1988;223:405–418.
191. Moutafis CD, Myant NB. Effects of nicotinic acid, alone or in combination with cholestyramine, on cholesterol metabolism in patients suffering from familial hyperbetalipoproteinaemia in the homozygous form. In: Gey KF, Carlson LA, eds. Metabolic Effects of Nicotinic Acid and Its Derivatives. Bern: H Huber, 1971:659–676.
192. Knopp RH, Ginsberg J, Albers JJ, et al. Contrasting effects of unmodified and time-release forms of niacin on lipoproteins in hyperlipidemic subjects: clues to mechanism of action of niacin. Metabolism 1985;34:642–650.
193. Steinberg D, Parthasarathy S, Carew TE. In vivo inhibition of foam cell development by probucol in Watanabe rabbits. Cardiology 1988;62:6B–12B.
194. Heel RC, Brogden RN, Speight TM, et al. Probucol: a review of its pharmacological properties and therapeutic use in patients with hypercholesterolemia. Drugs 1978;15:409–428.
195. Strandberg TE, Vanhanen H, Miettinen TA. Probucol in long-term treatment of hypercholesterolemia. Gen Pharmacol 1988;19:317–320.
196. Buckley MM-T, Goa KL, Price AH, et al. Probucol: a reappraisal of its pharmacological properties and therapeutic use in hypercholesterolemia. Drugs 1989;37:761–800.
197. Dachet C, Jacotot B, Buxtorf JC. The hypolipidemic action of probucol: drug transport and lipoprotein composition in type IIa hyperlipoproteinemia. Atherosclerosis 1985;58:261–268.
198. Kesaniemi YA, Grundy SM. Influence of probucol on cholesterol and lipoprotein metabolism in man. J Lipid Res 1984;25:780–790.
199. Bilheimer DW. Lipoprotein fractions and receptors: a role for probucol? Am J Cardiol 1986;57:7H–15H.
200. Naruszewicz M, Carew TE, Pittman RC, et al. A novel mechanism by which probucol lowers low density lipoprotein levels demonstrated in the LDL receptor-deficient rabbit. J Lipid Res 1984;25:1206–1213.
201. Steinberg D, Parthasarathy S, Carew TE, et al. Beyond cholesterol: modifications of low-density lipoprotein that increase its atherogenicity. N Engl J Med 1989;320:915–924.
202. Kita T, Nagano Y, Yokode M, et al. Probucol prevents the progression of atherosclerosis in watanabe heritable hyperlipidemic rabbit, an animal model for familial hypercholesterolemia. Proc Natl Acad Sci USA 1987;84:5928–5931.
203. Carew TE, Schwenke DC, Steinberg D. Antiatherogenic effect of probucol unrelated to its hypocholesterolemic effect: evidence that antioxidants in vivo can selectively inhibit low density lipoprotein degradation in macrophage-rich fatty streaks and slow the progression of atherosclerosis in the watanabe heritable hyperlipidemic rabbit. Proc Natl Acad Sci USA 1987;84:7725–7729.

204. Wissler RW, Vesselinovitch D. Combined effects of cholestyramine and probucol on regression of atherosclerosis in rhesus monkey aortas. Appl Pathol 1983;1:89–96.
205. Yamamoto A, Matsuzawa Y, Yokoyama S, et al. Effects of probucol on xanthomata regression in familial hypercholesterolemia. Am J Cardiol 1986;57:29H–35H.
206. Yamamoto A, Hara H, Takaichi S, et al. Effect of probucol on macrophages, leading to regression of xanthomas and atheromatous vascular lesions. Am J Cardiol 1988;62:31B–36B.
207. Iida H, Izumino K, Asaka M, et al. Effect of probucol on hyperlipidemia in patients with nephrotic syndrome. Nephron 1987;47:280–283.
208. Jackman WM, Friday KJ, Anderson JL, et al. The long QT syndromes: a critical review, new clinical observations and a unifying hypothesis. Prog Cardiovasc Dis 1988;31:115–172.
209. Davignon J. Medical management of hyperlipidemia and the role of probucol. Am J Cardiol 1986;57:22H–28H.
210. Miettinen TA, Huttunen JK, Naukkarinen V, et al. Long-term use of probucol In the multifactorial primary prevention of vascular disease. Am J Cardiol 1986;57:49H–54H.
211. Yokohama S, Yamamoto A, Kurasawa T. A little more information about aggravation of probucol-induced HDL-reduction by clofibrate. Atherosclerosis 1988;70:179–181.
212. Gordon DJ, Probstfield JL, Garrison RJ, et al. High-density lipoprotein cholesterol and cardiovascular disease. Circulation 1989;79:8–15.
213. Nestruck AC, Bouthillier D, Sing CF, et al. Apolipoprotein E polymorphism and plasma cholesterol response to probucol. Metabolism 1987;36:743–747.
214. Anderson JL, Schroeder JS. Effects of probucol on hyperlipidemic patients with cardiac allografts. J Cardiovasc Pharmacol 1979;1:353–365.
215. Walldius G, Carlson LA, Erikson U, et al. Development of femoral atherosclerosis in hypercholesterolemic patients during treatment with cholestyramine and probucol/placebo: probucol quantitative regression Swedish trial (PQRST): a status report. Am J Cardiol 1988;62:37B–43B.
216. Witztum JL, Simmons D, Steinberg D, et al. Intensive combination drug therapy of familial hypercholesterolemia with lovastatin, probucol, and colestipol hydrochloride. Circulation 1989;79:16–28.
217. Illingworth DR. Drug therapy of hypercholesterolemia. Clin Chem 1988;34:B123–B132.
218. Malloy MJ, Kane JP, Kunitake ST, et al. Complementarity of colestipol, niacin and lovastatin in treatment of severe familial hypercholesterolemia. Ann Intern Med 1987;107:616–623.
219. Illingworth DR, Bacon S. Influence of lovastatin plus gemfibrozil on plasma lipids and lipoproteins in patients with heterozygous familial hypercholesterolemia. Circulation 1989;79:590–596.
220. Dujovne CA, Harris WS. The pharmacological treatment of dyslipidemia. Annu Rev Pharmacol Toxicol 1989;29:265–288.
221. Hoeg JM, Maher MB, Bou E, et al. Normalization of plasma lipoprotein concentrations in patients with type II hyperlipoproteinemia by combined use of neomycin and niacin. Circulation 1984;70:1004–1011.

222. Samuel P, Holtzman CM, Goldstein J. Long-term reduction of serum cholesterol levels of patients with atherosclerosis by small doses of neomycin. Circulation 1967;35:938–945.

223. Samuel P. Treatment of hypercholesterolemia with neomycin—a time for reappraisal. N Engl J Med 1979;301:595–597.

224. Hoeg JM, Schaefer EJ, Romano CA, et al. Neomycin and plasma lipoproteins in type II hyperlipoproteinemia. Clin Pharmacol Ther 1984;36:555–565.

225. Miettinen TA. Effects of neomycin alone and in combination with cholestyramine on serum cholesterol and fecal steroids in hypercholesterolemic subjects. J Clin Invest 1979;64:1485–1493.

226. Kesaniemi YA, Grundy SM. Turnover of low density lipoproteins during inhibition of cholesterol absorption by neomycin. Arteriosclerosis 1984;4:41–48.

227. Council on Drugs. Evaluation of a hypocholesterolemic agent, dextrothyroxine sodium (choloxin). JAMA 1969;208:1014–1015.

228. Searcy RL, Hungerford DA, Low EMY. Effects of dextrothyroxine on serum lipoprotein and cholesterol levels. Curr Ther Res 1968;10:177–186.

229. Schwandt P, Weisweiler P. The effect of D-thyroxine on lipoprotein lipids and apolipoproteins in primary type IIa hyperlipoproteinemia. Atherosclerosis 1980;35:301–306.

230. Bantle JP, Hunninghake DB, Frantz ID, et al. Comparison of effectiveness of thyrotropin-suppressive doses of D- and L-thyroxine in treatment of hypercholesterolemia. Am J Med 1984;77:475–481.

231. Coronary Drug Project Research Group. The Coronary Drug Project: findings leading to further modifications of its protocol with respect to dextrothyroxine. JAMA 1972;220:996–1008.

232. Tikkanen MJ, Nikkila EA, Vartiainen E. Natural estrogen as an effective treatment for type-II hyperlipoproteinaemia in postmenopausal women. Lancet 1978;2:490–491.

233. Kushwaha RS, Hazzard WR, Gagne C, et al. Type III hyperlipoproteinemia: paradoxical hypolipidemic response to estrogen. Ann Intern Med 1977;87:517–525.

234. Falko JM, Schonfeld G, Witztum JL, et al. Effects of estrogen therapy on apolipoprotein E in type III hyperlipoproteinemia. Metabolism 1979;28:1171–1177.

235. Kovanen PT, Brown MS, Goldstein JL. Increased binding of low density lipoprotein to liver membranes from rats treated with 17α-ethinyl estradiol. J Biol Chem 1979;254:11367–11373.

236. Chao Y, Windler EE, Chen GC, et al. Hepatic catabolism of rat and human lipoproteins in rats treated with 17α-ethinyl estradiol. J Biol Chem 1979;254:11360–11366.

237. Coronary Drug Project Research Group. The Coronary Drug Project: initial findings leading to modifications of its research protocol. JAMA 1970;214:1303–1313.

238. Coronary Drug Project Research Group. The Coronary Drug Project: findings leading to discontinuation of the 2.5 mg/day estrogen group. JAMA 1973;226:652–657.

239. Ernster VL, Bush TL, Huggins GR, et al. Benefits and risks of menopausal estrogen and/or progestin hormone use. Prev Med 1988;17:201–223.

240. Barett-Connor E, Bush TL. Estrogen replacement and coronary heart disease. Cardiovasc Clin 1989;19:159–172.
241. Kane JP, and Malloy MJ. Treatment of hypercholesterolemia. Med Clin North Am 1982;66:537–550.
242. Lees AM, Mok HYI, Lees RS, et al. Plant sterols as cholesterol-lowering agents: clinical trials in patients with hypercholesterolemia and studies of sterol balance. Atherosclerosis 1977;28:325–338.
243. Schlierf G, Oster P, Heuck CC, et al. Sitosterol in juvenile type II hyperlipoproteinemia. Atherosclerosis 1978;30:245–248.

13
Life-Style and Lipids

ERICA FRANK

Overview

The relationship between life-style choices and lipids is different from the relationship between more purely biological parameters and lipids. Unlike the effects of pharmacokinetics, age, sex, or family history, life-style choices involve volition and factors that are hard to quantify, such as stress. Furthermore, animal models or double-blind studies are often irrelevant, unethical, or impossible. This has made difficult the production of good epidemiological data on life-styles and risk assessment.

Describing the effect of risk factors is usually only important if four conditions help separate facts from enthusiasm: if the effect is (1) consistently demonstrable, (2) statistically and (3) clinically significant, and (4) practicably remediable. This chapter demonstrates that although some good data exist (with findings that are also consistent with the usual recommendations of preventive medicine), much of the research on the effect of life-style choices on women's lipid levels is lacking in one or more of these areas.

Demonstrability

There are two aspects to the problem of demonstrability. The first is the reliability of individuals' single lipid values. Like measurements of blood pressure and glucose, true plasma lipid levels may vary due to such factors as patient exercise and eating. Lipid results may also vary with season, medications, position at time of blood drawing, duration of tourniquet application, choice of container anticoagulant, and specimen handling.[1-4] These issues are discussed in more detail in Chapter 4. The second problem of demonstrability is that of replicability of research findings. Given the purported importance of many suggested lipid-related risk factors for women, there are remarkably few good, large, prospective studies that control for confounding factors.

Statistical Significance and Scientific Rigor

Much that has been presented as "science" in the investigation of the health effects of life-style choices is the product of a practical world that does not always easily permit rigorous definitions and precise measurements of such parameters as "stress," or the enrollment of large sample sizes in long-term, prospective, unbiased, randomized, double-blind trials. These nonrigorously derived data then enter the realm of "facts" that perpetuate the myths created by faulty, poorly interpreted information.

Clinical Significance

Most research has been conducted on men, and its extrapolation to women is at best uncertain, and often demonstrably wrong. The end point, responsiveness of cardiovascular morbidity and mortality to lipid modification, is still uncertain in women since the best trials (the Multiple Risk Factor Intervention Trial,[5] Lipid Research Clinic Coronary Primary Prevention Trials,[6] and Helsinki Heart Study[7]) all studied the effects of dietary and pharmacological modifications only on men. This is particularly important in light of the finding that high density lipoprotein (HDL) is probably a stronger predictor of coronary heart disease (CHD) in women than in men,[8] and that, for any level of such major cardiovascular risk (such as total cholesterol, systolic blood pressure, or glucose intolerance), women seem to have lower morbidity than men.[9] Also, we have not yet explained the biological significance of many laboratory findings (such as the epinephrine release observed in stressful situations), or why overall mortality may not be reduced by lipid improvements.[3,5]

Remediability

Although life-style choices seem more malleable than genetic factors (such as the presence of familial hypercholesterolemia), theoretically modifiable risk factors may, in practice, actually prove very difficult to modify. Lipid-affecting life-style decisions are inextricably connected both to factors discussed elsewhere in this book (such as birth control pill use, diet, and obesity) and to many other intangible parameters for decisions (is a patient willing to commit to the effort required for an effective exercise program?). Modification of life-style choices (such as smoking cessation) requires considerably more patient effort than taking one lovastatin with dinner. The requirement of such effort may affect patients' noncompliance with suggested preventive measures, and may limit actual remediability of life-style choices.

Exercise

Exercise has been shown in both men and women to have acutely and chronically favorable effects on lipid levels.

Triglycerides are acutely reduced following intensive exercise in conditioned men.[10-12] There is also evidence of the benefits for both sexes of ongoing exercise on triglyceride levels,[13,14] including the ability of exercise to attenuate triglyceride elevations found with oral contraceptive use.[15] However, the evidence for women,[16] including middle-aged obese women,[17] is less conclusive than for men, and, for both men and women, the relationship between triglycerides and cardiovascular risk is unclear.

Exercise-related changes in total cholesterol are even more difficult to interpret since they involve both the increases in HDL levels and decreases in low density lipoproteins (LDL). Some investigators have found no significant relationship between exercise and total cholesterol (specifically in such anaerobic/static exercisers as weight-lifting men[18,19] and in weight-reducing obese middle-aged women[17]). Nonetheless, other investigators have reported significant total cholesterol changes in aerobically training men,[10,13,16] moderately (20 minutes of "aerobic dance" 3 times a week)[16] and rigorously (15+ miles/week) aerobically[13] training women, and anaerobically[18] training women.

Several studies have demonstrated decreased LDL levels in both male[10,12,13,18-20] and female[13,18] exercisers compared to controls. This has been shown for both sexes in both aerobic (running)[10,12,13] and anaerobic (weight-lifting)[18-20] exercise. Other studies have found, however, that women (specifically, moderately exercising[16] or obese middle aged-women[17]) may not be capable of exercise-related LDL reduction.

Although some researchers have found that HDL may be acutely elevable following intensive exercise in both men[11,12,21] and women,[21] others have not found this to be the case,[10] and most research has concentrated on the long-term effect of exercise on HDL. Increases in HDL have been shown in men performing anaerobic[19,20] and both low-intensity/long duration (walking postal workers) aerobic[22] and moderate- to high-intensity aerobic[13,14,23-25] activities.

Many studies have also demonstrated a positive relationship between amount of exercise and HDL levels in women. Significant improvements in HDL were found in young women who increased their weekly running from 15 to 47 and then 63 miles.[26] Similarly, female runners (averaging 31 miles/week) had significantly higher HDL levels than inactive female controls.[13] In a study of 47 inactive, 49 jogging (20 km/week), and 45 long-distance running (50 km/week) women, there were significant differences between joggers' and inactive women's, and long-distance runners' and joggers' HDL levels.[27] Another study found significant increases in HDL levels for inactive women who began a program of running for 30 minutes, 3 to 4 days per week.[14] Two other studies found no significant change in

HDL levels (in anaerobically training women[18] or weight-reducing middle-aged women[17]), but did find significant improvements in HDL:LDL ratios.

However, other studies of women have shown no HDL improvement for exercising women, although it is unclear why this is so. It is particularly questionable whether women are as sensitive as men to exercise-related HDL changes with only a moderate exercise program,[16,17,28] as the studies that failed to document a significant change in women's lipid levels generally had a lower dose of exercise exposure.

If these lipid (especially the HDL) changes are real, they may be attributable to a combination of increased exercise, lower total body weight (although some studies have controlled for this phenomenon, and one study found that decreased weight raised HDL levels only in cigarette smokers[29]), and decreased body mass index.[30-33] One suggested mechanism of action for lipid (especially HDL) changes is increased exercise-induced lipoprotein lipase activity. The reasons for this increase are uncertain, although it may involve either an elevated sensitivity to insulin or exercise-stimulated catecholamine release.[10,12,23,34,35] (Interestingly, although women may start with higher baseline lipoprotein lipase activity levels than men,[4] one study that bioassayed fat cell biopsies found that epinephrine-stimulated lipolysis increased with exercise more in men than in women.[36]) There are several other hypotheses for why cholesterol fraction levels change, including alterations in lipoprotein synthesis and degradation (other than lipoprotein lipase changes), and plasma volume shifts.[4]

In conclusion, much attention has been paid to whether there is an actual relationship between exercise and improved lipid profiles that is both real and independent of improvements in covariables such as lowered percent body fat. Most evidence supports a favorable effect of exercise on lipids, but, for women, moderate to intensive efforts may be necessary to produce significant improvements. In the clinical setting, therefore, we can tell female patients that exercise may improve their lipid profiles. However, perhaps most importantly, with *all* of these life-style choices patients can experience considerable "cross benefits"—improvements in areas other than lipid profiles. For cross benefits, then, as well as the lipid improvements and relatively low risks associated with this life-style intervention, we can recommend judicious exercise to our patients.

Ethanol

For the last few years, ostensible lipid improvement has been the best (and perhaps only well documented) health-improving reason for drinking. Although moderately used ethanol elevates triglycerides,[37] many studies have found that ethanol use raised HDL for both men[32,33,37,38] and women.[32] Ethanol may also increase lipoprotein lipase activity.[39] Additionally, it has been reported that with intermediate ethanol intake, apolipoprotein A-1 significantly increased[40] (even without significant changes in total HDL, HDL_2, or HDL_3), and that ethanol-related HDL elevations may be due to increased hepatic apoprotein A-1 synthesis.[38,39]

Nonetheless, despite some studies demonstrating that a favorable lipid profile is produced with low-dose ethanol consumption, it may be the case that only higher-dose,[39] that is, 75+ g (750 ml of wine)[37] per day of ethanol use will increase HDL_2; more moderate use (12.6 g or one 12-ounce beer/day)[40] may not affect total HDL or its subfractions, or may only increase the relatively lipid-poor HDL_3.[39,41] Another problem with many studies is that ethanol intake levels are notoriously under-reported, which may result in understating the ethanol dose that actually produced the HDL elevation.

There has been little examination of the effect of ethanol consumption on HDL levels in women. Although some investigators have found that in women, too, HDL levels may increase with ethanol use,[32,33,42] others have found that women may not be as sensitive as men to such changes,[41] especially regarding changes in HDL subfractions.[42]

We may therefore continue to advise patients that there is no definitive evidence of a health-promoting effect for ethanol, but there is substantial evidence of its ill effects.

Smoking

In the realm of life-style choices and their effect on lipids, smoking is, as elsewhere, the most unequivocal villain. Despite confounding variables (i.e., smokers may consume more ethanol than do nonsmokers) and the ethical impossibility of conducting a randomized trial, the data are strong.

Most studies have shown a significant inverse relationship between smoking and HDL for both men[30,33,43,44] and women.[33,44,45] Also, intriguingly, it has been suggested that children of smoking mothers have lower HDL_2 levels than those of nonsmokers (however, there was no attempt to separate genetic differences, prenatal exposure, passive smoking, or other environmental effects).[46]

Although data are strongest for HDL, we are not without data for other lipid fractions. There is evidence for cigarettes adversely affecting triglycerides,[30,31] LDL,[30] and very low density lipoproteins (VLDL),[30] although some studies found this data, especially for women, inconclusive.[30,42]

The mechanism of action for any differences (especially the well documented effect on HDL) is uncertain. It is possible that, at least for men, there is a positive association between cigarette use and both androstenedione and possibly testosterone levels, and no relationship to estradiol or estrone,[47] and this correlation might help provide an etiology for the ill effects of smoking on lipid levels. Happily, then, we need feel no conflict in continuing to recommend smoking cessation to all our patients.

Stress

Stress is the most difficult life-style area to evaluate effects of lipids. Stress is a difficult parameter to define clinically, and the implications of laboratory research are tenuous. There is, however, some information that is worth examining.

Some data suggest that women produce fewer catecholamines in response to stress, and this has been proposed to contribute to women's more favorable lipid profiles. A study that looked at both cognitive and physical (repeated venipuncture) stressors found greater male epinephrine reactivity to both of these types of stressors.[48] Regarding purely cognitive stressors, several studies have demonstrated that females, even as children,[49] exhibit similar baseline catecholamine levels when compared with males, but excrete significantly less epinephrine than do males exposed to identical intellectually stressful situations.[48,50–52]

There are, however, many potential confounding factors. For instance, are these situations actually as stressful for the women as the men? For example, it was found that more relationship-oriented and less examination achievement-oriented women may, unsurprisingly, show less increase in their epinephrine excretion during academically stressful activities than their more academically-oriented female peers. (The group of men was not separated in this fashion.) However, even when this relationship-oriented cohort was taken out of the male-female comparison group, the contrast between male and female epinephrine excretion was virtually unchanged.[50]

It is particularly unfortunate that convincing evidence on physiological reactivity is not yet available for postmenopausal women, since this is the time of highest female cardiovascular risk. A few disputed studies (most experiments have been small, nonrandomized, or performed only one time and by one investigator) have found that non-hormone-replaced, postmenopausal women may have more male-like catecholamine and cardiovascular responses in response to stress than their premenopausal or hormone-replaced controls. However, we cannot yet extrapolate clinical significance from these results. Hormonal shifts (as seen in women in their luteal phases and in postmenopausal women) may also produce more male-like cardiovascular and epinephrine responses.[52,53]

One study of particular interest examined directly the effect of differing stressors on lipid levels in women. In this investigation, Hazuda and colleagues[54] compared a group of Mexican-American and non-Hispanic white employed women with homemakers (stratifying for body mass index, blood pressure, cigarette smoking, exercise, caloric imbalance, ethanol intake, and use of oral contraceptives or other exogenous estrogens), and found no differences in total or LDL cholesterol levels, but a highly significant difference ($p \leq 0.001$, a difference of 4 mg/dl) in HDL and triglycerides (with employed women having higher HDL and lower triglycerides) between women working in and outside the home. These findings were true for both Mexican-American and non-Hispanic white workers, and were more pronounced in professional, managerial, sales, and clerical occupations than in blue-collar workers. Although these are fascinating findings, we are still left with the difficult task of interpreting these data. (For instance, do women working at home experience less stress or more than those working outside of the home?)

Even if we eventually definitively demonstrate that, in an experimental setting, males and females produce different quantities of catecholamines in response to stress, several pressing questions would remain. (1) Does this response reflect a usual reaction, or are stressors interpreted differently in an experimental setting? (2) Does this differential secretion rate *persist* over extended periods? One study found that, over a year's collection of urine samples (collected every 4 weeks), women and men did not differ significantly in total catecholamine excretion (although there were large interindividual and small intraindividual differences in excretion rates).[55] (3) What *actual effect* do catecholamines have on lipids? Although exercise-induced epinephrine elevations selectively mobilize needed lipids for fuel, it is unclear what effects stress-induced elevations have on lipids. Some older data suggest that total cholesterol does transiently increase (and triglycerides remain stable) in situations ranging from taking an exam to flying and to awaiting surgery. However, most of this information was obtained in the 1950s and 1960s, and generally not from female subjects.[56]

It may indeed be the case that there is gender dimorphism in physiological response to stressors, but the health implications are unclear. Given this tenuous information, we may conclude only that we have an intriguing and testable addition to the body of data that suggests that stress might be harmful to your health.

Conclusion

We should encourage life-style changes where the data are most compelling, the cross benefits to health factors other than lipids are greatest, and the risks are fewest. Although definitive data on the relationship between many life-style choices and lipid levels in women are lacking, there are sufficient data from lipid and other research fields to continue to discourage smoking and to recommend exercise. Although we cannot yet reject the possible salutary effect of ethanol on HDL and apoprotein A-1, in view of the many irrefutable health hazards associated with its abuse it remains imprudent for health-care providers to recommend alcohol intake. Finally, the effect of stress on lipids remains far too nebulous to affect recommendations.

Acknowledgments

The author wishes to thank Dr. J. Farquhar, Dr. S. Fortmann, and Dr. P. Wood of the Stanford Center for Research in Disease Prevention for reviewing this chapter.

References

1. Gordon DJ, Trost DC, Hyde J, et al. Seasonal cholesterol cycles: the Lipid Research Clinics Coronary Primary Prevention Trial placebo group. Circulation 1987;176(6):1224–1231.
2. Naito HK. Reliability of lipid and lipoprotein testing (I). Am J Cardiol 1985;56:6J–11J.
3. Corday E, Ryden L. Why some physicians have concerns about the cholesterol awareness program. J Am Coll Cardiol 1989;13(2):497–502.
4. Goldberg L, Elliot DL. The effect of exercise on lipid metabolism in men and women. Sports Med 1987;4:307–320.
5. Multiple Risk Factor Intervention Trial Group. Multiple Risk Factor Intervention Trial: risk factor changes and mortality results. JAMA 1982;248(12):1465–1477.
6. Lipid Research Clinics Program. The lipid research clinics coronary primary prevention trial results (II). JAMA 1984;251(3):365–374.
7. Frick MH, Elo O, Haapa V, et al. Helsinki heart study: primary prevention trial with gemfibrozil in middle-aged men with dyslipidemia. N Engl J Med 1987;317:1237–1245.
8. Crouse JR. Gender, lipoproteins, diet, and cardiovascular risk. Lancet 1989;i:318–320.
9. Lerner DJ, Kannel WB. Patterns of coronary heart disease morbidity and mortality in the sexes: a 26-year follow-up of the Framingham population. Am Heart J 1986;111(2):383–390.
10. Thompson PD, Cullinane E, Henderson LO, et al. Acute effects of prolonged exercise on serum lipids. Metabolism 1980;29(7):662–665.
11. Kantor MA, Cullinane EM, Herbert PN, Thompson PD. Acute increase in lipoprotein lipase following prolonged exercise. Metabolism 1984;33(5):454–457.
12. Dressendorfer RH, Wade CD, Hornick C, et al. High density lipoprotein-cholesterol in marathon runners during a 2-day road race. JAMA 1982;247(12):1715–1717.
13. Wood PD, Haskell WL, Stern MP, et al. Plasma lipoprotein distributions in male and female runners. Ann NY Acad Sci 1977;301:748–763.
14. Farrell PA, Barboriak J. The time course of alterations in plasma lipid and lipoprotein concentrations during eight weeks of endurance training. Atherosclerosis 1980;37:231–238.

15. Merians DR, Haskell WL, Vranizan KM. Relationship of exercise, oral contraceptive use, and body fat to concentrations of plasma lipids and lipoprotein cholesterol in young women. Am J Med 1985;78:913–919.
16. Brownell KD, Bachorik PS, Ayerle RS. Changes in plasma lipid and lipoprotein levels in men and women after a program of moderate exercise. Circulation 1982;65(3):477–484.
17. Lewis S, Haskell WL, Wood PD, et al. Effects of physical activity on weight reduction in obese middle-aged women. Am J Clin Nutr 1976;29:151–156.
18. Goldberg L, Elliot DL, Schutz RW, et al. Changes in lipid and lipoprotein levels after weight training. JAMA 1984; 252(4):504–506.
19. Hurley BF, Hagberg JM, Seals DR. Circuit weight training reduces coronary artery disease risk factors independent of changes in VO_2 max. Med Sci Sports Exer 1986;18(2)(suppl):S68–69. Abstract.
20. Johnson CC, Stone MH, Lopez-S A, et al. Diet and exercise in middle-aged men. Research 1982,81:695–701.
21. Lennon DLF, Stratman FW, Shrago E, et al. Total cholesterol and HDL-cholesterol changes during acute, moderate-intensity exercise in men and women. Metabolism 1983;32(3):244–249.
22. Cook TC, Laporte RE, Washburn RA, et al. Chronic low level physical activity as a determinant of high density lipoprotein cholesterol and subfractions. Med Sci Sports Exer 1986;18(6):653–657.
23. Hartung GH, Foreyt JP, Mitchell RE, et al. Relation of diet to high-density-lipoprotein cholesterol in middle-aged marathon runners, joggers, and inactive men. N Engl J Med 1980;302(7):357–361.
24. Nakamura N, Uzawa H, Maeda H, et al. Physical fitness: its contribution to serum high density lipoprotein. Atherosclerosis 1983;48:173–183.
25. Huttunen JK, Lansimies E, Voutilainen E, et al. Effect of moderate physical exercise on serum lipoproteins. Circulation 1979;60(6):1220–1229.
26. Rotkis T, Boyden TW, Pamenter RW, et al. High density lipoprotein cholesterol and body composition of female runners. Metabolism 1981;30(10):994–995.
27. Moore CE, Hartung GH, Mitchell RE, et al. The relationship of exercise and diet on high-density lipoprotein cholesterol levels in women. Metabolism 1983;32(2):189–195.
28. Frey MA, Doerr BM, Laubach LL, et al. Exercise does not change high-density lipoprotein cholesterol in women after ten weeks of training. Metabolism 1982;31(11):1142–1145.
29. Rabkin SW, Boyko E, Streja DA. Relationship of weight loss and cigarette smoking to changes in high-density lipoprotein cholesterol. Am J Clin Nutr 1981;34:1764–1768.
30. Freedman DS, Srinivasan SR, Shear CL, et al. Cigarette smoking initiation and longitudinal changes in serum lipids and lipoproteins in early adulthood: the Bogalusa heart study. Am J Epidemiol 1986;124(2):207–219.
31. Simons LA, Simons J, Jones AS. The interactions of body weight, age, cigarette smoking and hormone usage with blood pressure and plasma lipids in an Australian community. Aust NZ J Med 1984;14:215–221.
32. Linn S, Fulwood R, Rifkind B, et al. High density lipoprotein cholesterol levels among US adults by selected demographic and socioeconomic variables. Am J Epidemiol 1989;129:281–294.

33. Hubert HB, Eaker ED, Garrison RJ, et al. Life-style correlates of risk factor change in young adults: an eight-year study of coronary heart disease risk factors in the Framingham offspring. Am J Epidemiol 1987;125(5):812–831.
34. Wood PD, Haskell WL. The effect of exercise on plasma high density lipoproteins. Lipids 1979;14(4):417–427.
35. Nikkila EA, Taskinen M-R, Rehunen S, et al. Lipoprotein lipase activity in adipose tissue and skeletal muscle of runners: relation to serum lipoproteins. Metabolism 1978;27(11):1661–1671.
36. Despres JP, Bouchard C, Savard R, et al. The effect of a 20-week endurance training program on adipose-tissue morphology and lipolysis in men and women. Metabolism 1984;33(3):235–239.
37. Contaldo F, D'Arrigo E, Carandente V, et al. Short-term effects of moderate alcohol consumption on lipid metabolism and energy balance in normal men. Metabolism 1989;38(2):166–171.
38. Okamoto Y, Fujimori Y, Nakano H, et al. Role of the liver in alcohol-induced alteration of high-density lipoprotein metabolism. J Lab Clin Med 1988; 111:482–485.
39. Taskinen M-R, Nikkila EA, Valimaki M, et al. Alcohol-induced changes in serum lipoproteins and in their metabolism. Am Heart J 1987;113:458–464.
40. Moore RD, Smith CR, Kwiterovich PO, et al. Effect of low-dose alcohol versus abstention on apolipoproteins A-1 and B. Am J Med 1988;84:884–890.
41. Eichner ER. Alcohol, stroke and coronary artery disease. Am Fam Phys 1988;3:217–221.
42. Bush TL, Fried LP, Barrett-Connor E. Cholesterol, lipoproteins, and coronary heart disease in women. Clin Chem 1988;34(8B):B60–70.
43. Stubbe I, Eskilsson J, Nilsson-Ehle P. High-density lipoprotein concentrations after stopping smoking. Br Med J 1982;284:1511–1513.
44. Criqui MH, Wallace RB, Heiss G, et al. Cigarette smoking and plasma high-density lipoprotein cholesterol. Circulation 1980;62(suppl IV):70–76.
45. Fortmann SP, Haskell WL, Williams PT. Changes in plasma high density lipoprotein cholesterol after changes in cigarette use. Am J Epidemiol 1986; 124(4):706–710.
46. Bodurtha JN, Schieken R, Segrest J, et al. High-density lipoprotein-cholesterol subfractions in adolescent twins. Pediatrics 1987;79(2):181–189.
47. Dai WS, Gutai JP, Kuller LH, et al. Cigarette smoking and sex hormones in men. Am J Epidemiol 1988;128(4):796–805.
48. Frankenhaeuser M, Dunne E, Lundberg U. Sex differences in sympathetic-adrenal medullary reactions induced by different stressors. Psychopharmacology 1976;47:1–5.
49. Johansson G. Sex differences in the catecholamine output of children. Acta Physiol Scand 1972;85:569–572.
50. Rauste-von Wright M, von Wright J, Frankenhaeuser M. Relationships between sex-related psychological characteristics during adolescence and catecholamine excretion during achievement stress. Psychophysiology 1981;18(4): 362–370.
51. Collins A, Frankenhauser M. Stress responses in male and female engineering students. J Hum Stress 1978;4(2):43–48.
52. Manuck SB, Polefrone JM. Pathophysiologic reactivity in women. In: Baker

ED, Packard B, Wenger N, et al, eds. New York: Haymarket Doyma. 1987:164–171.

53. Hastrup JL, Light KC. Sex differences in cardiovascular stress responses: modulation as a function of menstrual cycle phases. J Psychosom Res 1984;28:475–483.

54. Hazuda HP, Haffner SM, Stern MP, et al. Employment status and women's protection against coronary heart disease. Am J Epidemiol 1986;123(4):623–640.

55. Johansson G, Post B. Catecholamine output of males and females over a one-year period. Acta Physiol Scand 1974;92:557–565.

56. Dimsdale JE, Herd JA. Variability of plasma lipids in response to emotional arousal. Psychosom Med 1982;44(5):413–430.

14
Lipids and Women's Health: Family Aspects

RICHARD E. GARCIA and DOUGLAS MOODIE

Considerable preventive medicine and anticipatory guidance can be provided for the family of a woman found to have hyperlipidemia. Precise etiological diagnosis of her lipid disorder enables the physician to give dietary advice and, when appropriate, genetic counseling. For the sake of this discussion, it is assumed that hypercholesterolemia is secondary to either dietary excess or genetic factors and that other causes such as liver or kidney disease, medications, or endocrine disorders, have been excluded. The purpose of this chapter is to discuss cholesterol surveillance and dietary advice for infants and children, the incidence of genetic dyslipidemias, and treatment issues for childhood hypercholesterolemia.

Overview

There is evidence that atherosclerosis begins during early life and that hypercholesterolemia plays a pivotal role in its evolution. The cholesterol hypothesis states that the higher the plasma cholesterol, the greater the incidence of coronary heart disease, and when the plasma cholesterol is reduced, the incidence of coronary heart disease decreases.[1] There is compelling evidence that early detection and treatment of hypercholesterolemia, a "heart healthy" diet, and avoidance of certain high risk coronary life style behaviors can significantly reduce the risk of ischemic heart disease in later life.

Two-thirds of Americans have atherosclerotic plaques in their arteries at the time of death, and one-half of the U.S. population die as a direct result of atherosclerosis in the form of stroke, myocardial infarction, or disease of the aorta. Fatty streaks are found in the aortas of infants.[2] Advanced coronary artery disease was observed at autopsy in 20- to 22-year-old soldiers who were killed in the Korean and Vietnam wars.[3,4] Cholesterol levels track well from 2 to 3 years of age into adulthood, and hypercholesterolemic children are likely to become hypercholesterolemic adults who are at risk for premature coronary heart disease.[5]

Screening

There has been disagreement as to whether all children should have a cholesterol screening test or only those from families with a history of premature heart attack or known hyperlipidemia.[6,7] A report of cholesterol screening of 6500 children in a suburban pediatric practice showed that 19% exceeded the 90th percentile and that nearly 50% of children with low density lipoprotein (LDL) cholesterol above the 95th percentile had no family history of elevated cholesterol or premature heart attack (< 55 years of age).[8] Figure 14–1 is a histogram depicting the distribution of the 6500 children studied. The bar at 100 includes all cholesterol levels less than 100 mg/dl ($n = 98$), and the bar at 300 includes all levels more than 300 mg/dl ($n = 19$). The mean cholesterol level for the group was 162 mg/dl, the 95th percentile was 214 mg/dl, and one standard deviation was 30 mg/dl. The authors thought, as a result of the study, that all children over 3 years of age should have a cholesterol test. It was further thought that children and adolescents should be routinely counseled to reduce cholesterol and saturated fat in their diet and to avoid high risk coronary life style behaviors, such as obesity, physical inactivity, and smoking.

Dietary Recommendation

The American Academy of Pediatrics, through its Committee on Nutrition, has offered advice for feeding young children.[9] There should be *no* fat restriction in the diet of children less than 2 years of age. When breast feeding is not possible, not successful, or stopped early, infant formula is the best alternative for providing nutritional requirements during the first 6 months of life. During the second 6 months, those babies who are eating one-third of their calories as a balanced mixture of cereal, fruits, vegetables, and meats may be given whole cow's milk. Beginning at 4 to 6 months of age, introduction of solid foods is recommended. Variety of food intake is the key to adequate and balanced nutrition at this time of life, and extremes of diet are to be avoided.

The Committees on Nutrition of the American Heart Association and the American Academy of Pediatrics closely agree on dietary recommendations for children over 2 years of age.[9,10] Maintenance of ideal body weight is desirable. Fat should comprise 30% of daily calories and should be evenly distributed among saturated, monounsaturated, and polyunsaturated fats. Baked goods, crackers, and chips should be prepared with unsaturated oils and egg whites, and no more than two to three egg yolks per week should be consumed. A cholesterol intake of 100 mg/1000 kcal/day (maximum 300 mg) is considered adequate.

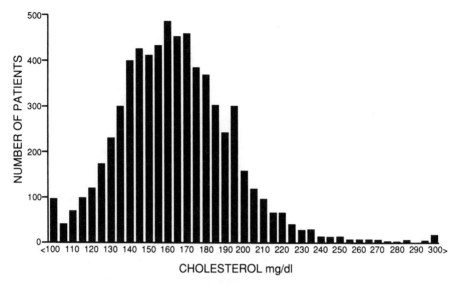

CHOLESTEROL mg/dl

FIGURE 14–1. Cholesterol screening in 6,500 children. (From Garcia RE and Moodie DS. Routine Cholesterol Surveillance in Childhood. Pediatrics 1989; Vol 84: No 5; 751–755. Reproduced by permission of Pediatrics.

Genetic Lipid Disorders

Hyperlipidemia due to genetic factors (primary hypercholesterolemia) is not rare.[11] Table 14–1 lists the common genetic lipid disorders and their incidence in the adult population.

Familial hypercholesterolemia is inherited as an autosomal dominant disorder with an incidence of 1:200 to 1:500 in the population. It is the most common genetic disorder associated with a clinical disease in man, occur-

TABLE 14–1. Common genetic lipid disorders

Type	Incidence (%)	Inheritance	Present in child	Early CAD
Familial hyper-cholesterolemia	0.2–0.5	Autosomal dominant	Yes	++++
Familial combined hyperlipidemia	1	Autosomal dominant	Young adult	+++
Polygenic hyper-cholesterolemia	1	Polygenic	Yes	++
Isolated low HDL cholesterol	2–3	Variable (some autosomal dominant)	Yes	++
Familial hypertri-glyceridemia	1	Autosomal dominant	Young adult	+

CAD = coronary artery disease.

ring ten times more often than neonatal hypothyroidism and 40 to 100 times more often than phenylketonuria. Heterozygous familial hypercholesterolemia is characterized by the presence of one-half the normal number of LDL-receptor sites on cell membranes. The serum cholesterol level is at least 240 mg/dl, and a first degree relative has a cholesterol above the 95th percentile or has had a premature myocardial infarction. Each child of a woman with this disorder has a 50% chance of inheriting the gene and manifesting the disease. Individuals with heterozygous familial hypercholesterolemia are at a 1:20 risk of ischemic heart disease by age 30 years and a 1:5 risk by 40 years; 85% have a myocardial infarction by age 60 years.[12] Homozygous familial hypercholesterolemia patients have essentially no LDL receptors, and their survival depends on liver transplantation and drug therapy.

Familial combined hyperlipidemia is estimated to occur in 1% of the adult population and is due to an autosomal dominant gene often not fully expressed until early adulthood. The basic abnormality is thought to be overproduction of hepatic apolipoprotein (apo) B, which results in excessive very low density lipoprotein (VLDL) particles of normal size. VLDL cholesterol is gradually converted to LDL cholesterol with apo B as its sole apolipoprotein. Triglycerides are removed via the action of lipoprotein lipase. As a result, one-third of such individuals have hypercholesterolemia, one-third have hypertriglyceridemia, and one-third have both.[13] One-half the offspring of a woman with this lipid disorder inherit the dominant gene and manifest the disease, although usually not until young adulthood. Her children should have periodic lipid profiles in order to diagnose the disease at an early age.

Polygenic hypercholesterolemia occurs in approximately 1% of the population and is considered to be due to inheritance of several genes that interact with each other and with environmental factors to influence the regulation of cholesterol metabolism.[14] First degree relatives of such patients have a significantly higher incidence of hypercholesterolemia than the general population. Cholesterol levels often persistently exceed 300 mg/dl. Children of women with this diagnosis should have periodic cholesterol tests to diagnose the disorder at an early age and institute appropriate management.

Familial hypertriglyceridemia occurs in approximately 1% of the adult population and is characterized by elevation of triglycerides alone.[15] It is due to an autosomal dominant gene that is frequently not fully expressed until adulthood, although 10 to 20% of affected individuals manifest the disorder during childhood. There appears to be both an excessive production of hepatic triglycerides and a mild defect in their removal from VLDL. Such patients do not have elevation of LDL cholesterol and frequently have low levels of high density lipoprotein (HDL) cholesterol. They are often obese and have had an excessive intake of alcohol. When this diagnosis is made in a woman, she should be counseled that 50% of her children are at risk for the disorder and should be appropriately screened at early ages.

Isolated reduced HDL cholesterol may occur in up to 3% of the population.[16] There are several causes for the disorder, though a significant number appear to be due to inheritance of an autosomal dominant gene with incomplete (20–30%) penetrance. The disease is diagnosed if the HDL cholesterol is less than 3 5 mg/dl. HDL cholesterol is responsible for reverse cholesterol transport, and its relative deficiency results in excessive cholesterol accumulation in peripheral tissues, most importantly the arterial tree. When a woman is found to have this lipid disorder, she should be counseled that her children are at risk and should have a lipid profile done at a relatively early age. Total cholesterol screening misses this disease, as such individuals are not hyperlipidemic.

Importance of Detection

Screening for lipid disorders is clearly a valuable and productive endeavor. Familial hypercholesterolemia, with an incidence of 0.2 to 0.5%, is the most common genetic disorder that eventually produces morbidity and mortality in Western society. Familial hypertriglyceridemia, polygenic hypercholesterolemia, and familial combined hyperlipidemia each affect 1%, and isolated low HDL cholesterol may occur in 3% of the population. Each of these lipid disorders significantly increases the risk of premature atherosclerotic heart disease. Hypercholesterolemia due to excessive dietary intake occurs in 3 to 5% of the population. The net result of these incidence data is that one adult in ten is likely to have a lipid abnormality.

There is a growing body of evidence that, if the incidence of atherosclerosis is to be significantly reduced, hypercholesterolemia and hypertension need to be detected at an early age and high risk coronary life-style behaviors (Table 14–2) must be avoided. Children at high risk for premature coronary heart disease are those who themselves have hypertension or diabetes, who smoke, or who have a first degree relative with a known lipid disorder or a myocardial infarction at less than 55 years of age.

The importance of hypercholesterolemia as a major risk factor for

TABLE 14–2. Coronary risk factors

Smoking
Obesity
Physical inactivity
Hypertension
Diabetes mellitus
Hypercholesterolemia
Male gender

coronary heart disease is no longer in doubt. Coronary heart disease mortality at a cholesterol level of 240 mg/dl is double that at the 200 mg/dl level.[17] No patient with a cholesterol level less than 150 mg/dl had a heart attack during 35 years of the Framington Heart Study, and 90% of individuals with a total cholesterol exceeding 300 mg/dl eventually do so.[18] Studies of hypercholesterolemic adult men have shown that for each 1% reduction of serum cholesterol there is a corresponding 2% reduction in the incidence of coronary artery disease.[19] Prevention of hypercholesterolemia during childhood surely reduces the risk of atherosclerotic heart disease in later life.

Current data suggest that all children over 3 years of age should have a cholesterol test and reduce their daily intake of cholesterol and saturated fats. Those children whose cholesterol exceeds the 95th percentile (200 mg/dl) should have a lipid profile. If their LDL cholesterol exceeds the 95th percentile (130 mg/dl), more careful follow-up and dietary intervention with the advice of a nutritionist is indicated. Diets with a cholesterol intake of less than 200 mg/day, fat intake less than 30% of calories, and a polyunsaturated fat/saturated fat ratio of more than 1:1 are difficult to comply with, and long-term effects on growth and development are not fully known.

Treatment

A major reduction in the risk of coronary heart disease is likely to require a major reduction of serum cholesterol in those children with LDL cholesterol levels that exceed the 95th percentile despite dietary intervention. Long-term, well designed, controlled studies involving large numbers of severely hypercholesterolemic children are required before specific recommendations can be made regarding drug therapy in the childhood population. Appropriate children for drug therapy include those with LDL cholesterol levels above 190 mg/dl and those above 160 mg/dl with two major coronary risk factors. A therapeutic goal for LDL cholesterol of 160 mg/dl for the former and 130 mg/dl for the latter population seems realistic and attainable.

Cholestyramine and colestipol are likely to be the frontline drugs for therapy of childhood hypercholesterolemia. They act by binding cholesterol in the gut and interfering with its reabsorption via the enterohepatic circulation. Niacin interferes with hepatic VLDL production, and lovastatin blocks the rate-limiting enzyme in cholesterol synthesis, 3-hydroxy-3-methyl coenzyme A (HMG CoA) reductase. Major current problems of drug therapy for hypercholesterolemic children include cost, compliance, and concerns about long-term metabolic effects. Safer and better tolerated medications will be forthcoming, and studies to document the efficacy of pharmacotherapy for childhood hypercholesterolemia are currently being designed. There is a strong possibility that coronary heart disease is largely preventable by avoiding hyperlipidemia and high risk coronary life-style behaviors during early life.

References

1. Kwiterovich PO. Commentaries, biochemical, clinical, epidemiologic, genetic, and pathologic data in the pediatric age group relevant to the cholesterol hypothesis . Pediatrics 1986;78:349–359.
2. Reisman M. Atherosclerosis and pediatrics. J Pediatr 1965;66:1´17.
3. Enos WF, Holmes RH, Boyer J. Coronary disease among United States soldiers killed in action in Korea: preliminary report. JAMA 1953;152:1090–1093.
4. McNamara JJ, Molot MA, Stremple JF. Coronary artery disease in combat casualties in Viet Nam. JAMA 1971;216:1185–1187.
5. Laver RM, Lee J, Clarke WR. Factors affecting the relationship between childhood and adult cholesterol levels: the Muscatine Study. Pediatrics 1988;82:309–318.
6. Orchard TJ, Donahue RP, Kuller LH, et al. Cholesterol screening in childhood: does it predict adult hypercholesterolemia? The Beaver County experience. J Pediatr 1983;103:687–691.
7. AAP Committee on Nutrition: Indications for cholesterol testing in children. Pediatrics 1988;83:141–142.
8. Garcia RE, Moodie DS. A case for routine cholesterol surveillance in childhood. Unpublished data, 1989.
9. AAP Committee on Nutrition. Prudent lifestyle for children: dietary fat and cholesterol. Pediatrics 1986;78:521–524.
10. Position statement. Diagnosis and treatment of primary hyperlipidemia in childhood: a joint statement for physicians by the Committee on Atherosclerosis and Hypertension in Childhood of the Council of Cardiovascular Disease in the Young and the Nutrition Committee, American Heart Association. Circulation 1986;74:1181A–1188A.
11. Motulsky AG. Medical intelligence: current concepts in genetics; the genetic hyperlipidemias. N Engl J Med 1976;294:823–827.
12. Goldstein JL, Brown MS. Familial hypercholesterolemia. In: Stanbury JB, ed. The Metabolic Basis of Inherited Disease. 5th Ed. New York: McGraw-Hill, 1983:672–712.
13. Glueck CJ, Fallot R, Buncher CR, et al. Familial combined hyperlipoproteinemia: studies in 91 adults and 95 children from 33 kindreds. Metabolism 1973;22:1403–1420.
14. Goldstein JL, Hazzard WR, Schrott HG, et al. Hyperlipidemia in coronary heart disease. I. Lipid levels in 500 survivors or myocardial infarction. J Clin Invest 1973;52:1533–1543.
15. Weidman WH. Cardiovascular risk modification in childhood: hyperlipidemia. Editorial. Mayo Clin Proc 1986;61:910–913.
16. Schaefer EJ. Clinical, biochemical, and genetic features in familial disorders of high density lipoprotein deficiency. Arteriosclerosis 1984;4:303–322.
17. Stamler J, Wentworth D, Neaton JD, et al. Is relationship between serum

cholesterol and risk of premature death from coronary heart disease continuous and graded? Findings in 356,222 primary screenees of the Multiple Risk Factor Intervention Trial (MRFIT). JAMA 1986;256:2823–2828.

18. Castelli WP. Epidemiology of coronary heart disease: the Framingham Study. Am J Med 1984; [vol 76, issue 2A]: 4–12.
19. Lipid Research Program. The Lipid Research Clinics coronary primary prevention trial results. I. Reduction in incidence of coronary heart disease. JAMA 1984;251:351–364.

15
Conclusion: A Comprehensive Approach to Women's Health

GEOFFREY P. REDMOND

There is little disagreement that health care should promote the patients overall health rather than confine its concern to the presence or absence of particular diseases. Accomplishing this goal is not easy, however. Most of us have, of necessity, been trained as specialists and cannot possibly have detailed knowledge of every area that may be important to the health of each of our patients. It is especially difficult when two disparate areas are suddenly found to be related on both basic and clinical levels as has happened with female reproductive medicine and lipidology. The only solution to this problem is for each physician to have at least some familiarity with those matters outside this speciality that pertain to the overall health of the patients he or she sees. Thus the lipidologist must learn some reproductive endocrinology in order to properly care for female patients, and a gynecologist must become more familiar with lipid abnormalities. This book has attempted to present the necessary background in these formerly separate disciplines. It remains only to summarize briefly how the present state of knowledge can be applied to the comprehensive care of female patients.

What should be done to determine cardiovascular risk in women and favorably alter it? The first step is to be aware that assessment of cardiovascular risk factors is as important for women as for men, as amply documented in this book. History taking includes attention to diet as well as other health behaviors, e.g., smoking and exercise, that affect cardiovascular health. A family history of cardiovascular disease and diabetes should be ascertained. Physical examination always includes weight, but there are other findings that pertain to future cardiovascular risk, notably acanthosis nigricans, hirsutism, android habitus, and other signs of androgenization. These findings are far more common than the classic signs of hyperlipidemia, such as xanthomas. A lipid profile should be performed periodically in all women. Those who have acanthosis nigricans or android obesity should also have a glucose tolerance test with simultaneous insulin levels. Although the cost-effectiveness of these procedures has not yet been rigorously quantitated, it is clearly in the interest of the individual patient that they be carried out.

Detailed guidelines exist[1] for when complete lipid profiles should be obtained based on the total cholesterol level and family history. The author has reservations about these guidelines as they apply to women. First, it is high density lipoprotein (HDL) and not total cholesterol that correlates best with cardiovascular risk in women. An individual woman with a mildly elevated total cholesterol level may have a markedly increased HDL level and a favorable risk ratio or a low HDL level and an unfavorable risk ratio. Total cholesterol measurement does not discriminate these situations. Unless HDL is also measured, many women with unfavorable patterns go undiagnosed. The guidelines do not call for a lipid profile being done with a total cholesterol level of less than 240 mg/dl unless there are other risk factors present.[1] The present author has seen many women in his practice with a total cholesterol of less than 240 mg/dl but unexpectedly low HDL levels, giving an unfavorable risk ratio. He believes female patients thus deserve a lipid profile that includes triglycerides, HDL, and calculation of low density lipoprotein (LDL) at least every 2 to 5 years.

Another limitation of the guidelines is the emphasis on LDL as the primary cholesterol subfraction to be used for treatment decisions. With the use of new agents such as lovastatin, it may be easier to correct a high LDL level than a low HDL level. Although lowering the LDL with lovastatin also lowers total cholesterol (TC), resulting in a better TC/HDL ratio, it is unclear that this change has the same significance in women as it does in men. The point is not that the guidelines should be ignored and treatment withheld but that it is unclear that this approach will turn out to be the best one when our knowledge is more complete.

The selection of a similar cutoff point in both men and women of 35 mg/dl for treatment for low HDL is also of concern. This point is discussed in Chapter 4 from a somewhat different perspective. This level represents the 10th percentile for women and the 25th percentile for men. The justification for this difference is that the risk in women is lower and therefore the HDL level is further below baseline for a comparable increase in coronary heart disease risk. Although it spares some women exposure to treatment, it also denies them its benefits. The question can be asked whether women should be treated when they get to the same absolute level of risk at which men are treated or at the level at which they lose some of their female advantages but still have less risk than men. This issue is in part philosophical but also scientific, as the risk and benefits of cholesterol alteration in women are less clear. It seems appropriate to establish distinct guidelines for men and women based on their different lipid metabolism. More complete scientific information to support more specific criteria should become available as trials now planned or in progress are completed.

Enthusiasm for limiting lipid intake or lowering levels that may apply to adolescents and adults should not be uncritically applied to children. For most of us the issue is avoiding overnutrition; but in the case of the fetus and young child, undernutrition represents more of a hazard. Cholesterol and triglycerides should not be unduly restricted in the diets of small children. The same concerns apply to nutrition during pregnancy. In general, during pregnancy lipid lowering should not be carried out with medication or radical dietary alteration. The effect of an unfavorable cholesterol pattern occurs over years rather than months. Therefore there appear to be potential hazard and little advantage in using lipid-owering agents in pregnant women.

The physician who treats women or children is in an excellent position to educate regarding appropriate diet for the entire family. There has been a clear trend toward lowered consumption of saturated fat in the American population. These data are counter to the prejudice of many physicians that their patients are unwilling to alter their dietary habits. Measurement of lipid levels may provide an opportune moment for discussion of these matters. An experienced dietitian can be of immense help in suggesting ways to lower cholesterol and saturated fat within the family's particular cultural and personal views regarding food. Standardized materials cannot substitute for this personal approach. We were all taught to begin our inquiries of patients by ascertaining their "chief complaint." Although this approach is an indispensable part of the patient-physician interaction, it is clear that medicine has moved far beyond a narrow concern with acute problems to promotion of health and well-being over the life span. Recent years have brought a recognition that lipid intake and metabolism is of great importance for future health. The additional time and expense required to measure the lipid profile and discuss it with the patient appears to be well justified by the potential benefits.

Reference

1. Goodman DS, Expert Panel. Report of the national cholesterol education program expert panel on detection, evaluation and treatment of high blood cholesterol in adults. Arch Intern Med 1988;148:36–69.

Index